Gerontologic
Nursing
Wholistic Care of the Older Adult

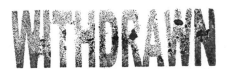
0815113315

Gerontologic Nursing
Wholistic Care of the Older Adult

Second Edition

Mary M. Burke, RN, DNSc, GNP-C
Associate Professor
Nurse Practitioner Program
George Washington University
Washington, DC

Mary B. Walsh, RN, MSN, FAAN
Associate Professor, Retired
School of Nursing
The Catholic University of America
Washington, DC

With 100 illustrations

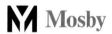 Mosby

St. Louis Baltimore Boston Carlsbad Chicago Naples New York Philadelphia Portland
London Madrid Mexico City Singapore Sydney Tokyo Toronto Wiesbaden

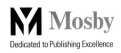
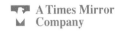

Publisher: Nancy Coon
Editor: Michael S. Ledbetter
Associate Developmental Editor: Cecily Barolak
Project Manager: Dana Peick
Senior Production Editor: Stavra Demetrulias
Designer: Amy Buxton
Manufacturing Supervisor: Karen Lewis

A NOTE TO THE READER:

The author and publisher have made every attempt to check dosages and nursing content for accuracy. Because the science of pharmacology is continually advancing, our knowledge base continues to expand. Therefore we recommend that the reader always check product information for changes in dosage or administration before administering any medication. This is particularly important with new or rarely used drugs.

SECOND EDITION

© **1997 by Mosby-Year Book, Inc.**

Previous edition copyrighted 1992.

Printed in the United States of America
Composition by Carlisle Communications, Ltd.
Lithography/color film by Color Dot Graphics, Inc.
Printing/binding by R.R. Donnelley and Sons, Inc.

Mosby-Year Book, Inc.
11830 Westline Industrial Drive
St. Louis, Missouri 63146

International Standard Book Number
0-8151-1331-5

96 97 98 99 00 / 9 8 7 6 5 4 3 2 1

CONTRIBUTORS

to Second Edition

Mary Beth Bigley, MSN, ANP-C
Assistant Professor of Health Care
 Science
George Washington University
Washington, DC

Francis J. Burke, JD
Attorney
Washington, DC

**Mary M. (Mickie) Burke,
 RN, DNSc, GNP-C**
Associate Professor
Nurse Practitioner Program
George Washington University
Washington, DC

**Caroline Bagley Burnett,
 RN, ScD**
Clinical Associate Professor
 of Nursing
Georgetown University
Division of Cancer Prevention
 and Control
Lombardi Cancer Center
School of Nursing
Washington, DC

Charles A. Cefalu, MD, MS
Director of Geriatrics and
 Associate Professor
Department of Family Medicine
Georgetown University School of
 Medicine/Providence Hospital
Washington, DC

Helene M. Clark, RN, PhD
Assistant Professor
School of Nursing
The Catholic University of America
Washington, DC

Sister Maureen Duffy, MS, RD
Clinical Dietician
Providence Hospital
Washington, DC

Theresa Ferlotti, RN, MSN, GNP
Staff Nurse/Clinician II
Georgetown University Medical
 Center
Washington, DC

Barbara Galen, MSN, CANP
Rockville, MD

Myrtle R. McCulloch, EdD, RD
Assistant Professor of Nursing
Georgetown University School
 of Nursing
Washington, DC

**B. Joan McDowell, PhD,
 CRNP, FAAN**
Associate Professor of Nursing
University of Pittsburgh
Pittsburgh, Pennsylvania

Karen Ehlke Reilly, ScD
Project Director
Allied Technology Group, Inc.
Rockville, Maryland

Helen T. Roach, RN, MSN
Critical Care Clinical Educator
Georgetown University Medical
 Center
Washington, DC

**Sister Maria Salerno, OSF, DNSc,
 RNCS, NP**
Associate Professor
Director Primary Care
 ANP Program
Codirector FNP Program
School of Nursing
The Catholic University of America
Washington, DC

Susan E. Sherman, RN, MA
President
Independence Foundation
Philadelphia, PA

Sheila M. Sparks, RN, DNSc, CS
Assistant Professor
School of Nursing
Georgetown University
Washington, DC

Patricia Stockton, M. PHIL
Research Associate
Department of Psychiatry, Division
 of Psychosocial Research
Georgetown Medical Center
Washington, DC

Catherine A. Swanson, RN, MSN
Case Manager
Lung Cancer
Lombardi Cancer Center
Georgetown University Medical
  Center
Washington, DC

**Sister Carol Taylor, RN, CSFN,
  PhD Candidate, MSN**
Assistant Professor, Humanities
Clinical Ethicist
Health Care Ethicist
Holy Family College
Philadelphia, Pennsylvania

**Mary B. Walsh, RN, MSN,
  FAAN**
Associate Professor, Retired
School of Nursing
The Catholic University of America
Washington, DC

CONTRIBUTORS

to First Edition

Kathleen Adams, RN, MSN, CANP
Adjunct Assistant Professor
Nurse Practitioner Program
George Washington University
Washington, DC

Mary Beth Bigley, RN, MSN, CANP
Cardiovascular Nurse Specialist
Arlington Hospital
Arlington, Virginia

Kathryn L. Burgio, PhD
Research Assistant Professor
  of Medicine
Assistant Professor of Nursing
University of Pittsburgh–
  Falk Clinic
Pittsburgh, Pennsylvania

Mary M. Burke, RN, DNSc, CRNP
Assistant Professor
School of Nursing
Georgetown University
Washington, DC

Helene M. Clark, PhD, RNC
Assistant Professor
School of Nursing
The Catholic University
  of America
Washington, DC

Janice C. Hallal, RN, DNSc
Associate Professor
School of Nursing
The Catholic University
  of America
Washington, DC

M. Anne Hart, MSG, MPA
District of Columbia Long Term
  Care Ombudsman
Legal Counsel for the Elderly
Washington, DC

Jean Johnson, RN, MSN, NPC
Associate Professor
Department of Health Care
  Sciences
George Washington University
Washington, DC

Carol N. Knowlton, RN, MSN
Assistant Dean for Student Affairs
School of Nursing
The Catholic University
  of America
Washington, DC

B. Joan McDowell, CRNP, PhD, RNC
Research Assistant Professor
  of Medicine
Assistant Professor of Nursing
University of Pittsburgh
Pittsburgh, Pennsylvania

Mary Eletta Morse, RN, MSN, GNPC
Geriatric Clinical Nurse Specialist
Alexandria Hospital
Alexandria, Virginia

Helen T. Roach, RN, MSN
Clinical Educator
Nursing Education and Research
Georgetown University Hospital
Washington, DC

Claudia Schlosberg, JD
Dixon Implementation
  Monitoring Committee
Mental Health Law Project
Washington, DC

Sandra C. Sewell, RN, MSN
Program Manager,
  Care Management
Gerontological Center
Suburban Hospital
Bethesda, Maryland

Sheila Sparks, RN, DNSc
Assistant Professor
School of Nursing
Georgetown University
Washington, DC

Patricia Stockton, BSc, MCSP
Research Associate
Department of Psychiatry
  and Center on Aging
Georgetown University
Washington, DC

Catherine A. Swanson, RN, MSN, NPC
Clinical Educator
Nursing Education and Research
Georgetown University Hospital
Washington, DC

Kyriake Valassi, PhD
Professor of Nutritional
  Biochemistry
School of Nursing
The Catholic University
  of America
Washington, DC

Mary B. Walsh, RN, MSN,
  FAAN
Associate Professor, Retired
School of Nursing
The Catholic University
  of America
Washington, DC

Sister Paul Gabriel Wilhere, RN,
  MEd
Nursing Home Consultant,
  Long Term Care
Pittsburgh, Pennsylvania

To Frank and Paul,
spouses extraordinaire,
who provided patience, humor, and support
throughout the two editions of this text

PREFACE

When the authors/editors prepared the first edition of this text, the recognition of increased numbers of older adults was more true then than it is now. The difference is, there are so many more older adults in the population now (see Chapter 1), and their needs are greater in number today and are wider in variety than they were upon publication of the first edition. In view of the changes in the population today, the authors/editors felt it necessary to update the data that were presented at that time, as well as to incorporate new data that are now available about older adults.

The subtitle of the original text has been adjusted to exclude "care of the frail elderly"; however, the content of this text will continue to address the needs of the frail elderly, while not making them the sole or primary focus. The new subtitle, "Wholistic Care of the Older Adult," highlights a change in focus to include all older adults who may be healthy *or* ill; their needs will be considered throughout the text. The nurse's role in assisting older persons to prevent illness for as long as possible, and to remain as independent as possible, despite alterations in health in whatever form they appear, will also be incorporated into the text. The basic assumption throughout the text will be that of health and independence, while maintaining a realistic tone. Utilization of all of one's talents and abilities will be the thrust, with the hope that the achievements of the older persons will far exceed those predicted or projected by others.

The focus of this text is on the gerontologic knowledge that is needed by those health care professionals who are responsible for promoting and maintaining the health of older adults. Primarily, the intent is to provide information for the student of nursing that will increase the student's ability to provide quality care for the older person. While the idea of "student" places the emphasis on the beginning learner, this can have various connotations. It is possible that the beginning student will be the high school graduate who has just entered a baccalaureate nursing program; or, this beginning student may be one of several types of students who has transferred to a nursing major from an educational program with various types of preparation. The ultimate goal of such a learner is to become a health caregiver for the older person whose concern is to maintain or restore health and/or to ameliorate illness. While this is the primary focus for the development of content for this text, it is quite possible that other persons can benefit from the knowledge presentation; that is, graduate students in nursing programs, or nurses who are employed in various settings as they care for older patients.

■ Organization

Each of the chapters that addresses clinical content does so with a selection of content that the authors/editors believe is crucial to the care of gerontologic patients/persons. The contributors for these chapters have been selected according to their professional expertise in the appropriate area.

The nursing process framework is the structure for each of the clinical chapters. Elements of the nursing process are considered to be: assessing, diagnosing, planning and identifying outcomes, implementing, and evaluating.

In view of the locations where gerontologic patients or older persons live, the settings for the care of the older person include:

the acute care setting
the nursing home setting
the community or personal home.

The second edition has updated all existing chapters; furthermore, in response to readers' comments and the changing health care system, five new chapters have been added: The Transition Years, Drug Therapy in Older Adults, Bowel Elimination, Cancer in the Older Adult, and Ethical Perspectives. The scope of the book has been adapted to accommodate the emphasis on the early years of aging and the enhancement of the health of the older adult.

The first five chapters address the demography of the older population today, critical elements of gerontologic nursing, the theories about aging that guide the care of older adults, the psychosocial components of the transitional years, and the pharmacodynamics of the care of older adults.

Fourteen clinical chapters deal with the predominant issues and problems that are presently faced by older persons. These include an update of the following topics that were presented in the first edition: sexuality, sensation, integument, regulation, cardiovascular, respiration, mobility, urinary incontinence, nutrition, sleep, cognition, and safety. In addition to these twelve topics, there are two additional chapters about cancer and bowel elimination.

Finally, the last four chapters are presented as a cluster of content dealing with the topics of grief, legal issues, ethics, and some dreams and fears about the future for older adults.

Clusters of topics are similar to the groups of data that were presented in the first edition. The content under each chapter heading has been updated according to the experiences of the authors, and according to the reports of progress and change as defined in the literature. Research reports are included as they have been reported in the extant literature. The progress of health care may appear to proceed too slowly as we live out the changes and improvements that are swirling around us as we function in the care of older adults. However, in retrospect, examining the past five years is quite revealing and surprising. It is encouraging to note the number of studies that have been initiated and completed in the area of gerontologic nursing. It is heartening to see a rise in interested and well-prepared health personnel to care for the older citizen. It gives one a true boost in spirits to become aware of the improved stature that gerontology and gerontologic nursing have acquired in a relatively brief time. This is also to say that much more needs to be done by all who now function in this critical specialty, but this is to say that much has been done and much is underway.

■ Features

Various features throughout the text, both new and included from the first edition, are utilized to enhance content and serve as useful teaching tools. **Learning Objectives** at the beginning of each chapter identify key areas to be discussed. **Aging Alerts,** integrated throughout the text, highlight important aging considerations. Assessment criteria, age-related changes, pharmacology, lab and diagnostic testing, pathology, and risk factors are included in numerous **tables and boxes.**

To incorporate the wholistic approach of this edition, two new features have been added: **Health Promotion boxes** in the clinical chapters include suggestions for the nurse to encourage healthy behaviors in older adults; and *Healthy People 2000 Objectives* highlight goals for health promotion and disease prevention.

■ Instructor's Resource Manual

The **Instructor's Resource Manual** has been created in response to great demand for such an ancillary. This IRM follows the text chapter by chapter and includes chapter outlines and overviews; Teaching Suggestions for Classroom and Practice Applications and Critical Thinking Exercises to aid students in applying what they have learned; Chapter Review Questions/Activities; and a Test Bank.

■ Acknowledgments

To accept the challenge of editing a textbook on Gerontologic Nursing is quite adequate to show any person(s) how inadequate each of us is to function alone. The greater the information about the subject matter, the greater is our dependence on our peers and colleagues. There are wonderful and impressive people in the health care profession who are anxious to share with others the information gained through experience. Sharing this information with peers and colleagues is quite beneficial to the knowledge base of all of us. We are truly indebted to our co-workers, to our students, and to our patients. A special word of thanks to Sister Paul Gabriel, who has been our mentor and model for many years. They have all contributed to increasing our knowledge base about gerontologic nursing—and for this we are grateful. For all those persons who have pursued research studies, large and small, we thank you for reporting the results of your efforts so that all of us will gain from your experiences. Keep up the good work!

Accessibility to the published data about gerontologic nursing is essential for those who are involved with the care of older adults. Several persons are outstanding in this respect for this edition. Nellie Lee Powell, at the School of Nursing Library at The Catholic University of America, continues to be supportive and valuable to the production of printed data; we could not have proceeded without her. Amy Holloway at George Washington University was a great help in the development of computer illustrations and the reference librarians at the George Washington Himmelfarb library were extremely helpful. We would also like to acknowledge Debbie Drake, Mary Reuther Herring, and Cora Zembrzuski for their helpful suggestions for revising the manuscript. We thank you all.

This book may be written by authors/editors and their names appear on the cover and chapters, but the people behind the scenes are the ones who deserve the kudos. We were most fortunate with our experience with the Mosby staff. We would like to continue to thank Linda Duncan, our editor on the first edition. Our current editor, Michael Ledbetter, provides us with encouragement, understanding, and always graciousness. We couldn't have had a better editor. But the best is saved for last: Cecily Barolak, Associate Development Editor, was always there when we needed anything. What to do? Where to send it? How to say it? Who will do it? The list goes on and on, but Cecily, with her calm and friendly way, was never rushed, always available, and able to listen.

Our families are still with us, quite a feat through two editions. We love them all and thank them for their patience, and are grateful for their encouragement.

Mary M. Burke
Mary B. Walsh

CONTENTS

Gerontologic
Nursing
Wholistic Care of the Older Adult

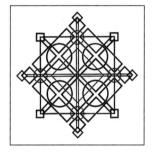

Grow old along with me!
The best is yet to be,
The last of life, for which the first was made.

ROBERT BROWNING

The Older Adult Population

■ Learning Objectives

On completion of this chapter, the reader will be able to do the following:

1. Define the older adult population, recognizing stereotypes applied to this population.
2. Recognize the complexity of factors that influence the lives of older adults—including health maintenance, available care during illness or disability, and current health care financing and services—and the significance of environmental factors that include geographic location and features of the individual's community and home.
3. Describe sociologic, economic, and educational trends among older adults.
4. Recognize current demographic trends among older adults in the United States, identifying present and predictive trends.

■ Background

A statement of a 5-year-old kindergartner in Silver Spring, Maryland: "My teacher [26] is really old, like you, Mom [41]." A statement of a 73-year-old man in Milwaukee, Wisconsin: "I certainly am looking forward to my wedding next month! No, I'm not old yet." These two statements illustrate how varied and relative is the concept of age. When speaking of age, every person has a subjective view of the term *old*. The multitude of differences among older adults makes it both difficult and unwise to generalize traits as applicable to all older adults. In the conceptualizing and speaking of old age and older adults, terms and specific individuals or groups must be defined

clearly. Vague labels, such as "old," "elderly," or "senior citizen," suggest stereotypes that are misleading and inappropriate when applied to individuals within the labeled populations.

In the United States, further misinterpretation results from linking the concept of retirement to specific ages or age groups. Stereotypes regarding retirement may have been somewhat justifiable in the mid-1800s, when Bismarck announced the first nationwide pension plan for the German people. He decided that retirement would be mandated at age 65 and that a pension plan would be available to all retirees. Bismarck's action actually affected few Germans (Mitchell, 1971) because in the mid-nineteenth century few people ever reached age 65. Today quite the opposite is true. Not only are there greater numbers of people living to age 65 and beyond, but the social contributions of those in their 60s, 70s, and 80s are quite significant. For example, one in five of those over 75 help their children or grandchildren in daily living activities (Commonwealth Fund, 1992). As life expectancy continues to increase, employers are revising their ideas and policies about retirement and even soliciting the expertise of older adults. The chronologic age for retirement now varies widely. Although early retirement may be unavoidable for people in some occupations, such as dancers or pilots, retirement age remains virtually undefined for people in less physical occupations, such as writers, artists, or accountants. Fullerton (1993) projected that the labor force made up of those 55 years old and older would increase by more than 38% between 1992 and 2005.

Many view older adults as frail or feeble, with limited capacity for making contributions society would view as beneficial. Unfortunately, the common perception of aging and older adults often differs sharply from the reality of aging. A Commonwealth Fund study (1992), *The Nation's Great Overlooked Resource: The Contributions of Americans 55+,* found that almost 38 million Americans over age 55 contribute to American society; their contributions are estimated to equal those of 20 million full-time employees. One in 5 contribute a sizable portion to their children's or grandchildren's income; only 1 in 20 receive a sizable portion from their children or grandchildren. Impressions and interpretations about older adults can vary widely, depending on one's beliefs, knowledge, experience, orientation, and age. The astute and objective observer will view each aging person according to individual talents, abilities, and state of health, thereby minimizing or avoiding misconceptions about aging.

Although the astute observer looks past aging generalities and focuses on the unique individual, there are times when it is useful to view older adults as a group or special population. The special population can be defined in terms of common characteristics and social situations. For example, the health care planner must make generalizations about the older adult population when defining health care financing or health care delivery alternatives for those over 65. Decisions regarding allocation of social goods are often based on population groups and their needs. An understanding of some common group characteristics of those 65 and older is useful in decision making and understanding human needs. Three alternative social structures, aimed at describing human needs, will be discussed here.

Human life processes continue throughout the life span. Individuals of any age experience a spectrum of human needs. For example, anyone, regardless of age, experiences fundamental physiologic needs, as well as needs for safety and security, love and belonging, self-esteem, and self-actualization (Maslow, 1970). The relative significance of each need and the hierarchic relationships among these needs are shown in Maslow's hierarchy (Figure 1-1). (Extensive illustration and discussion of Maslow's interpretation of human needs is presented in Ebersole & Hess, 1994.) The most basic needs are physiologic; life

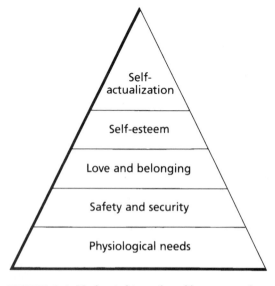

FIGURE 1-1 Maslow's hierarchy of human needs.

cannot continue without these needs being met. The psychosocial need of self-actualization is at the top of Maslow's pyramid.

Galtung (1980) suggests a second approach to the identification and analysis of human needs. Basic human needs are differentiated, according to two pairs of interrelated factors, as material versus nonmaterial needs and as actor-dependent versus structure-dependent needs. The first pair of factors concerns the needs of an individual's body versus those of the mind. There is a clear delineation between material and nonmaterial needs. For example, a material need might be housing, whereas freedom might be a nonmaterial need. The second pair of factors is related to the means by which needs are satisfied, or source of satisfaction. This involves the social context of human needs. Human need satisfaction depends on either the actor or the structure of the need situation. Actor-dependent needs depend on the motivation and capacity of some *one* person to satisfy those needs. Structure-dependent needs are met by satisfiers built into the social structure itself, without being dependent on particular persons. Table 1-1 illustrates the typology of human needs suggested by Galtung.

A third approach in describing human needs is one that arranges human needs in specific clusters. Yura and Walsh (1988) arranged a selected group of human needs according to three clusters, adapting the work of Galtung and others. They classify human needs as follows:

TABLE 1-1 Galtung's typology of human needs

Source of satisfaction	Material needs	Nonmaterial needs
Actor dependent	Security needs	Freedom needs
Structure dependent	Welfare needs	Identity needs

Adapted from Galtung, J. (1980). The basic human needs approach. In K. Lederer (Ed.), *Human needs*. Cambridge, MA: Oelgeschlager, Gunn, and Hain.

Survival needs
Closeness needs
Freedom needs

These are particularly useful ways of grouping and labeling human needs when dealing with the family and with the community (Table 1-2).

Human needs continue to exist throughout the life of each person, with multiple variables affecting the intensity of these needs as a person grows older. Because health is perceived as a major factor in realizing a satisfactory, high-quality life, most older adults devote a reasonable amount of energy to achieving the highest level of health possible. Being over 65 years old does not by any means prohibit participation in a variety of activities that promote and encourage healthy living. The range and variety of activities continue to exist, with perhaps the intensity of the activity adjusted according to individual endurance.

This text makes some generalizations about older adults, yet readers are encouraged to avoid overgeneralizing about all older people. Instead, readers are urged to meet each older person as an individual, to treat each person in a wholistic manner, and to consider each as a unique person with particular needs, desires, talents, and interests. This approach recognizes the challenge, the excitement, and the satisfaction of living and working with older adults.

■ Definition of Older Adults

For purposes of this text, *older adults* are people 65 years old or older. In 1993 older adults made up almost 13% of the U.S. population, numbering almost 33 million (American Association of Retired Persons [AARP], 1994). By the year 2000 older adults are projected to make up approximately 20% of the U.S. population, with a greater racial diversity. The term *65 and older* describes individuals with a broad spectrum of ages, health statuses, and general capacities. Not only does the term *older adult* apply to the married, employed 68-year-old; it also applies to the single, 92-year-old nursing home resident. Age subcategories are sometimes useful in further describing

TABLE 1-2 Human needs

Survival needs	Closeness needs	Freedom needs
Activity	Acceptance	Autonomy
Adaption	Appreciation	Beauty
Air	Belonging	Challenge
Elimination	Confidence	Conceptualization
Fluids intake	Humor	Freedom from pain
Gas interchange	Love, being loved	Self-control
Nutrition	Personal recognition	Self-fulfillment
Protection from fear	Sexual integrity	Spiritual experience
Perception of reality	Tenderness	Territoriality
Rest, leisure	Wholesome body image	Value system
Safety		
Sensory integrity		
Skin integrity		
Sleep		

Adapted from Yura, H., & Walsh, M. B. (1988). *The nursing process.* E. Norwalk, CT: Appleton and Lange.

the population known as *older adults* and are presented accordingly in this text.

As a normal process of aging, changes occur that slow nerve impulses, lengthen healing time, and reduce the body's ability to fend off disease (Schaie and Willis, 1986). Although physical, mental, and sensory impairments do increase with age, severe and disabling limitations are still relatively rare among older people. The fear of disability is greater than the incidence of disability, and if unchecked, this fear can handicap the lifestyle of a person. Anxiety and fear about health problems become greater as people get older. These concerns should not be ignored, but neither should they be magnified. The best antidote for such fears is to provide accurate information, education, and reassurance regarding the health problems—many of them treatable—and to focus on the most active and fullest life possible. Emphasis should be on the positive ways to maintain health. Neglect of problems can quickly lead to loss of function, and older adults can rapidly become unnecessarily dependent as a result of such neglect. On the other hand, a focus on healthy aging enables older adults to maximize their human potential and enjoy the "golden years."

■ Myths and Stereotypes

Myths and stereotypes perpetuate erroneous ideas regarding aging, as shown in Box 1-1. Reaching age 65 does not provide automatic entry into inactive frailty. In fact, the onset of aging is a gradual, subtle process, varying in rate and intensity by individual. Aging is not an abrupt change, nor is it a sure and steady retrogression from good health to poor health (Abdellah, 1989). Rather, it is a developmental stage of life, with challenges and opportunities that may vary by issue but that are similar in principle to those of other developmental stages.

Although the number of chronic ailments does increase as people grow older, these ailments do not necessarily inhibit or impair every older person. Some people do become more frail as they get older, but many do not. For example, George Burns was 95 years old in 1991, and he had already scheduled a personal performance for his one-hundredth birthday. Another celebrated oldster, similarly visible to the general public, is actor Bob Hope, 92 years old in 1995, continuing his Christmas tradition of performing for U.S. troops by traveling to the Persian Gulf.

BOX 1-1 NATIONAL INSTITUTE ON AGING: WHAT IS YOUR AGING IQ?

TRUE OR FALSE?

 1. Baby boomers are the fastest growing segment of the population.
 2. Families don't bother with their older relatives.
 3. Everyone becomes confused or forgetful if they live long enough.
 4. You can be too old to exercise.
 5. Heart disease is a much bigger problem for older men than for older women.
 6. The older you get, the less you sleep.
 7. People should watch their weight as they age.
 8. Most older people are depressed. Why shouldn't they be?
 9. Older people should not have screening tests for cancer. Why bother?
10. Older people take more medications than younger people.
11. People begin to lose interest in sex around age 55.
12. If your parents had Alzheimer's disease, you will inevitably get it.
13. Diet and exercise reduce the risk of osteoporosis.
14. As your body changes with age, so does your personality.
15. Older people might as well accept urinary accidents as a fact of life.
16. Suicide is mainly a problem for teenagers.
17. Falls and injuries "just happen" to older people.
18. Everybody gets cataracts.
19. Extremes of heat and cold can be especially dangerous for older people.
20. "You can't teach an old dog new tricks."

ANSWERS

 1. **False.** There are more than 3 million Americans over the age of 85. That number is expected to quadruple by the year 2040, when there will be more than 12 million people in that age group. The population age 85 and older is the fastest growing age group in the United States.
 2. **False.** Most older people live close to their children and see them often. Many live with their spouses. An estimated 80% of men and 60% of women live in family settings. Only 5% of the older population live in nursing homes.
 3. **False.** Confusion and serious forgetfulness in old age can be caused by Alzheimer's disease or other conditions that result in irreversible damage to the brain. But at least 100 other problems can bring on the same symptoms. A minor head injury, high fever, poor nutrition, adverse drug reactions, and depression also can lead to confusion. These conditions are treatable, however, and the confusion they cause can be eliminated.
 4. **False.** Exercise at any age can help strengthen the heart and lungs and lower blood pressure. It also can improve muscle strength and, if carefully chosen, lessen bone loss with age. See a physician before beginning a new exercise program.
 5. **False.** The risk of heart disease increases dramatically for women after menopause. By age 65 both men and women have a one-in-three chance of showing symptoms. But risks can be significantly reduced by following a healthy diet and exercising.
 6. **False.** In later life it's the quality of sleep that declines, not total sleep time. Researchers have found that sleep tends to become more fragmented as people age. A number of reports suggest that older people are less likely than younger people to stay awake throughout the day and that older people tend to take more naps than younger people.

Continued

BOX 1-1 NATIONAL INSTITUTE ON AGING: WHAT IS YOUR AGING IQ?—cont'd

7. **True.** Most people gain weight as they age. Because of changes in the body and decreasing physical activity, older people usually need fewer calories. Still, a balanced diet is important. Older people require essential nutrients just like younger adults. You should be concerned about your weight if there has been an involuntary gain or loss of 10 pounds in the past 6 months.

8. **False.** Most older people are not depressed. When it does occur, depression is treatable throughout the life cycle using a variety of approaches such as family support, psychotherapy, or antidepressant medications. A physician can determine whether the depression is caused by medication an older person might be taking, by physical illness, by stress, or by other factors.

9. **False.** Many older people can beat cancer, especially if it's found early. Over half of all cancers occur in people 65 and older, which means that screening for cancer in this age group is especially important.

10. **True.** Older people often have a combination of conditions that require drugs. They consume 25% of all medications and can have many more problems with adverse reactions. Check with your doctor to make sure all drugs and dosages are appropriate.

11. **False.** Most older people can lead an active, satisfying sex life.

12. **False.** The overwhelming majority of people with Alzheimer's disease have not inherited the disorder. In a few families, scientists have seen an extremely high incidence of the disease and have identified genes in these families that they think may be responsible.

13. **True.** Women are at particular risk for osteoporosis. They can help prevent bone loss by eating foods rich in calcium and exercising regularly throughout life. Foods such as milk and other dairy products, dark green leafy vegetables, salmon, sardines, and tofu promote new bone growth. Activities such as walking, biking, and simple exercises to strengthen the upper body also can be effective.

14. **False.** Research has found that, except for the changes that can result from Alzheimer's disease and other forms of dementia, personality is one of the few constants of life. That is, you are likely to age much as you've lived.

15. **False.** Urinary incontinence is a symptom, not a disease. Usually it is caused by specific changes in body function that can result from infection, diseases, pregnancy, or the use of certain medications. A variety of treatment options is available for people who seek medical attention.

16. **False.** Suicide is most prevalent among people age 65 and older. An older person's concern with suicide should be taken very seriously, and professional help should be sought quickly.

17. **False.** Falls are the most common cause of injuries among people over age 65. But many of these injuries, which result in broken bones, can be avoided. Regular vision and hearing tests and good safety habits can help prevent accidents. Knowing whether your medications affect balance and coordination also is a good idea.

18. **False.** Not everyone gets cataracts, although a great many older people do. Some 18% of people between the ages of 65 and 74 have cataracts, and more than 40% of those between 75 and 85 have the problem. Cataracts can be treated very successfully with surgery; more than 90% of people say they can see better after the procedure.

19. **True.** The body's thermostat tends to function less efficiently with age, making the older person's body less able to adapt to heat or cold.

20. **False.** People at any age can learn new information and skills. Research indicates that older people can obtain new skills and improve old ones, including learning how to use a computer.

From U.S. Department of Health and Human Services, Public Health Service, National Institutes of Health (1991).

Julia Child, at the age of 82, continues with public appearances and book publishing. At the age of 85, Jacques Cousteau will set sail next year to explore and film the rivers and coast of China.

■ Complex Factors in the Lives of Older Adults

HEALTH AND ILLNESS

Health can be defined in various ways. The World Health Organization defines health as "a state of complete physical, mental, and social well-being and not merely the absence of disease and infirmity" (Brockington, 1975, p. 5). Pender (1982) defines *wholistic health* as the "actualization of human potential through purposeful, self-initiated behavior, satisfying relationships with others, and competent personal care." The National Council on Aging (1994) talks of organizational, political, and economic instruments affecting behavior and environment geared to preventing, delaying, or minimizing disease or disability while promoting independence. Many other definitions of health can be found in the literature, and each definition reflects the purpose and orientation of the author. Some view health as it relates to illness or disease rather than emphasizing the positive dimensions of health. Other authors view health positively, identifying it as a normal, expected state in people of any age. They view coping with illness or disease as an associated state, but not the dominant state of existence.

Healthy aging programs, an increased understanding of the aging process, and advances in health care technology all have contributed to increased longevity. The life expectancy of someone born in 1992 was 28 years longer than that of someone born in 1900 (AARP, 1994). Centenarians, those who reach the age of 100 years, have more than doubled during the 1980s (Taeuber, 1993). Many more older adults are living healthier lives. Conversely, as a result of modern medicine's ability to arrest disease stages, many older adults are living with various types of chronic ailments and illnesses. For impaired older adults, a focus on their strengths often assists them in achieving goals once conceptualized as unattainable. Most people are familiar with the negative cycle associated with the inability to perform an activity. The lack of accomplishment is followed by discouragement and depression, which is then followed by increased inability to perform activities, and finally by complete withdrawal from the activity. A positive cycle works in the same way. Goal achievement in activities leads to encouragement and a positive self-image, which, in turn, enhances identification and achievement of future goals.

Facilitating a positive cycle becomes increasingly important as older adults live longer (Table 1-3). In 1990 there were over 3 million Americans 85 years old and older. By the year 2050 the U.S. Bureau of the Census has projected that the number of Americans 85 years old and older will have increased to over 17 million. Furthermore, in 1985 25,000 Americans were 100 years old or older. By the year 2050 the number of Americans 100 years old and older is expected to be over 1 million ("**The Facts of Life,**" 1987) (Figure 1-2). These life expectancy figures underscore the importance of highlighting the health, abilities, and strengths of people moving into the seventh, eighth, and even ninth decades of life. The importance of enhancing the quality of life cannot be overemphasized.

Maintaining a positive attitude may be particularly difficult as older adults adapt to changes in health that accompany the aging process. There is little risk of people in their 20s and 30s suffering a chronic disease such as arthritis or osteoporosis. From the age of 40 on, however, the risk doubles exponentially about every 5 years (Table 1-4). By the time a person reaches age 85, there is also a one-in-three chance that that person will have dementia, immobility, incontinence, or other age-related disabilities.

To enhance a positive attitude among older adults by minimizing disabilities related to older

TABLE 1-3 Actual and projected growth of the older population: 1900 to 2050*

Year	Total population all ages	55 to 64 years		65 to 74 years		75 to 84 years		85 years and over		65 years and over	
		Number†	%	Number†	%	Number†	%	Number†	%	Number†	%
1900	76,303	4,009	5.3	2,189	2.9	772	1.0	123	0.2	3,084	4.0
1910	91,972	5,054	5.5	2,793	3.0	989	1.1	167	0.2	3,950	4.3
1920	105,711	6,532	6.2	3,464	3.3	1,259	1.2	210	0.2	4,933	4.7
1930	122,775	8,397	6.8	4,721	3.8	1,641	1.3	272	0.2	6,634	5.4
1940	131,669	10,572	8.0	6,375	4.8	2,278	1.7	365	0.3	9,019	6.8
1950	150,967	13,295	8.8	8,415	5.6	3,278	2.2	577	0.4	12,270	8.1
1960	179,323	15,572	8.7	10,997	6.1	4,633	2.6	929	0.5	16,560	9.2
1970	203,302	18,608	9.2	12,447	6.1	6,124	3.0	1,409	0.7	19,980	9.8
1980	226,505	21,700	9.6	15,578	6.9	7,727	3.4	2,240	1.0	25,544	11.3
1990	249,657	21,051	8.4	18,035	7.2	10,349	4.1	3,313	1.3	31,697	12.7
2000	274,815	23,988	8.7	18,258	6.6	12,339	4.5	4,289	1.6	34,886	12.7
2010	298,109	34,378	11.5	21,235	7.1	12,767	4.3	5,702	1.9	39,705	13.1
2020	322,602	41,959	13.0	31,680	9.8	15,467	4.8	6,480	2.0	53,627	16.6
2030	344,951	36,866	10.7	37,865	11.0	23,592	6.8	8,381	2.4	69,839	20.2
2040	364,349	38,079	10.5	33,683	9.2	28,689	7.9	13,221	3.6	75,588	20.7
2050	382,674	42,620	11.1	35,217	9.2	26,008	6.8	17,652	4.6	78,876	20.6

From U.S. Bureau of the Census, Decennial Censuses of Population (for 1900-1980). U.S. Bureau of the Census, Projections of the Populations of the United States, by Age, Sex, and Race: 1983 to 2080. Current Population Reports, Series P-25, no. 1092, November 1992.

*Projections are middle series.

†Numbers in thousands.

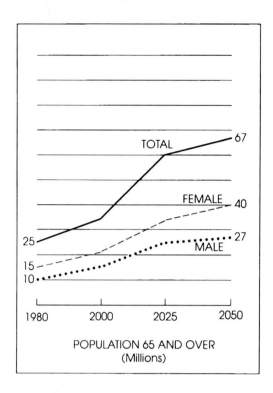

POPULATION 65 AND OVER
(Millions)

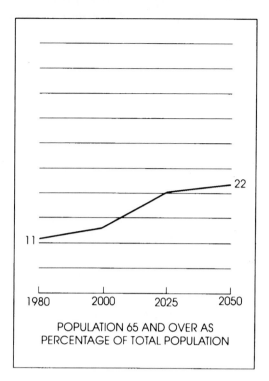

POPULATION 65 AND OVER AS
PERCENTAGE OF TOTAL POPULATION

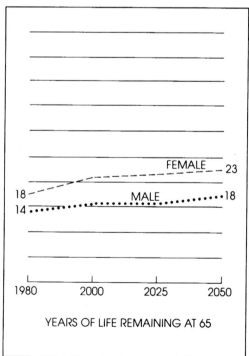

YEARS OF LIFE REMAINING AT 65

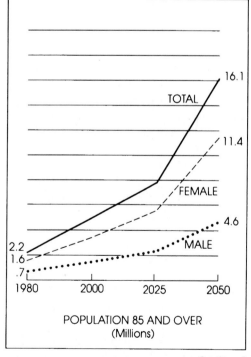

POPULATION 85 AND OVER
(Millions)

Continued

FIGURE 1-2 Projected demographic trends for the elderly, 1980-2050. (From U.S. Bureau of the Census.)

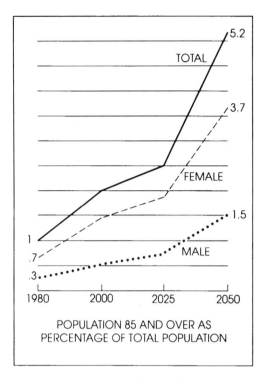

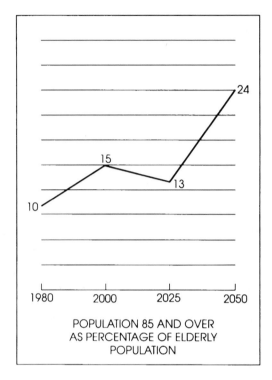

FIGURE 1-2, cont'd. For legend see p. 9.

age, Perry and Butler (1988) suggest earmarking research dollars for reducing frailty, improving health, and increasing independence among older adults. Given the common, but incorrect, belief that not much can be done to alter the aging process, coupled with the competition for research initiative dollars, aging research often loses out to other programs. Unless research dollars are directed toward minimizing older adult disabilities, recognizing the costliness of disabilities in terms of both social good and human suffering, Perry and Butler predict, for example, that Alzheimer's disease victims will increase fivefold by the middle of the next century. Unless advances are made relating to conditions associated with nursing home admissions, such as incontinence, memory loss, and immobility, there will be up to 6 million older Americans in nursing homes by the middle of the twenty-first century, as compared to 1.8 million residents in 1990. Perry and Butler plead for reducing or

eliminating "costly medical procedures, lengthy hospital stays, and financially draining long-term care."

Some research initiatives are presently underway that attempt to address these issues. For example, the Health Care Financing Administration (HCFA), within the U.S. Department of Health and Human Services, sponsors demonstrations aimed at integrating acute and long-term care benefits for older adults. The Program of All-inclusive Care for the Elderly (PACE) incorporates both acute and long-term care services for frail older adults available through Medicare and Medicaid, through a team case management approach (Vladeck et al., 1993). Another HCFA demonstration is the Social Health Maintenance Organization, which provides a wide range of support care for functionally limited Medicare recipients. HCFA's EverCare demonstration is aimed at managing the special acute care needs of the institutionalized older adult population.

TABLE 1-4 Prevalence of selected reported chronic conditions, by age, during 1987

Chronic conditions	Number of cases*	Rate per 1000 persons				
		Under 18 years	18 to 44 years	45 to 64 years	65 to 74 years	75 years and over
Heart conditions	19,656	22.2	40.7	126.1	284.7	322.2
Chronic bronchitis	12,749	62.1	40.4	56.9	86.9	58.2
Arthritis	31,438	2.8	52.8	273.3	463.6	511.9
Diabetes	6,641	2.0	11.9	56.4	98.3	98.2
Diseases of urinary system	6,769	7.3	27.8	39.6	54.8	67.7
Orthopedic impairment	27,725	35.8	135.4	155.0	154.9	182.0

From U.S. National Center for Health Statistics. (1990). *Vital and health statistics* (Series 10).
*Numbers in thousands.

Some gerontologists believe that the ability to reset the biologic clock, that is, to delay or eliminate the decline caused by aging, may be on the horizon. New information about aging is constantly being uncovered, and present-day advances in immunology and molecular aging genetics have provided valuable insights into the aging process. With reasonable, perhaps only modest, extensions of technology, there may be early resolution of problems associated with immobility, osteoporosis, and incontinence. Doubling the present monetary allotment for osteoporosis research could conceivably eliminate this major health problem, which now afflicts approximately 90% of women over the age of 75. Postponement of health deficits associated with aging has a threefold benefit: (1) the individual's health status improves, thus increasing the quality of life; (2) society's health care costs decrease; and (3) older adults' contributions to society increase, resulting in an increase in total social good. An increase in an older adult's health expectancy through reductions in chronic and disabling conditions is closely associated with an increase in enjoying the later years in life (Perry and Butler, 1988). Though one may tire of frequent references to *the improvement or maintenance of a high quality of life,* continued discussion of this term and its meaning to older adults is appropriate—even essential. As health care

providers continue to strive to increase life expectancy, of equal concern is adding quality of life to later years.

Mortality data both answer longevity questions and raise related concerns among health care delivery personnel and health policy researchers. Projections for future health care delivery and categoric financial allocation depend on data generated from current experiences and events. Various studies and reports address these concerns. One such study was prepared by K. G. Manton (1986) to determine (1) whether people are living past age 85 because better medical care and new treatments are helping those with chronic health problems to live longer and (2) whether people who live to age 85 and beyond are, on average, healthier.

One of Manton's observations was the large gain in life expectancy for those at age 85. Between 1960 and 1980, 85-year-old white men gained almost 1 year in life expectancy and 85-year-old white women gained almost 2 years in life expectancy (Tables 1-5 and 1-6). The health policy and social implications of this sizable increase are considered to be enormous. For example, this suggests a significant increase in the population who will be entitled to receive Social Security benefits. In fact, in 1995 the Social Security Administration was made an independent federal agency to increase administrative efficiency

TABLE 1-5 Expectation of life at birth, 1960 to 1988, and projections, 1990 to 2010*

Year	Total			White			Black and other			Black		
	Total	Male	Female	Total	Male	Female	Total	Male	Female	Total	Male	Female
1960	69.7	66.6	73.1	70.6	67.4	74.1	63.6	61.1	66.3	—	—	—
1970	70.8	67.1	74.7	71.7	68.0	75.6	65.3	61.3	69.4	64.1	60.0	68.3
1975	72.6	68.8	76.6	73.4	69.5	77.3	68.0	63.7	72.4	66.8	62.4	71.3
1976	72.9	69.1	76.8	73.6	69.9	77.5	68.4	64.2	72.7	67.2	62.9	71.6
1977	73.3	69.5	77.2	74.0	70.2	77.9	68.9	64.7	73.2	67.7	63.4	72.0
1978	73.5	69.6	77.3	74.1	70.4	78.0	69.3	65.0	73.5	68.1	63.7	72.4
1979	73.9	70.0	77.8	74.6	70.8	78.4	69.8	65.4	74.1	68.5	64.0	72.9
1980	73.7	70.0	77.4	74.4	70.7	78.1	69.5	65.3	73.6	68.1	63.8	72.5
1981	74.2	70.4	77.8	74.8	71.1	78.4	70.3	66.1	74.4	68.9	64.5	73.2
1982	74.5	70.9	78.1	75.1	71.5	78.7	71.0	66.8	75.0	69.4	65.1	73.7
1983	74.6	71.0	78.1	75.2	71.7	78.7	71.1	67.2	74.9	69.6	65.4	73.6
1984	74.7	71.2	78.2	75.3	71.8	78.7	71.3	67.4	75.0	69.7	65.6	73.7
1985	74.7	71.2	78.2	75.3	71.9	78.7	71.2	67.2	75.0	69.5	65.3	73.5
1986	74.8	71.3	78.3	75.4	72.0	78.8	71.2	67.2	75.1	69.4	65.2	73.5
1987	75.0	71.5	78.4	75.6	72.2	78.9	71.3	67.3	75.2	69.4	65.2	73.6
1988, preliminary	74.9	71.4	78.3	75.5	72.1	78.9	71.5	67.4	75.5	69.5	65.1	73.8
1990, projected[†]	75.4	71.8	78.8	76.1	72.7	79.4	69.1	64.5	73.6	71.2	67.0	75.2
1995, projected[†]	76.3	72.8	79.7	76.8	73.4	80.2	—	—	—	72.4	68.8	76.0
2000, projected[†]	77.0	73.5	80.4	77.5	74.0	80.9	—	—	—	73.5	69.9	77.1
2005, projected[†]	77.6	74.2	81.0	78.1	74.6	81.5	—	—	—	74.6	71.0	78.1
2010, projected[†]	77.9	74.4	81.3	78.3	74.9	81.7	—	—	—	75.0	71.4	78.5

From U.S. National Center for Health Statistics. *Vital statistics of the United States* (unpublished date).

*Data are annual, except as noted. Life expectancy is expressed in years; beginning in 1970, it excludes deaths of nonresidents of the United States, see also *Historical statistics: Colonial times to 1970* (Series B 107-115).

[†]From U.S. Bureau of the Census. *Current population reports* (Series P-25, No. 1018). Based on middle mortality assumptions.

12

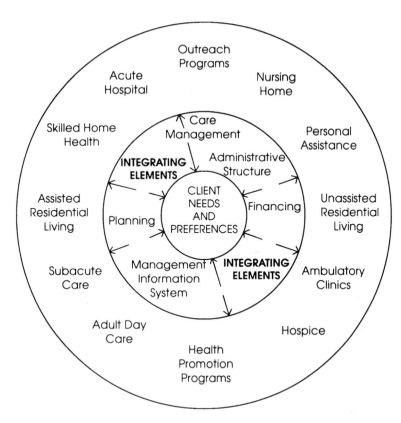

FIGURE 1-7 Example of a continuum for long-term care. (From Catholic Health Association's Task Force on Long Term Care Policy. [1988]. *A time to be old, a time to flourish—The special needs of the elderly-at-risk.* St. Louis.)

facility-focused delivery system or (2) as a patient-centered delivery system. Often the former focus is used, integrating services that focus on the facility's financial and management interests. Figure 1-8 depicts a hierarchic arrangement of integrated services in an acute care hospital. This arrangement is frequently referred to as a continuum of care, but it has little concern for individual choice. The structure requires the patient to move through all levels of care without being able to select the one or more needed services.

If the health care continuum in a health care facility is to be driven by individual need and choice, the initial step required is to perform a community assessment. The community assessment focuses on determining which services are needed by the older adult population. Once the appropriate services are identified, the next step is to ensure the availability of and access to needed services for older adults and their caregivers in the community. Figure 1-9 suggests one possible array of services that might be available to older adults. Realistically, a total patient-focused system that incorporates existing health care delivery facilities may not be financially possible, regardless of older adults' needs. The challenge of constructing a realistic patient-focused system that integrates existing health care services focuses on (1) determining community need

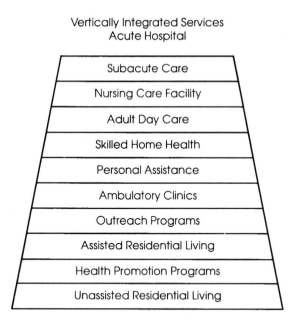

Vertically Integrated Services
Acute Hospital

Subacute Care

Nursing Care Facility

Adult Day Care

Skilled Home Health

Personal Assistance

Ambulatory Clinics

Outreach Programs

Assisted Residential Living

Health Promotion Programs

Unassisted Residential Living

FIGURE 1-8 Vertically integrated model of service acquisition. (From Catholic Health Association's Task Force on Long Term Care Policy. [1988]. *A time to be old, a time to flourish—The special needs of the elderly-at-risk.* St. Louis.)

that maximizes health benefits of older adults and (2) minimizing the financial risk to health care providers who choose to integrate, while maximizing the participants' return to ensure their continued interest. The ultimate challenge is to define and deliver "cost effective, quality of life" services.

THE ENVIRONMENT

What are the geographic location patterns of older adults? How can their physical environment be described, and what are the associated factors influencing their location choices? What are some of the housing alternatives available to older adults, especially as they age and become limited with respect to instrumental activities of daily living (IADLs)?

As people grow older, and especially as some of their functional abilities are altered, they usually seek accommodations that will be comfortable and safe. They look for homes and neighbor-

hoods that will enable them to meet their needs with as much independence as possible. Older adults consider a variety of factors that influence comfort, safety, and independence in making decisions about where, how, and with whom they will live. Table 1-13 illustrates, generally, the living arrangements experienced by selected age groups.

Older adults are less likely to change residences than members of any other age group. In 1992 only 5% of older adults had moved since the previous year, as compared to 19% of those under 65 (AARP, 1994). Older adults often prefer to remain in their own home environment, especially if it is conducive to comfortable, safe, and conveniently independent living. Within the residence, comfort may require easy access (e.g., no entry stairs), ease of movement within the residence (e.g., one level), and easy maintenance.

As it becomes more difficult for the older adult to live comfortably and independently with these arrangements, alternative living arrangements may be desirable. Assisted living communities enhance independence by providing social and physical support where necessary. For further discussion of these issues, see the section on housing.

In addition to considerations related to individual residence, the overall community also affects the older adult's choice of a living environment. Several factors affect the desirability of the community in which the residence is located—many of these factors particularly affect the relative independence of an older adult:

Safety considerations are paramount. Some older adults are unable to move about in their neighborhoods because of high crime rates. This is especially true in some urban areas.

A desire to live near family members may be the deciding factor in determining where to live.

Limited finances for moving may prohibit relocation or may mandate relocation to a less expensive residence.

Availability of transportation or easy access to community resources contributes to convenient living. Proximity to health care services, shop

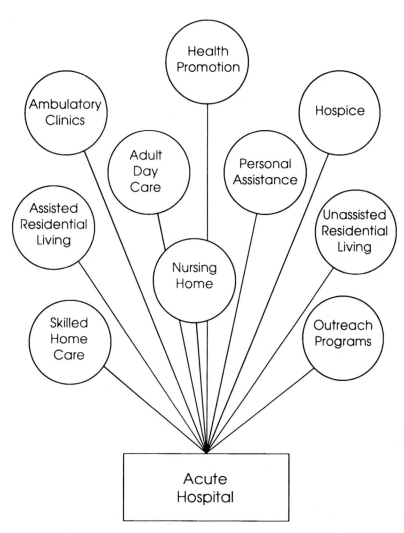

FIGURE 1-9 System development from the client's perspective. (From Catholic Health Association's Task Force on Long Term Care Policy. [1988]. *A time to be old, a time to flourish—The special needs of the elderly-at-risk.* St. Louis.)

ping, groceries, businesses, and recreational facilities greatly enhances the desirability of a community.

Geographic location

For some older adults, the warm climates of selected southern states are appealing. In 1993 over half of all older adults lived in nine states: California (over 3 million), Florida (over 2 million), New York (over 2 million), Pennsylvania (over 1 million), Texas (over 1 million), Ohio (over 1 million), Illinois (over 1 million), Michigan (over 1 million), and New Jersey (over 1 million) (AARP, 1994) (Figure 1-10). Older adults are less likely to live in central cities and more likely to live in suburbs; yet they are 3 times as

TABLE 1-13 Living arrangements of the elderly: 1990 and 1980 (In thousands. Noninstitutional populations)

Living arrangement and age	1990 Number			1990 Percent distribution			1980 Number			1980 Percent distribution		
	Total	Men	Women	Total	Men	Women	Total	Men	Women	Total	Men	Women
65 years and over	29,566	12,334	17,232	100.0	100.0	100.0	24,157	9,889	14,268	100.0	100.0	100.0
Living												
Alone	9,176	1,942	7,233	31.0	15.7	42.0	7,067	1,447	5,620	29.3	14.6	39.4
With spouse	16,003	9,158	6,845	54.1	74.3	39.7	12,781	7,441	5,340	52.9	75.2	37.4
With other relatives	3,734	953	2,782	12.6	7.7	16.1	3,892	832	3,060	16.1	8.4	21.4
With nonrelatives only†	653	281	372	2.2	2.3	2.2	417	169	248	1.7	1.7	1.7
65 to 74 years	17,979	8,013	9,966	100.0	100.0	100.0	15,302	6,621	8,681	100.0	100.0	100.0
Living												
Alone	4,350	1,042	3,309	24.2	13.0	33.2	3,750	797	2,953	24.5	12.0	34.0
With spouse	11,353	6,265	5,089	63.1	78.2	51.1	9,436	5,285	4,151	61.7	79.8	47.8
With other relatives	1,931	528	1,401	10.7	6.6	14.1	1,890	436	1,454	12.4	6.6	16.7
With nonrelatives only†	345	178	167	1.9	2.2	1.7	226	103	123	1.5	1.6	1.4
75 to 84 years	9,354	3,562	5,792	100.0	100.0	100.0	7,172	2,708	4,464	100.0	100.0	100.0
Living												
Alone	3,774	688	3,086	40.3	19.3	53.3	2,664	505	2,159	37.1	18.6	48.4
With spouse	4,145	2,537	1,607	44.3	71.2	27.7	2,977	1,882	1,095	41.5	69.5	24.5
With other relatives	1,237	264	974	13.2	7.4	16.8	1,394	271	1,123	19.4	10.0	25.2
With nonrelatives only†	198	73	125	2.1	2.0	2.2	137	50	87	1.9	1.8	1.9
85 years and over	2,233	758	1,475	100.0	100.0	100.0	1,683	560	1,123	100.0	100.0	100.0
Living												
Alone	1,051	213	838	47.1	28.1	56.8	653	145	508	38.8	25.9	45.2
With spouse	505	356	150	22.6	47.0	10.2	368	274	94	21.9	48.9	8.4
With other relatives	567	160	406	25.4	21.1	27.5	608	125	483	36.1	22.3	43.0
With nonrelatives only†	110	29	81	4.9	3.8	5.5	54	16	38	3.2	2.9	3.4

From Saluter, A. F., U.S. Bureau of the Census. (1991, May). *Marital status and living arrangements: March 1990* (Current Population Reports, Series P-20, No. 450). Washington, DC: U.S. Government Printing Office. Table L.
†1980 data include a small number of persons in unrelated subfamilies.

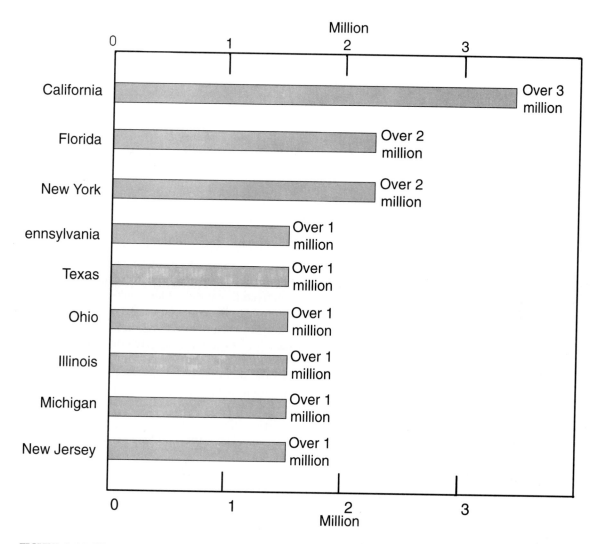

FIGURE 1-10 Nine states with the highest proportion of people 65 years old and over, 1990. States are ranked largest to smallest. (From U.S. Bureau of the Census, *Current Population Reports,* Series P-25, 1990.)

likely to live in a metropolitan area as in a nonmetropolitan area (Taeuber, 1993).

During the 1980s the greatest increase in the older adult population was in the western states and southeastern coastal states (Taeuber, 1993). By the year 2010 approximately 56% of the projected 39 million older adults will live in one of ten states—California, Florida, New York, Texas, Pennsylvania, Illinois, Ohio, New Jersey, North Carolina, or Michigan. Since the 1960s the southern and western areas of the United States have been popular areas for relocation upon retiring. This just-retired population tended to be healthy and economically secure. Since the 1970s these locations have gained popularity among the older old, a population that is typically less healthy. However, these regions may not have planned for delivering health care to a changing population.

Although older adults are less likely to change residence than are members of other age groups, some do change geographic locations for various reasons. In an AARP profile (1994), the majority of older adults (75%) who did move, moved to another location in the same state. Some older adults move their residence to be nearer other family members, especially their own children. However, one group of older adults in the profile somewhat facetiously suggested that older parents moved in order to live *further* from their children. Typically healthy and socially active, these older adults could have been illuminating their desire to avoid some of the tasks and responsibilities associated with their child's younger family, preferring to "reap the rewards" retirement years bring.

Housing

As the twenty-first century approaches, the number of older adults increases in proportion to the total U.S. population. One opportunity will be that of creatively defining alternative and accessible residence options for an adult population with a wide range of functional capabilities. Included in this population are those who require assistance with IADLs. This accounts for 45% of those who are 85 or over and who are noninstitutionalized (U.S. Bureau of the Census, 1992) and for the 1.7 million nursing home residents (Table 1-14 and Figure 1-11).

There is a wide range of living arrangements among older adults. Of the older adult, noninstitutionalized, 1990 population, 69% lived in family settings (10 million men and 9.9 million women). About 13% of people over age 65 were living with children, siblings, other relatives (excluding spouses), or nonrelatives, many of whom were under age 65. The number of older people living

TABLE 1-14 Nursing home population, by U.S. region: 1980 to 1990 percentage change*

U.S. region	1980	1990	Percentage change
Total	1,426	1,721	24.2
Northeast	327	399	22.0
Midwest	472	545	15.3
South	397	558	40.8
West	230	270	17.3

From U.S. Bureau of the Census.
*Numbers in thousands.

alone increased by 72% between 1970 and 1987, about 1½ times the growth rate for the older population in general. Approximately 9.2 million noninstitutionalized older adults lived alone in 1990, 7.2 million women and 1.9 million men. A relatively small number (1.3 million) and percentage (5%) of people age 65 or older lived in nursing homes in 1985. In 1987 1% of people 65 to 74 years old lived in nursing homes, as did 6% of people between ages 75 and 84, and 22% of people 85 years of age and over. The probability of being admitted to a nursing home increases with age. The typical nursing home resident is an older woman, with four out of five residents 75 years of age or over (Taeuber, 1993).

The American Association of Retired Persons, always at the forefront of addressing the needs of senior citizens, publishes a variety of literature aimed at facilitating exploration and decision making regarding residence options. Most older adults choose to remain in their own home environment if the specialized services they need can be made available to them. An AARP publication, *Staying at Home: A Guide to Long-Term Care and Housing,* includes data to assist people in deciding whether home care is plausible and whether specialized services can be brought to the home. For example, if an older adult needs help around the house, a potential service might be a homemaker or home health aide to help with chores or personal care. AARP

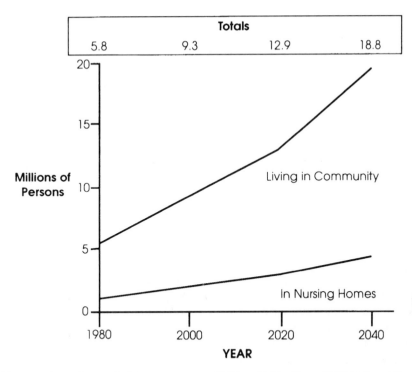

Totals			
5.8	9.3	12.9	18.8

FIGURE 1-11 Older Americans in need of long-term care, 1980 to 2040. (From 1982 National Long-term Care Survey and 1977 National Nursing Home Survey and Social Security Administration Projections.)

also provides suggestions for requesting home health services and paying for long-term care, and lists specific criteria for evaluating the quality of the available services. The search for basic information might begin with a call to the Eldercare locator, a toll-free service aimed at linking older adults and their families to information about available resources (1-800-677-1116; 9 AM to 5 PM EST).

Continued residence in one's own home is only one alternative as one grows older. As the number of older adults and the need for assistance in the ADL's grow, so do the range and types of residence options. At one extreme is the continuing care retirement community (CCRC), offering a wide range of services from housekeeping to nursing care. CCRCs are one alternative for older adults needing assistance with daily living tasks. Care focuses on the older adult's needs and the desire to live in a safe and

clearly—often physically—defined community environment. Another type of assisted living arrangement is the assisted living facility or board and care home. This type of arrangement offers daily assistance services for older adults, short of nursing home care. Congregate housing is another residence option. Older adults may have their own apartment, but congregate housing focuses on group living, with shared meals, planned activities, and daily housekeeping service provided. Another type of living arrangement, offering less direct support with daily living activities, is the elder cottage housing opportunity (ECHO). These are typically self-contained, barrier-free units placed in the yard of a single-family house. Home sharing is another type of living arrangement that offers little direct support with ADLs. As the name *home sharing* implies, two or more unrelated older adults share common areas of a house or apartment.

A newer concept in residence options is retirement communities constructed right on university campuses. Even in college towns where retirement communities do not exist, college campuses have been attracting increased numbers of retirees in recent years. Building a life-care community where retired faculty and alumni can reside has appeal for both retirees and property owners. One advantage for the property owner (often the university or college itself) is that people who are seeking places for retirement may offset the loss created by the shrinking pool of 18-year-olds. The retirees may feel a natural affection for returning to the environment where they spent many enjoyable days. Retirees may wish to take advantage of cultural and educational opportunities while reflecting on past memories. In addition, continuing contributions from the retirees may be both experiential and financial. Retirees can continue to teach and share their expertise and experience in a variety of ways in the educational setting, also possibly making financial contributions in the form of alumni gifts and bequests. An educational institution associated with a medical school and/or a nursing school may have an additional reason to be attracted to this arrangement. Having many retirees available close to the learning center makes for an ideal situation for geriatric-gerontology educational programs. The eventual outcome of these new ventures remains to be seen, but to many, this arrangement has a special appeal (Lewin, 1990). As the need for housing for older adults increases in the twenty-first century, it seems likely that there will be additional innovative and creative means developed for meeting this basic need.

■ Sociologic Concerns, Economics, and Intellectual Abilities

SOCIOLOGIC CONCERNS

As older adults enter their retirement years, the majority are relatively healthy and receive retirement income from previous paid employment (Neugarten, 1978). Currently, older men retire earlier than they did 40 years ago (Taeuber, 1993). In 1950 almost 70% of men 55 years of age and over were working; in 1990 this figure decreased to under 40%. Over 45% of men 65 and older were working in 1950; in 1990 only 16% of men 65 and older were working.

Women's retirement patterns follow a similar decreasing trend. However, a policy expert panel on aging suggests that this trend may not continue (Wilson, et al., 1994). Improvements in older adults' health status, the desire to stay active, and economic constraints limiting one's choice to retire early all contribute to the likelihood of future older adults staying in the work force.

Despite these retirement projections for future older adults, the number of healthy, young retirees currently continues to grow. As a result, older adults have the opportunity to explore a wide range of activities. For example, older adults may choose to travel, attend recreational or educational events, or participate in relaxing and satisfying hobbies for which they could never find time before. They can also pursue another career, which may be similar to, or completely different from, the one from which they have just retired. Opportunities to do volunteer work abound. The expertise and experience of older adults are invaluable, making them unique contributors in countless situations.

As the pool of healthy older adults continues to grow, the social perception of hiring older workers is changing. The results are increases in new and innovative job opportunities for older adults. Concerns about older adults' productivity are proving to be unfounded, based on the experiences of companies that employ older adults. The Days Inns of America experiment in hiring older workers as reservations agents was highly successful from a cost-benefit standpoint (McNaught & Barth, 1992). Older workers remained on the job longer than younger workers; they received higher wages because they stayed on the job longer; and although they spent more time talking to callers, they were more successful in booking reservations than younger workers.

Another "do it yourself" chain experimentally staffed only older workers and found it to be very successful, with no adverse effects on profitability (Hogarth & Barth, 1991). Travelers Corporation, a large financial services company, found that older adults were the answer to maximizing the company's staffing efficiency with highly productive temporary workers (McNaught & Barth, 1991). Even the McDonald's fast-food chain developed a "McMasters' Program," which enables retired adults to fill the dearth of available employees (Beck, 1990). Often employment opportunities provide more than career enhancement or pure economic gains. The jobs also provide a means of increasing the older adult's self-esteem or satisfying the human need for social contacts.

Many companies and employers are taking innovative approaches to hiring older adults, matching the needs of their business to the expertise of older adults who wish to be employed. T. Franklin Williams suggests that this trend toward continuing employment will increase in the twenty-first century: "We're going to see more and more second and third careers" (Beck, 1990).

Depending on their state of health and underlying motivation, many retirees spend much of their time in a volunteer role. Policy experts in aging state that the growing number of healthy older adults represents an abundant volunteer resource pool (Wilson et al., 1994). On average, 25 hours per week are freed up as a result of retirement for males; 18 hours per week for females. Maintaining an active role in their community is a stimulating and attractive way of life for many older adults. For example, elementary schools recruit retirees to teach and tutor in special programs (e.g., day reading programs and evening computer classes). AARP currently funds a grant aimed at involving older adults as mentors and tutors in public elementary schools in Montgomery County, Maryland. Both children and retirees enjoy these interactions, which serve to enrich intergenerational understanding. This type of experience fosters a positive, regenera-

tive cycle. The more active and involved older adults become, the healthier they are. The longer they remain healthy, the more active and involved they can remain. Most contemporary public services offer a wide range of attractive volunteer opportunities for older adults.

Another sociologic concern relates to the "sandwich generation," those older adults who bear the responsibility both for their children and for their aging parents. They are sandwiched between two dependent generations. This relatively new role for older adults is becoming increasingly common as the baby boom generation ages. It quite likely could become the norm for future older adults (Beck, 1990) (Figure 1-12). The baby boomers of today will constitute a large number of older adults tomorrow. They potentially will be more physically and financially independent and will be better educated than today's typical older adult. As a result of this, and of living longer, they will more likely be in the role of caregiver for both their children and their parents. Many American families may even see four generations living at one point in time by the year 2000. A national survey found that "sandwich generation" adults see themselves as making substantial transfers of both time and money to their frail, older parents, with women providing help in terms of time and men most likely providing financial help.

Many older adults are self-sufficient and are able to maintain healthy independence. These are the older adults who will be responsible for caring for their older parents. More older adults in their early retirement years will face the responsibility of caring for their very old, frail parents or relatives (Taeuber, 1993). As longevity increases, it is inevitable that some parents will live to see their children retire. They may even seek the assistance of their retired children for some type of support. The difficulties of these responsibilities for the older adult sandwich generation can be onerous. For example, consider the situation of an older, single adult with two grown children who also has aging parents living nearby. The adult is the only child living near the

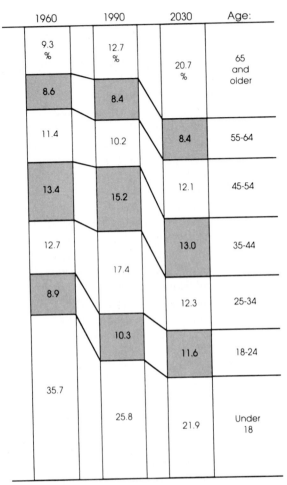

FIGURE 1-12 Age distribution of total U.S. population. (From U.S. Bureau of the Census.)

parents, and the parents' health is beginning to fail. Furthermore, the adult's children still require assistance (in terms of time and money). The result is intense pressure and sometimes devastating stress on the adult, who must juggle twilight career responsibilities (which may increase because of increased financial pressures), providing assistance to the children, and filling the caretaker role for aging parents. An added challenge may involve searching for adequate resources and support services to assist in fulfilling multiple responsibilities.

Not the least of the problems encountered in this type of situation is the psychologic task of role reversal faced when the adult child must care for dependent parents. As the dependency of the aging parent increases, the adult child increasingly assumes the caregiver role. This may set the stage for increasing psychologic dependence on the part of the parent. Role reversal may be consciously recognized and perpetuated, unconsciously recognized and perpetuated, or consciously recognized and limited. Some adult children report negative feelings, resulting in strained relationships among family members. Many adult children are able to develop significant emotional bonds with their aging parents and report, in spite of difficulties, a high level of personal satisfaction and acceptance of their filial responsibilities.

The sandwich generation problems coming to light in the 1990s will surely increase in future decades. Some statistics indicate that as of the beginning of the 1990s, about 5 million Americans were spending some of their time caring for a parent. By the year 2010 that number is likely to double.

ECONOMICS

In the past, one could perhaps make generalizations about anyone over 65 and be fairly accurate. The number of people over 65 was relatively small compared to all other age groups. Quite often there were social restrictions on older adults' roles and functions. However, as we observe increases in the proportion of older adults and changes in their health status, quality of life, social choices, and economic diversity, society's concept of those over 65 changes. Broad generalizations about anyone over 65 become very difficult to make. There is greater economic status variation among older adults than ever before. It is impossible to describe older adults in terms of a broad economic statement that might apply to every older adult.

Some view older people as being quite comfortable economically, a view supported by several reports that give evidence of financial security among a sizable number of older adults. For example, J. B. Quinn (1990) states that members of the pre–World War II generation married in their early 20s, had children, and by age 50, finished paying for their children's college tuition. They then focused on saving for their own retirement 10 to 15 years down the road. The standard of living of pre–World War II older adults is in sharp contrast with the experiences of the baby boomer older adults. Competition for job openings and security, delays in marriage, delays in having children, increasing longevity, and caretaker responsibilities for frail parents all contribute to quite a different economic experience for retiring older adults today. Personal savings and retirement benefits amounts may be reduced in the future, putting more of an economic burden on retired older adults (Taeuber, 1993).

The professional literature and daily news stories report a concern for older baby boomers and for the responsibility they will bear in caring for parents and grandparents. Though some older baby boomers are indeed heavily burdened by the care they must provide to aging parents, one should not conclude that all older adults excessively burden their adult children. In fact, many older parents actually help their adult children by providing down payments for a home purchase or tuition assistance for their grandchildren. Many older adults may find themselves in the comfortable position of being able to reap the rewards of their diligent work and the frugality they exercised in their younger years. Contrary to concerned reports regarding the older baby boomers, others have concluded that the older generation holds unprecedented wealth. Because aging parents today are less likely than those of previous generations to need financial assistance from their children, some conclude that most older adults are wealthy.

These conflicting and extreme conclusions illustrate how stereotypes of older adults often lead to erroneous generalizations. For example, many people who write about older adults in America describe them as poor, hopeless, helpless, sick, and downtrodden—objects of pity and public charity. On the other hand, a more recent stereotype is that older adults in America are rich, greedy, self-serving, and self-centered, needing no help from their family, the U.S. government, or anyone else. Before jumping to either conclusion, it behooves the observer to be very discriminating when defining the older population (Quinn, 1990). The fact is, both kinds of older adults exist. All seek the assurance of adequate and reliable retirement income that can "spell the critical difference between dignity and despair" (AARP & Pacific Presbyterian Medical Center of San Francisco, 1989). Although many older adults can expect to be financially comfortable in their retirement years, many others live in poverty or at least near the poverty level, which seriously compromises their sense of dignity.

Income generally decreases after retirement, but the income after retirement is relatively stable because so many older adults receive Social Security payments (Taeuber, 1993). Social Security benefits represent the largest share of income for people age 85 and older (Figure 1-13). Although the primary source of income for older adults remains Social Security, there are several other income sources: property, pensions, personal savings, investments, earnings, and a variety of financial assets. Social Security income and pension benefits accounted for approximately 45% of the total household income of older adults in 1986 (Taeuber, 1993). However, not every older citizen has the benefit of all or even several of these sources. Older adults are more likely than those 25 to 64 years old to receive welfare assistance (Taeuber, 1993). Differences in income are best explained by the following factors: former occupational status, educational attainment, work history, age, sex, race, ethnicity, marital status, and living arrangements (Taeuber, 1993).

Economic facts of life for older adults in the United States during the late 1980s and early 1990s included the following:

In 1989 11.4% of people 65 and over lived in poverty. That is, their weekly income was $120

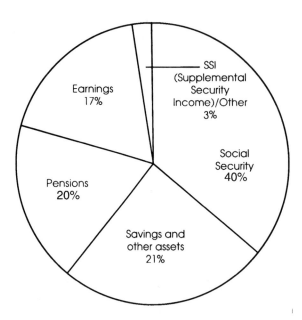

FIGURE 1-13 Sources of income for people 85 years old and older. (From U.S. Department of Health and Human Services, Social Security Administration, and Office of Research and Statistics. [1994]. *Income of the aged chartbook, 1992* [SSA Pub. No. 13-11727]. Washington, DC: U.S. Government Printing Office.)

or less for single-person households and $152 for two-person households. This was 8% lower than the poverty income figures for single-person households 15 to 64 years old and 11% lower than the poverty income figures for two-person households 15 to 64 years old (Taeuber, 1993).

Between 17% and 28% of white women 85 years of age or older in 1990 were living in poverty (Taeuber, 1993). The rate increased to between 15% and 55% for black women. Poverty levels were greater for women, minorities, older adults living alone, and the very old.

In 1990 over 27% of married-couple households of 65- to 69-year-olds received annual incomes of less than $20,000. The percentage increased to over 32% for married-couple households 70 to 74 years old and to over 40% for married-

couple households 75 years old and over (Taeuber, 1993).

In 1990 the mean monthly private pension income (not including Social Security) was $652. Six out of ten older adults receiving private pension income were men. About one third of those living alone received private pension income (Taeuber, 1993).

Examination of the economic status of older adults in the United States results in a wide diversity of views. Economic and demographic statistics can support conflicting conclusions. One may find statistics supporting either the belief that older adults are very rich or that they are very poor, depending upon the statistical parameters presented and/or omitted (Table 1-15 and Figure 1-14).

In a qualitative report about "the other side of easy street," the Villers Foundation set out to separate fact from fiction and to identify what is reality for older adults versus what are myths about their economic status. At the heart of the report is a plea to eliminate the disparity between the rich and the poor, no matter their age. Goals for all ages are the elimination of poverty, providing access to health care, and creating availability of shelter (Bethell, 1987).

The Villers report examines some of the myths incorrectly describing the economics of old age. One such myth is that there is not very much poverty among older adults, as a result of their above-average income. They are believed to live better than those younger than age 65. Differences in describing who is poor and who is not would be eliminated given clear definitions and measurements of poverty. The existing poverty index has been criticized because it fails to consider poverty as a relative concept (Stone, 1989). If criteria for identifying those who are living in poverty were applied to all age groups consistently, the poverty rate among older adults would increase markedly. Because children are a large percentage of the population and there is a high rate of poverty among children, the rate of

TABLE 1-15 Persons 65 years old and over who were below poverty level, by selected characteristics: 1970 to 1987*

	Number below poverty level (in thousands)					Percentage below poverty level				
	1970	1979†	1985	1986	1987	1970	1979†	1985	1986	1987
Total, 65 years and over‡	4,793	3,682	3,456	3,477	3,491	24.6	15.2	12.6	12.4	12.2
White	4,011	2,911	2,698	2,689	2,597	22.6	13.3	11.0	10.7	10.1
Black	735	740	717	722	808	47.7	36.3	31.5	31.0	33.9
Hispanic§	—	154	219	204	247	—	26.8	23.9	22.5	27.4
In families	2,013	1,380	1,173	1,164	1,247	14.8	8.4	6.4	6.2	6.5
Householder	1,188	822	708	716	751	16.5	9.1	7.0	7.0	7.2
Male	980	629	498	520	533	15.9	8.4	6.0	6.1	6.1
Female	209	193	210	196	218	20.1	13.0	12.1	11.8	12.6
Other members	825	559	465	448	496	13.0	7.6	5.6	5.2	5.7
Unrelated individuals	2,779	2,299	2,281	2,311	2,241	47.2	29.4	25.6	25.2	24.0
Male	549	428	402	412	416	38.9	25.3	20.5	19.6	19.3
Female	2,230	1,871	1,879	1,899	1,825	49.8	30.5	27.0	26.8	25.4
Total, 60 years and over	5,977	4,753	4,677	4,547	4,657	21.3	13.9	12.3	11.7	11.8

From U.S. Bureau of the Census. *Current population reports* (Series P-60, No. 61). And unpublished data.

*Persons as of March of following year. Based on old processing procedures; therefore data will not agree with other tables.

†Population controls based on 1980 census.

‡Beginning in 1979, includes members of unrelated subfamilies not shown separately; for earlier years, unrelated subfamily members are included in the "In families" category.

§Hispanic persons may be of any race.

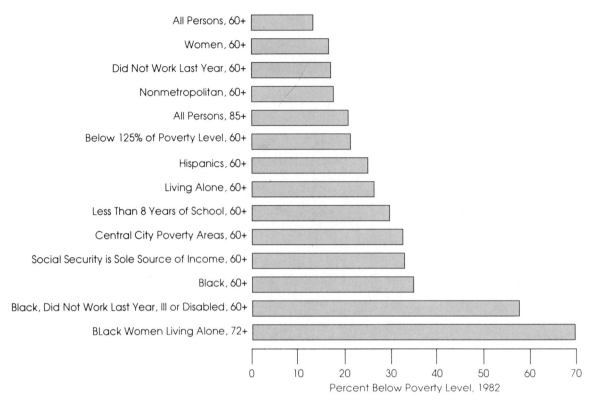

FIGURE 1-14 Percent below poverty level by selected population group. Poverty remains high for some groups. (From U.S. Bureau of the Census.)

poverty among adults who have no children is calculated as being lower than it would be if children were not considered. If only adults were considered, it could be concluded that poverty among older adults is a more serious problem than it appears to be when all age groups are considered (Bethell, 1987).

In 1989 the U.S. Bureau of the Census defined the monetary cutoff for poverty as $6240 per year for an older individual and $7904 for older couples. Some contend that this defines poverty too narrowly. A broader definition of poverty should consider availability of resources such as "basic services, decision-making power, and dignity" (Stone, 1989, p. 22). For example, the cost of health care among older adults is an

additional factor that should be considered when determining the level of poverty. Older adults spent approximately 15% of their income on health care in 1985. If the poverty level were adjusted to consider these out-of-pocket health costs, the poverty rate among older adults would rise further (Stone, 1989).

INTELLECTUAL ABILITIES AND OPPORTUNITIES IN CONTINUING EDUCATION

When considering sociologic information, one must bear in mind that what is known about a group of people may not be true of many individuals within that group. Like many other groups, the aging population defies overgeneralization. The emphasis on youth in the United States further fuels the tendency to stereotype the aging population. However, these stereotypes are being challenged as the number of older adults increases. For example, shoe advertisements depict active older adults. And it is not unusual to turn on the television and see older adults skydiving. But there remain uphill challenges to dispelling many of the myths about aging. Among the most pernicious of these is the prevailing myth that intellectual abilities automatically decline with age. Schaie (1983) has taken steps to dispel this myth by conducting a longitudinal study of about 4000 participants who have been tested throughout the study's 30 years. Schaie and the other researchers at Pennsylvania State University have concluded that "in the absence of disease, those [people] who have maintained a very high level of interaction with their environment" do not demonstrate a decline in mental skills or knowledge as they age. The "use it or lose it" principle appears to apply to the maintenance of high levels of intellectual performance, as well as to muscular strength (Keller, 1986).

Many older adults still "use it" and are far from "losing it," contradicting the stereotypes of being sick, poor, and lonely. These older adults are more concerned about seizing opportunities for learning and enjoying life than some younger people are prepared to believe. As early as 1978 Birren said the following: "I am forecasting a graying of the university where persons of all ages will be seeking knowledge about the conditions of life. They will be an informed and eager group, interested in extending their options in life as well as contemplating the meaning of their own life with a measure of maturity unique to themselves."

In the future, education systems will have to revamp their offerings, schedules, and resources to accommodate the decreasing numbers of younger people and the increasing numbers of older people. Some of the older people will be seeking skills and knowledge applicable to new and different careers. This knowledge will complement their existing experience and skills gleaned from past careers and will build new skills for new frontiers. Other older adults, rather than seeking career-related skills, will pursue further education for the sheer pleasure of learning.

Gerontologic literature contains very little information about the kind of reaction the older student can expect from the traditional university community. Without solid evidence regarding the experiences of older adult students, there was once a fear that faculty might be biased against the older person. Hays conducted a research study (supported by the Andrus Foundation) at Wichita State University in Kansas related to this issue. He found just the opposite to be true (AARP, 1989-1990). As a result of this study, the first longitudinal data base was established about older student behavior, with a focus on students ages 60 and older. Data were collected over a 6-year period. Data were obtained by encouraging older people to audit selected classes and then by interviewing the older adults auditing these classes. Findings indicated that over 75% of the faculty members whose classes were audited found that older adults were better motivated than younger students and learned just as quickly. Three out of five faculty members felt that older students contributed positively to the classes. The study also helped university officials to better understand the older student and relieved university officials' concerns regarding the cost associated with enrolling older students—the costs were found to be minimal (AARP, 1989-1990).

Older students enroll in programs for a variety of reasons—to pursue different or additional degrees, to enhance their careers, to increase their earning capabilities, or for the simple pursuit of knowledge. These various reasons for continuing education may influence which of several educational options an older adult chooses. Four options offer special advantages for many older learners:

1. Some universities open their enrollments to interested retirees who are not in degree

programs, giving open slots in selected courses. These non–degree-seeking older students register, enroll in the courses, and participate in all the same requirements and activities as the younger students.

2. The Elderhostel program exemplifies an exciting opportunity to learn. This Boston-based, nonprofit program provides an environment where older citizens are stimulated intellectually. The plan follows the tradition of hosteling as practiced in Europe. Older people live on a college or university campus and attend classes, usually for a 1-week period, to experience the life and learning of the college student. The fee for this educational experience is modest—about $250 per week for room, board, and tuition. The Elderhostel concept is based on the belief that retirement offers a time of opportunity for the older person to engage in and enjoy new experiences and new challenges.

3. The Older Adult Service and Information System (OASIS), in operation since 1982, is a partnership between governmental departments of aging, usually at a county level, and businesses, usually those located in shopping centers or shopping malls. Volunteers offer their services to provide instruction for interested older adults who learn about health care, creative writing, music appreciation, wood carving, physical fitness, dancing, and any number of creative recreational activities.

4. Full- or part-time summer programs are especially attractive to older adults who look forward to traveling and new activities in the summer months. Educators are becoming increasingly concerned that schools and classrooms may not be well utilized between the month of graduation and the beginning of a new school year. Providing opportunities for interested and motivated older adults allows the classrooms to be used constructively and enables the faculty and teachers to pursue gainful employment between academic semesters.

Whether the older student pays a full- or part-time tuition or even a reduced or discounted tuition, the gray-haired student is becoming a welcome sight on campus. The older students' interest and enthusiasm make an excellent climate for fostering teaching and learning. They stimulate and motivate younger learners and facilitate the creation of an exciting, productive, competitive atmosphere.

■ Demography of Aging in the United States

FACTORS INFLUENCING DEMOGRAPHIC TRENDS

A predictive demographic profile of older adults is paramount to a policymaker's accurate planning for the short- and long-term needs of the older adult population. Anyone involved in delivering services or care for older adults needs specific information regarding factors such as age, gender, race, living arrangements, and marital status. Articles and publications (especially from the U.S. Department of Commerce, Bureau of the Census) about aging and older adults often include these types of statistical data. In filtering through these data and assessing predictions, one must astutely gauge the accuracy of the underlying assumptions associated with predictive modeling (McFarland, 1978). Demographers often mention two factors associated with predicting trends among older adults:

1. Incidence of disease
2. Rate of aging

Reduction of the incidence of disease would lead to reduced mortality rates and an increase in the number of older adults. This projection assumes that health practices will improve, which, in turn, will contribute to the control of disease. Lifestyle changes are most directly associated with reductions in disease, typically those related to diet and exercise. Examples of lifestyle changes are the reduction or elimination of smoking and use of alcohol or drugs; increased physical activity; improved dietary habits; and annual (or more frequent) physical examinations that include health screening for early disease detection and treatment planning.

Control of the rate of aging is a bit more complex than reducing the incidence of disease. It involves first understanding the genetic and environmental factors associated with the aging process. This includes an understanding of such things as the aging body's physiologic (e.g., immune, endocrine) systems. The second step is to apply this understanding to deterring the effects of the aging process (Neugarten, 1978). The National Institute on Aging within the National Institutes of Health is responsible for conducting and supporting biomedical, social, and behavioral research and for disseminating information related to the aging process and diseases of older adults (National Institute on Aging [NIA], 1994).

CHANGING DEMOGRAPHICS AMONG OLDER ADULTS

In 1993 there were 32.8 million persons in the United States age 65 or over. This was 12.7% of the total U.S. population, or about one in eight persons. Since 1900 the number of people age 65 and over has increased more than 10 times and the percentage has tripled (AARP, 1994). The population can also be tracked by breaking out age categories for older adults. In 1990 approximately 7% of the U.S. population was between 65 and 74 (about 18 million persons). This was over 8 times the number of people in this age group in 1900. In 1990 approximately 4% of the U.S. population was between 75 and 84 years old and approximately 1.2% was 85 years old or older. These numbers were 12 times and 23 times, respectively, the numbers in 1900 (AARP & Pacific Presbyterian Medical Center, 1989; Taeuber, 1993) (Table 1-16 and Figure 1-12).

Population growth by age category is projected based on current birth and death data.

TABLE 1-16 Total population, by age: 1960 to 1991

Year	Total	65 to 74 years	75 years and over
1960	180,671	11,053	5,622
1975	215,973	13,971	8,779
1985	239,279	17,009	11,531
1988	246,329	17,897	12,470
1991	252,503	18,548	13,497

From U.S. Bureau of the Census. *Current population reports* (Series P-25, Nos. 519-917).

The U.S. Bureau of the Census provides such data and generates forecasting models that estimate future U.S. population growth. The older adult population is expected to continue to grow in the future, slowing somewhat in the 1990s because of the smaller number of births during the 1930s. However, an accelerated increase is forecast between 2010 and 2030, when the baby boom generation reaches age 65 (AARP, 1994). At that time, 77 million persons (one third of the current U.S. population) will be senior citizens (Beck, 1990). Based on current data and trends, demographers project that there will be almost 80 million older adults in the United States by the year 2030 (or over 20% of the total U.S. population). This is almost 3 times the number of older adults that were in the United States in 1980 (AARP, 1994). The age groups made up of people over 55 will be the only U.S. age groups to experience significant growth in the next century, especially if current fertility and immigration levels remain stable (AARP & Pacific Presbyterian Medical Center, 1989).

The total population of the United States is expected to rise from 249 million in 1990 to 345 million in 2030 and 383 million in 2050. Following this peak, it is predicted that a slow decline in numbers will occur until 2080, when the population will stabilize.

Other changes in population in the United States will create subtle but certain alterations in the workplace, education, and health care. Some businesses, professions, and industries will expand. For example, as the population ages, deaths will outnumber births, so the funeral business and associated industries (e.g., casket companies, cemeteries, florists, and funeral equipment suppliers) will expand. Total birth rates will drop, and there could be labor shortages in those industries in which labor supplies depend on young workers. Factors, unknown at the present, could alter these scenarios. For example, technologic breakthroughs could dramatically change the manner and shape of current business and industry practices.

In the future the health care system will be challenged to provide institutional care for those who need it. At present, this is usually the very old person with comorbidity and significant disabilities. The health care system will also be challenged to promote healthy aging directives among older adults. Those who are interested in assisting older adults in maximizing their quality of life will have to provide creative programs and novel initiatives to meet the unique needs of the increasingly complex mix of older individuals.

Gender

Women make up the majority of the expanding number of older adults and are more likely than men to live alone, to be poor, and to suffer from long-term chronic illnesses. In 1990 there were about 67 men age 65 and over for every 100 women age 65 and over. This was approximately 18.5 million older adult women and about 12.5 million older adult men. The ratio of men to women in 1990 was 81:100 for people 65 to 69 years of age; 74:100 for people 70 to 74 years of age; 64:100 for people 75 to 79 years of age; 53:100 for people 80 to 84 years of age; and 39:100 for people 85 years of age and older (Taeuber, 1993) (Figure 1-15).

Racial and ethnic groups

Studies of the racial and ethnic characteristics of older populations depict the following: In 1993 about 86% of people age 65 and over in the United States were white, non-Hispanics; 8% were African American; 3% were of Hispanic origin; 2% were Asian or Pacific Islander; and less than 1% were American Indian or Native Alaskan (AARP, 1994) (Figure 1-16). Haub (1990), of the Population Reference Bureau, predicts that the dramatically lower birth rates among whites will partially account for some dramatic changes in the United States' racial and ethnic mix in the future. By the year 2080 Haub suggests that white, non-Hispanic Americans will be on the verge of losing their majority to the current three largest minority groups: African Americans, Asian Americans, and Hispanics. This prediction suggests a change from that of a U.S. Bureau of the Census 1988 report estimating a U.S. population of 245 million in 2080, with 84.4% being white, 12.3% black, and 3.3% "other races" (Asians, Pacific Islanders, Native Americans, and Eskimos and other Alaskan Native Americans).

Marital status

In 1993 about 77% of older adult men were married, as compared to 42% of older adult women. Almost half of the older adult women were widows (48%, or 8.6 million). This was 5 times the number of older adult widowers (1.8 million). Approximately 5% of older adults were divorced (1.6 million). The number of divorced older adults has increased 3 times as fast as the entire older adult population since 1980 (AARP, 1994). This trend is quite likely to continue into the future. Approximately the same percentage of older adult men and older adult women had never married (5%) (AARP & Pacific Presbyterian Medical Center, 1989).

Education

As the baby boom generation reaches old age, it will enjoy an educational advantage over other

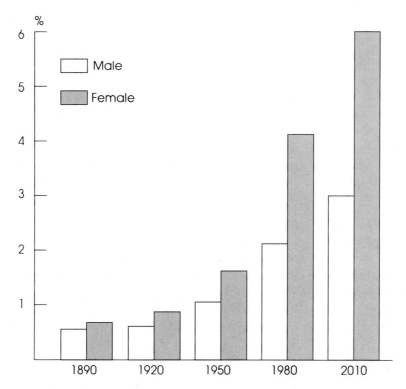

FIGURE 1-15 Percentage of total U.S. population (male and female) age 75 years and older. (From U.S. Bureau of the Census.)

older generations. The goal of parents in the early part of the twentieth century was to see their children complete high school. By midcentury the goal was to complete the first or second level of a college or university education. In 1993 approximately 12% of older adults had a bachelor's degree (AARP, 1994). This percentage varied considerably by race. In the latter years of the twentieth century the number of doctoral-prepared people has increased phenomenally. When the twenty-first century begins, older adults are predicted to be recipients of various types of education, received in a variety of settings, with multiple applications.

The education level of older adults has increased in the last 20 years. The percentage of older adults who have completed high school increased from 28% in 1970 to 60% in 1993 (AARP, 1994).

Still greater changes are expected for the next generation of aging Americans—those students who entered first grade in 1991, with expected high school graduation in the year 2003. By 2003 a world of change is predicted. The following list highlights just a few of the facts that will confront the high school graduate, class of 2003 ("What the Class . . ." 1988):

The body of available knowledge will have doubled 4 times since 1988. They will have been exposed to more information in 18 years than their grandparents were exposed to in a lifetime.

POPULATION CHANGES -- 1980 to 2030

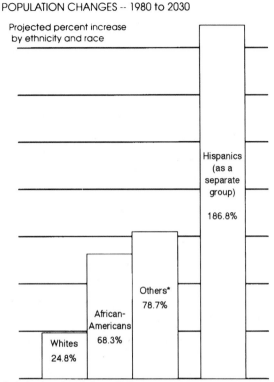

Projected percent increase
by ethnicity and race

Hispanics
(as a
separate
group)

186.8%

Others*
78.7%

African-
Americans
68.3%

Whites
24.8%

Includes American Indians, Eskimos,
plus Aleuts, Asian, and Pacific Islanders

FIGURE 1-16 Population changes related to cultural diversity, 1980-2030.

Only 15% of jobs will require a college education but nearly all will require job-specific training.

In three families out of four, both spouses will have full-time jobs.

Salaries for women will have grown from within 70% of men's salaries in 1988 to within 90% of men's salaries.

Of the people in the United States, 118,000 will be older than 100 (in 1988 there were 26,000 centenarians).

Life expectancy

The U.S. Department of Health and Human Services reports that someone born in 1900 was expected to live to be 47 years of age. Someone born in 1988 could expect to live to an average age of 74 years or more (Figure 1-17).

The number of people age 85 and older is expected to double by the year 2010 and to triple by the year 2025. So the fastest growing segment of the population will continue to be people over 85 years of age. In 1988 1 in every 15 persons was more than 85 years old. By 2030 1 in every 10 persons will be more than 85 years old (Fisk, 1988). There are several implications to be considered as one ponders these statistics:

Most of the nursing home residents who are 85 and older require some assistance with at least one activity of daily living, and many have three or more dependencies.

These include activities such as eating, bathing, dressing, getting out of bed, and going to the bathroom.

Projected increases in the number of older adults and the very old resulting from the baby boom generation raise concerns regarding available services and personnel to care for this population.

People will be old much longer in the future, because of increasing life expectancy.

Four-generation families will be the norm by the year 2000, with some families having great-great-grandparents in their midst. This prediction has serious implications for family finances. Will money be spent on college tuition for children or on some type of eldercare for aging parents or grandparents?

Members of the sandwich generation will be faced with caring for their own children while caring for their parents as well.

Because of changing demographic statistics, some policy experts believe that in the future the United States will be run by older adults. The population cohort of younger people is shrinking. Instead of those under age 35 making up 55% of the population as they did in 1989, their percentage will drop to 41% by the year 2030. There will be more than a million people over the age of 100 by the year 2050 and nearly 3 million between 95 and 99 years old.

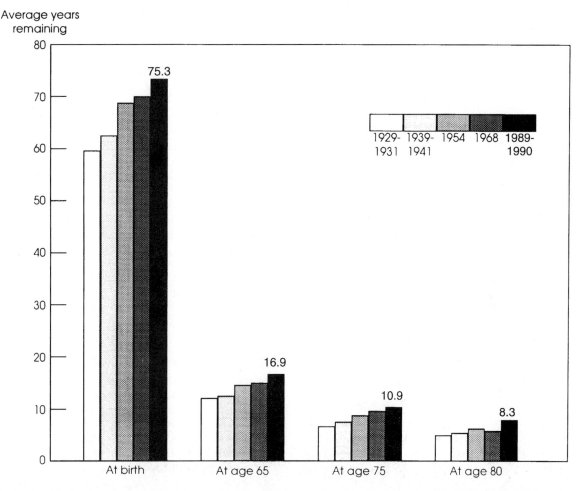

FIGURE 1-17 Average remaining lifetime at birth, age 65, age 75, and age 80; 1929-1931, 1939-1941, 1954, 1968, and 1989-1990. (From U.S. Bureau of the Census.)

■ Summarizing Major Trends Among the Older Adult Population

The following statements summarize major trends among the older adult population (Taeuber, 1993):

1. Currently there are more older adults than ever before in history.
2. Older adults are an increasing proportion of the U.S. population.

3. The increase in older adults will be steady until 2011, when the baby boomers turn 65.
4. Older adult women outnumber older adult men.
5. More people will survive to older ages in the future.
6. As more people survive to older ages, more will experience chronic disease disabilities.
7. Concern over identifying appropriate care for the older adults will increase, and the

young-old will experience new opportunities in extended careers and retirement activities.

8. The population of older adults will be more racially diverse.
9. The educational attainment of older adults will increase significantly.
10. Although currently some older adults are economically secure, there remains a sub-population of the oldest old with high rates of poverty.

Many questions remain that require continued study of older adults. Many are related to predictions in the demographics of aging. In the future, how many older adults will be young-old and how many will be old-old? How healthy will they be? Other research relates to social structure and older adults. How will the quality of their life be described? What are alternative living arrangements for the very old? Still other research is related to genetic and environmental issues. Will projections that consider disease control promote more healthful living and facilitate a healthier, more active and independent lifestyle? Will expanding knowledge of genetic and environmental factors associated with aging result in increases in years and quality of life? What alterations in diet and exercise yield the largest return in an older adult's life? Perhaps the most important research question relates to improving the quality of life as a whole, no matter when it ends.

Most policymakers now acknowledge that the wave of the future will be mightily swayed by senior power, sometimes referred to as the "gerontocracy." Though few experts agree as to the extent to which older adults will influence future trends and events, few would dispute that older adults will surely have a large and multifaceted impact on society.

REFERENCES

Abdellah, F. (1989). Foreword. In M. E. O'Brien, *Anatomy of a nursing home: A new view of resident life*. Owings Mills, MD: National Health Publishing.

American Association of Retired Persons. (1989, December-1990, January). AARP older students, quick studies. *Modern Maturity, 32*(6), 97.

American Association of Retired Persons. (1994). *A profile of older Americans* (Brochure No. PF3049 [1294]-D996). Washington, DC: Program Resources Department.

American Association of Retired Persons & Pacific Presbyterian Medical Center of San Francisco. (1989). *Aging in America*. Washington, DC: American Association of Retired Persons.

Beck, M. (1990, Winter-Spring). The geezer boom. *Newsweek,* pp. 62-68.

Besdine, R. W., & Rose, R. M. (1982). Aspects of infection in the elderly. In C. Eisdorfer (Ed.), *Annual review of gerontology and geriatrics*. New York: Springer.

Bethell, T. N. (Ed.). (1987). *On the other side of easy street: Myths and facts about the economics of old age*. Washington, DC: Villers Foundation.

Birren, J. (1978). A gerontologist's overview. In L. F. Jarvik (Ed.), *Aging into the twenty-first century: Middle-agers today*. New York: Gardner Press.

Brockington, F. (1975). *World health*. New York: Churchill Livingstone.

Buck, J., & Klemm, J. (1992). Recent trends in Medicaid expenditures. *Health Care Financing Review: Medicare and Medicaid Statistical Supplement,* 123-54. Baltimore: U.S. Department of Health and Human Services, Health Care Financing Administration, ORD.

Catholic Health Association's Task Force on Long Term Care Policy. (1988). *A time to be old, a time to flourish—The special needs of the elderly-at-risk*. St. Louis: Author.

Commonwealth Fund. (1992). *The nation's great overlooked resource: The contributions of Americans 55+*. New York: Commonwealth Fund, Americans over 55 at Work Program.

Ebersole, P., & Hess, P. (1994). *Toward healthy aging: Human needs and nursing response* (4th ed.). St. Louis: Mosby.

The facts of life in older America. (1987, October-November). *Modern Maturity, 30*(5), 13.

Fisk, C. F. (1988). Address to the surgeon general's workshop. In *Health promotion and aging*. Washington, DC: U.S. Department of Health and Human Services, Public Health Service.

Fullerton, H. N. (1993, November). Another look at the labor force. *Monthly Labor Review,* pp. 31-40.

Galtung, J. (1980). The basic needs approach. In K. Lederer (Ed.), *Human needs* (pp. 55-130). Cambridge, MA: Oelgeschlager, Gunn, and Hain.

Gilford, D. M. (Ed.). (1988). *The aging population in the twenty-first century.* Washington, DC: National Academy Press.

Guralnik, J. M., LaCroix, A. Z., Everett, D. F., & Kovar, M. G. (1989, May 26). *Aging in the '80s: The prevalence of comorbidity and its association with disability* (Advance data from Vital and Health Statistics of the National Center for Health Statistics, No. 170). Washington, DC: U.S. Department of Health and Human Services, Public Health Service, Centers for Disease Control.

Haub, C. (1990, July 8). 2050: Standing room only? *Washington Post Outposts,* p. C3.

Helbing, C. (1992). Medicare program expenditures. *Health Care Financing Review: Medicare and Medicaid Statistical Supplement,* 123-54. Baltimore: U.S. Department of Health and Human Services, Health Care Financing Administration, ORD.

Hogarth, T., & Barth, M. (1991). Costs and benefits of hiring older workers: A case study of B & Q. *International Journal of Manpower, 12*(8), 5-17. MCB University Press.

Keller, A. S. (1986, November 18). Exercising the mind. *Washington Post Health/Aging,* p. 10.

Lewin, T. (1990, February 19). Retirees return to campus in housing trend for elderly. *New York Times,* p. A1.

Manton, K. G. (1986). Cause of specific mortality patterns among the oldest old: Multiple causes of death trends 1968 to 1980. *Journal of Gerontology, 41*(2), 282-289.

Maslow, A. H. (1970). *Motivation and personality* (2nd ed.). New York: Harper and Row.

McFarland, D. D. (1978). The aged in the twenty-first century: A demographer's view. In L. F. Jarvik (Ed.), *Aging into the twenty-first century: Middle-agers today.* New York: Gardner Press.

McNaught, W., & Barth, M. (1991). *Using retirees to fill temporary labor needs: The Travelers' experience* (Background Paper Series, No. 5). New York: Commonwealth Fund, Americans over 55 at Work Program.

McNaught, W., & Barth, M. (1992, Spring). Are older workers "good buys"?—A case study of Days Inns of America. *Sloan Management Review, 33*(3), 53-63.

Mitchell, A. (1971). *Bismarck and the French nation.* New York: Pegasus.

Moon, M. (1993). *Medicare now and in the future.* Washington, DC: Urban Institute Press.

National Council on the Aging. (1994). Promotional literature regarding the Health Promotion Institute. Washington, DC: Author.

National Institute on Aging. (1994). *Aging research: Practice, promise, and priorities.* Washington, DC: National Institutes of Health.

Neugarten, B. L. (1978). The future and the young-old. In L. F. Jarvik (Ed.), *Aging into the twenty-first century: Middle-agers today.* New York: Gardner Press.

Older, slower-growing America predicted. (1989, February 1). *Washington Post,* p. B4.

Pender, N. J. (1982). *Health promotion in nursing practice.* Norwalk, CT: Appleton-Century-Crofts.

Perry, D., & Butler, R.N. (1988, December 20). Aim not just for longer life, but extended "health span." *Washington Post Health,* p. 16.

Quinn, J. B. (1990, Winter-Spring). Growing old frugally [Special issue]. *Newsweek,* pp. 102-105.

Schaie, K. W. (1983). The Seattle longitudinal study: A 21-year exploration in psychometric intelligence in adulthood. In K. W. Schaie (Ed.), *Longitudinal studies of adult psychological development.* New York: Guilford.

Schaie, K. W., & Willis, S. L. (1986). *Adult development and aging* (2nd ed.). Boston: Little, Brown.

Stone, R. I. (1989). *The feminization of poverty among the elderly.* Rockville, MD: U.S. Department of Health and Human Services, Public Health Service, National Center for Health Services Research and Health Care Technology Assessment.

Taeuber, C. (1993). *Sixty-five plus in America* (Current Population Reports, Special Studies, No. P23-178RV). Washington, DC: U.S. Department of Commerce, Economics, and Statistics Administration, Bureau of the Census.

U.S. Bureau of the Census. (1990). *Persons in institutions and other group quarters.* (1980 Census of Population, No. PC80-2-4D; 1990 Census of Population and Housing, Summary Tape File 1A). Washington, DC: Author.

U.S. Bureau of the Census. (1992a). *Population projections of the United States, by age, sex, race, and Hispanic origin: 1992 to 2050* (Current Population Reports, No. P25-1092). Washington, DC: U.S. Government Printing Office.

U.S. Bureau of the Census. (1992b). *Sixty-five plus in America* (Current Population Reports, Special Studies,

No. P23-178RV). Washington, DC: U.S. Government Printing Office.

U.S. Department of Health and Human Services. (1990). *The Medicare handbook* (DHHS Pub. No. HCFA 10050). Washington, DC: U.S. Department of Health and Human Services, Health Care Financing Administration.

U.S. Department of Health and Human Services. (1993a). *Health Care Financing Review: Medicare and Medicaid Statistical Supplement.* Washington, DC: U.S. Department of Health and Human Services, Health Care Financing Administration.

U.S. Department of Health and Human Services. (1993b). *Vital and health statistics: Health data on older Americans—United States, 1992.* (DHHS Pub. No. [PHS] 93-1411). Washington, DC: Public Health Service, Centers for Disease Control and Prevention, National Center for Health Statistics.

Vladeck, B., Miller, N., & Clauser, S. (1993). *The changing face of long-term care. Health Care Financing Review* (Vol. 14, No. 4). Baltimore.

Watson, W. (1982). *Aging and social behavior.* Monterey, CA: Wadsworth.

What the class of '00 needs to know. (1988, July 3). *Washington Post Magazine,* p. 11.

Wilson, L., Simon-Rusinowitz, L., & Marks, L. (1994). *Policy issues and trends influencing employment and volunteerism in the next generation of older Americans: Views from policy experts* (Project summary). College Park: University of Maryland, Center on Aging.

Yura, H., & Walsh, M. B. (1988). *The nursing process.* E. Norwalk, CT: Appleton and Lange.

Yurick, et al. (1984). *The aged person and the nursing process.* Norwalk, CT: Appleton-Century-Crofts.

BIBLIOGRAPHY

American Association of Retired Persons. (1986). *A home away from home.* Washington, DC: Author.

American Association of Retired Persons. (1987). *A handbook about care in the home.* Washington, DC: Author.

American Association of Retired Persons. (1988). *Tomorrow's choices.* Washington, DC: Author.

American Public Health Association. (1989). Nursing home data report is released to the public. *Nation's Health, 19*(1), 5.

Atchley, R. C. (1980). *The social forces in later life: An introduction to social gerontology* (3rd ed.). Belmont, CA: Wadsworth.

Comfort, A. (1978). A biologist laments and exhorts. In L. F. Jarvik (Ed.), *Aging into the twenty-first century: Middle-agers today.* New York: Gardner Press.

Dychtwald, K., & Flower, J. (1989). The challenges and opportunities of an aging America. In K. Dychtwald (Ed.), *Age wave.* Los Angeles: Jeremy P. Tarcher.

Jarvik, L. F. (Ed.). (1978). *Aging into the twenty-first century: Middle-agers today.* New York: Gardner Press.

LaRue, A., & Jarvik, L. F. (1978). Aging and intellectual functioning: Great expectations? In L. F. Jarvik (Ed.), *Aging into the twenty-first century: Middle-agers today.* New York: Gardner Press.

Lawrence, B. (1990, March 6). An oasis of education for seniors. *Prince George's Journal,* p. A6.

National Institute on Aging. (1993). *The health and retirement study—Preliminary findings.* Washington, DC: National Institutes of Health.

Rivlin, A. M., & Wiener, J. M. (1988). *Caring for the disabled elderly.* Washington, DC: Brookings Institution.

Rosenwaike, I. (1985). *The extreme aged in America: A portrait of an expanding population.* Westport, CT: Greenwood Press.

Rowan, T. (1989, May 11). The grim effects of loneliness. *Catholic Standard,* p. 2.

Theories of longevity—The search for the fountain of youth. (1986, February-March). *Bostonia,* pp. 29-32.

U.S. Department of Health and Human Services. (1991). *What's your aging I.Q.?* (NIH Pub. No. 1991-281-837/40019). Washington, DC: Public Health Service.

U.S. Department of Health, Education, and Welfare. (1977). *A staff report: Public policy and the frail elderly* (DHEW Pub. No. 79-2059). Washington, DC: Office of Human Development Services, Federal Council on Aging.

World Health Organization. (1946). *Constitution of the World Health Organization.* New York: Author.

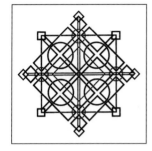

If I can stop one heart from breaking, I shall not live in vain.
If I can ease one life the aching, or cool one pain,
Or help one lonely person into happiness again
I shall not live in vain.

EMILY DICKINSON

Gerontologic Nursing

■ Learning Objectives

On completion of this chapter, the reader will be able to do the following:

1. Discuss the history of gerontologic nursing.
2. Describe the current status of gerontologic nursing.
3. Identify the importance of the nursing process, including nursing diagnosis.
4. Recognize several conceptual or theoretic frameworks for nursing.
5. Describe the results of the leadership efforts of the American Nurses' Association in defining standards for gerontologic nursing, initiating and maintaining nursing certification, and defining the nature and scope of nursing.
6. Recognize the contributions of the teaching nursing homes.

■ Historical Overview of Gerontologic Nursing

The nursing profession has developed dramatically during the second half of the twentieth century, partly because of a tremendous increase in the knowledge of human physiology, biochemistry, medicine, medical technology, and pharmacology. In like manner, gerontologic nursing has undergone major changes, especially because of the changing demographics of the U.S. populations. The nursing profession and the gerontologic nursing specialty have enjoyed tremendous professional development during recent decades; many challenges have been faced and many are yet to be defined, but all are accepted as legitimate obstacles that can be overcome.

One purpose of this chapter is to consider several perspectives of gerontologic nursing. Box 2-1 highlights selected events and people in the history of nursing that have had a significant influence on the development of nursing in general, and on gerontologic nursing in particular. Because history helps us understand our present state of development, it behooves all of us occasionally to reflect on the past. Although some would have preferred that the rate of change and development of new ideas in nursing had been faster, a careful and thoughtful analysis of historic

BOX 2-1 EVENTS AND PEOPLE WHO HAVE INFLUENCED GERONTOLOGIC NURSING

Florence Nightingale (1820–1910)—Nursing gained stature as a profession with professional goals:

- To care for the patient as a person
- To approach patient care wholistically, emphasizing the patient's physical, psychologic, and spiritual needs
- To promote wellness, as well as to provide care during illness
- To provide care according to a plan based on scientific principles and practices

Early twentieth century (1900-1940)

- Nursing was task oriented.
- Nurses followed hospital regulations and physicians' orders.
- There was little autonomy in nursing.
- Nurse actions were reactive rather than proactive.
- Gerontologic nursing was minimal; older adults were not as numerous in the population as they are today.
- Care of ill patients was the primary focus.
- Little or no attention was given to health maintenance.
- Older adults were cared for in hospitals or in nursing homes, and no deliberate plans were made for the older person to return home.
- Little attention was given to rehabilitation.

Housing for older adults (before 1930)—Few facilities existed for the older adults who were destitute or without family; many older adults lived on "poor farms."

Social Security Act (1935)—This welcome legislation made funds available to older adults who were needy or who had limited financial resources.

World War II and postwar years (1940-1960)

- The population of older adults began to gradually increase.
- While emphasis on care during illness continued, nurses increasingly gave attention to wellness activities such as exercise, nutrition, ambulation, and rehabilitation for patients of all ages.
- Nursing education programs moved into institutions of higher education.
- Educational grants and funding for professional nurses became available.

Latter twentieth century (1960-1995)

- Theories of nursing evolved.
- Critical care nurses entered the health care system.
- Cardiac surgery, recovery rooms, and critical care units became integral parts of acute care systems.
- Technology advances included ventilators, cardiac and hemodynamic monitoring, and computerized documentation.
- Medicare and Medicaid payment and regulations and diagnosis-related groups (DRGs) were introduced.
- Nurse practitioners entered the health care system.
- Master's and doctoral education in nursing increased.
- Cycles of oversupply and shortages of nurses were recognized.

BOX 2-2 POINTS OF VIEW ABOUT GERONTOLOGIC NURSING

- An opportunity to exercise professional skills, to apply clinical knowledge in practice, and to use clinical decision-making skills
- An opportunity to be creative and to use initiative in providing patient care
- An opportunity to care for older adults in various settings, such as community clinics, the patient's own home, the nursing home, and the acute care hospital
- An opportunity to collaborate with other health care disciplines in the planning and implementation of care for older adults
- An opportunity to teach and to support older adults in performing activities of daily living and in maintaining their independence
- An opportunity to appreciate the wisdom of older adults and to be enriched as they share memories of their life experiences
- A specialty that has a poor image among many professional nurses
- Often equated with employment and nursing practice exclusively in nursing homes, which is frequently viewed negatively
- Often, lower wages than those received by nurses in nongerontologic specialties
- Indirect reimbursement for nursing services
- Limited opportunities for career advancement
- Limited opportunities for collaborating with peers because of fewer colleagues in this specialty than in others
- Limited assignment of nursing students to gerontologic nursing as part of their educational practice

---

events suggests that nursing has progressed at a reasonable pace when compared with other professions. What is most important, advances in nursing are still continuing.

In addition to significant strides in the development of the nursing profession generally, gerontologic nursing in particular has become an important and legitimate specialty in professional nursing. The development of this specialty can be more fully understood by comparing pros and cons of gerontologic nursing. On the one hand, gerontologic nursing offers a variety of challenging opportunities for professional development. On the other hand, nurses who choose to care for older adults are just beginning to receive the professional recognition and rewards they deserve. Elaboration on the perceptions of this specialty are presented in Box 2-2.

While fully recognizing that the professional nurse continues to face many uphill challenges as

the care of older adults becomes more complex, this chapter examines recent progress in nursing. Specific benchmarks of progress are identified, as are relationships between nursing generally and the specialty of gerontologic nursing. In the future, nurses will be able to rely on the foundation of professional gerontologic nursing that is currently being established and to build on this foundation so that care of older adults will be less frustrating in the future than it has been in the past.

Since midcentury, several events in nursing stand out as important turning points in the profession:

In the 1960s

- The nursing process was defined.
- Theoretic-conceptual frameworks of nursing were developed.

In the 1970s

- Nursing diagnoses were identified.
- Nursing certification was established and nursing standards were defined.

In the 1980s

- Nursing was defined in a social policy statement.
- Teaching nursing homes were developed as models for care.

In the 1990s (to date)

- A White House Conference on Aging was held, the first since 1981.
- The Biennial Nurse Theorist Conference was held in 1993.
- Revisions of the social policy statement for nursing were published, as was a statement of the standards and scope of gerontologic nursing.

These events have established nursing as a respected profession among the health care disciplines and have moved nursing into roles that are both respected by health care colleagues and peers and appreciated by patients and families who seek and receive the services provided by nurses. The remainder of this chapter describes these key events of the 1960s, the 1970s, the 1980s, and the first half of the 1990s.

■ In the 1960s

During the 1960s two important developments occurred that continue to have an impact on nursing:

1. The nursing process was defined.
2. Theoretic-conceptual frameworks for nursing were enunciated.

DEFINITION OF THE NURSING PROCESS

During the 1960s, nursing was defined as a scientifically based problem-solving process. Many nurses welcomed this defining statement about how nurses perform patient care. The nursing process was defined clearly and specifically so that colleagues in the health care profession could understand it; this helped to establish clearer lines of communication among nurses and colleagues than had existed previously.

Two mid-1960s publications were instrumental in spelling out the nursing process as the base on which nursing has continued to build. One report was issued by the Western Interstate Commission of Higher Education (WICHE), in which the nursing process was defined as "that which goes on between the patient and the nurse in a given setting" (Lewis et al., 1967, p. 6). It identified components of the process as being perception, communication, interpretation (assessment), intervention (nursing action), and evaluation.

The second publication was a report of an 8-week continuing education program that defined and discussed *The Nursing Process: Assessing, Planning, Implementing, Evaluating* (Yura & Walsh, 1967). These two history-making publications set the stage for defining the essence of nursing as being a process "central to all nursing actions . . . applicable in any setting." It is flexible and adaptable, and it provides "a base from which all systematic nursing actions can proceed" (Yura & Walsh, 1983, p. 1). All nursing specialists, including gerontologic nurses, rely on the framework of the nursing process. Nurses adapt specific components of the process according to the needs and the traits of the population for whom they are caring in each nursing situation.

For purposes of this text the nursing process is made up of the following steps: (1) collecting data about the patient to identify real or potential problems (assessment), (2) on the basis of the data collected, arriving at a conclusion about the patient's needs (diagnosis), (3) specifying the goals toward which patient care will be directed (outcome identification), (4) developing plans to prevent or to solve the patient problems that have been identified (planning), (5) putting the plans into action (implementation), and (6) determining to what extent the plans and actions were effective in preventing or resolving the identified problems and diagnoses (evaluation).

Over the past 30 years different authors have used various labels to present, discuss, and apply the nursing process. Despite differences in labeling, all recognize the process as scientific, orderly, and systematic. The crucial common feature of all descriptions of the process is that all the aforementioned activities are included in the process, whatever the terminology being used. The present text does not explicate the various differences among the numerous descriptions of this process. Interested readers who would like a more comprehensive description of the many perspectives on this problem-solving process are urged to obtain a text that addresses the nursing process in detail.

The following pages describe each component of the nursing process in terms of the nurse's role and responsibility in using the nursing process to assess, diagnose, identify outcomes, plan, implement, and evaluate the care of the older person.

Characteristics of the nursing process

The logical problem-solving process of nursing requires nurses to collect and analyze data about the patient. Having reached conclusions about the patient's health status, the nurse informs the patient and the caregivers about the patient's health-related needs, desires, concerns, and problems. Based upon the data gathered about the patient, the nurse determines the goals to be achieved, sets priorities regarding these goals, plans and carries out appropriate strategies and interventions, and then reexamines the situation to ensure that the patient's problems will be resolved.

Nurses possess three kinds of qualifications for satisfactorily applying the nursing process: knowledge, technical skills, and interpersonal skills. An extensive repertoire of sound *knowledge* provides a solid foundation from which all aspects of the process can proceed. *Technical skills* enable the nurse to carry out the activities that constitute the craft of nursing. The nurse's *interpersonal skills* allow the establishment of good relationships between the nurse and the older person. To achieve this goal, there needs to be clear communication, trust, and mutual respect in the intimate and vital situations of nursing care. With full understanding of their responsibility for care of older adults in any setting, professional nurses establish and maintain the following:

1. Honest, clear communications with the patient, caregivers, and family members
2. A sense of mutual trust between the patient and the nurse
3. The patient's confidence in the ability of nursing personnel to meet needs and to help with problem prevention and solution

Preparation for initiating the nursing process

To facilitate communication between the nurse and the patient, the nurse should arrange seating and body positioning that optimize eye-to-eye contact with the patient. If the patient is sitting in a chair, the nurse should arrange a chair to sit nearby. It may be necessary to adjust furniture to facilitate comfortable eye contact if the patient is lying down or sitting in a low seat. A nurse who stands or sits above the eye level of the patient may intimidate the patient or otherwise hinder the nurse-to-patient communication.

Seating arrangements should allow the nurse to face the patient. This enables communication via facial expressions and gestures, clear reception of verbal inquiries and messages, and observation of the facial features and moving lips of the speaker. This is especially important for the older person who may have some hearing impairment or some difficulty in speaking audibly and distinctly. Though neither communicator may be proficient in lipreading, the communication will be enhanced by these visual cues.

Regarding the placement of light fixtures, the nurse should be positioned so that the light falls on the nurse's face. Again, this aids the patient in observing facial expressions and interpreting the messages being communicated by the nurse.

One of the major goals of this preparation is to establish a sense of trust between the nurse and the patient. Through the adept use of interpersonal skills, mutual respect can be established, which can set the stage for a trusting, comfortable relationship. This kind of nurse-patient relationship can be critical to maintaining a high quality of life for older patients who may be experiencing numerous insults and difficulties.

In addition to physically preparing the setting for the nursing process, the nurse mentally prepares for interactions with patients. A hurried, anxious nurse may neglect subtle signs being given by the patient or may overwhelm the patient with more information than the patient can absorb. The pace of communication and data collection must be appropriate for the particular nurse-patient interaction. It is important for the patients that the nurse speak clearly and slowly so that patients can grasp what is being said. Adequate time should be allowed for the patients to respond to questions. The nurse communicates, by words and actions, that the patients are important and that the information being given is important. When initiating the nursing process, the nurse must foster the patient's comfort and trust that the patient's strengths will be recognized and fostered to prevent problems from developing and to solve any identified health problems. Once rapport is established, the patient and nurse can smoothly begin the assessment data-collecting activities.

Assessment

The nurse reviews the older patient's situation for the purpose of collecting data about the patient, particularly to identify the strengths and limitations (actual and potential) of the individual. These data that are gathered by the nurse lead to the nursing diagnoses that will guide the patient's care.

The nurse gathers data based on an overall plan for the assessment. The nurse selects an appropriate assessment form or some other organizational plan, which has been developed by the nurse or by the gerontologic nursing team, to guide data collection. This plan uses a theoretic framework to guide nursing practice in the applicable setting. The nurse's values and philosophy about life and about nursing are inherent in this framework.

During the assessment the nurse guides the dialogue and directs questions and comments to the patient to collect the information necessary for determining the patient's needs. Throughout this process the nurse acknowledges each older person as a unique individual, subject to the same environmental insults experienced by younger people, and possibly even more sensitive to these insults than are younger people. Therefore the nurse should allow time for the patient to communicate, both in replying to the nurse's questions and in asking questions of the nurse. An effective assessment is a dialogue, not a monologue. As in any communication experience, the participants *take time to listen* to each other.

If family members are available and are knowledgeable about the patient's needs and interests, they should be included in the assessment discussion, given the full consent and approval of the patient. Family involvement can produce positive results for the patient, the family, and the nurse. This type of exchange provides insight about the family's perspective and allows the nurse to observe and assess the kinds of relationships that exist within the patient's family. For example, does a family member interrupt a cognitively alert patient's responses, providing answers before the patient has had an opportunity to do so?

Some older patients may have lived alone for many years and may have had limited social activities. If this is the case, the patient may relish the presence of the nurse as an interested person who is asking about the patient's needs and desires; this may stimulate an interest in more communication than was anticipated. When this occurs, the nurse will be challenged to use creative interpersonal skills in directing the patient's verbalizations to those areas of assessment that will provide the kinds of data

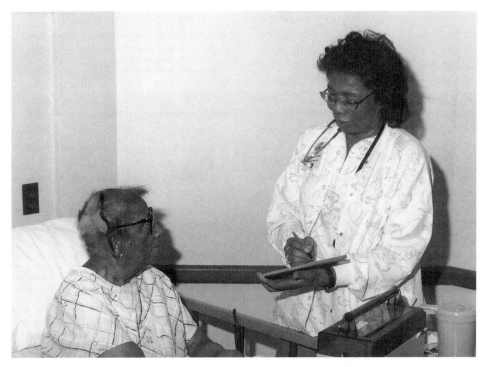

Nurse gathering assessment data. *Courtesy Loy Ledbetter, St. Louis.*

needed for nursing diagnosis. The nurse should also include the observation of this perceived social need in the assessment data; it will be significant information to use in planning the care of this person, because the opportunity to converse with an interested person may well be therapeutic in itself.

Nursing diagnosis

Nursing diagnosis is a clinical judgment about individual, family, or community responses to actual or potential health problems or life processes. Nursing diagnoses provide the basis for selection of nursing interventions to achieve outcomes for which the nurse is accountable (Gordon, 1994).

Following the collection of data during assessment, the nurse analyzes and logically clusters the data. When the data have been organized, the nurse determines the strengths and the needs of the patient to determine the nursing diagnoses.

The three major components of the nursing diagnosis are (1) the problem, (2) the etiology of the problem, and (3) the signs or symptoms of the problem, referred to collectively as *PES* (Gordon, 1994). The problem (P) occurs in the health state of the older person. This can be an actual problem or a potential problem. The nurse identifies potential problems as a result of inquiry and observation about the patient's habits, practices, and nutrition, and other factors that contribute to or detract from health.

The etiology (E) comprises those influences in the patient's environment that contribute to the person's identified health problems. The signs or symptoms (S), or defining characteristics of the problem, are those objective and subjective clues that the nurse observes and detects and that lead the nurse to the nursing diagnosis.

Some of these defining characteristics are based on group consensus about probable associations rather than on hard data about known links; intensive research remains to be done in this area. The developing of research-based diagnoses for each PES based on accurate clinical data depends on the nurse's prudent judgment. Clinical judgment and decision making facilitate the development of accurate nursing diagnoses. These skills are especially significant for gerontologic nurses, who find a limited number of research publications to guide the development of these very important dimensions of nursing.

Outcome identification

To influence health outcomes, the nurse and the health care team derive the expected outcomes of care from the nursing diagnoses. It is the patient's care that is being planned, and the patient's choices and decisions must be given primary consideration. If the patient is unable to participate in defining the goals to be achieved, the family members (as appropriate) may speak for the patient.

The group should specify both short-range ("proximate") goals and long-range ("ultimate") goals, including general time lines within which to meet these goals. For example, if the older patient is in an acute care setting, an immediate goal may be to orient the patient to the new surroundings. A long-range goal may be to enable the patient to walk around in the hospital unit without getting lost. The health care team may decide that this should be accomplished by the end of 24 hours of hospitalization. Identification of these goals, stated in measurable terms and including a reasonable time estimate, will be important for moving the patient toward wellness. The goals also are consistent with the diagnosis-related group, or DRG, criteria that influence the length of time available for the patient, depending on the patient's diagnosis and progress.

In addition to defining expected outcomes, the nurse and the health care team will also set priorities to determine which of the identified problems to address first. Assuming that more than one nursing diagnosis is specified, it usually is not possible to resolve all diagnoses simultaneously. To assist with priority setting, the patient should indicate which problem is most troublesome and should be resolved first. With input from the patient and the family, the nurse considers which of the problems is most important from a health care standpoint. For example, if a nursing home patient is dehydrated, resolution of this deficit will assume a higher priority than will the resolution of a problem related to inadequate socialization.

Planning

The purpose of planning is to determine what can be done to help the patient achieve optimal wellness; it involves reviewing the goals, setting priorities, and designing methods to resolve the problems that were identified by the nursing diagnoses. The nurse leads these care-planning activities. In addition, the patient, family members, and other health care personnel who play a role in the patient's health maintenance may be involved in the planning.

Once the goals are determined and the priorities are set, the planning team designs the means by which to resolve the problems (diagnoses). If the patient has a problem with constipation, for example, the planning team will discuss the foods that will encourage elimination and the activities in which the older person can engage to stimulate intestinal peristalsis.

Throughout the planning discussions, the patient's perceptions must be considered. The other members of the planning team may identify a problem and a plan for resolution quite differently than would the patient. The final plan is more likely to be implemented and to succeed when the team considers the patient's views and reactions to the other team members' ideas, suggestions, and proposals.

Careful, deliberate planning, based on the assessment data and valid nursing diagnoses, is critical to the successful outcome of patient care activities. Through astute perception, knowledgeable observation, and effective communication, the nurse and the other team members can prescribe a plan that will meet the needs of the older patient. In the past, nurses have largely used intuition to guide their plans and decisions about patient care, but nurses now use patient data, scientific processes, and their own intellectual skills to determine the direction of that care. This is very important with all patients, but especially significant in the care of the older person whose age may play an important role.

Implementation

Implementation involves the initiation and completion of the actions necessary for accomplishing the goals that were defined in the planning sessions. By definition, this is the action phase of the nursing process: someone *does* something to address the problems that the older adults are experiencing. The people who perform the activity may be the patients themselves, family members, nurses, or other designated members of the health team. The team will determine who is responsible for the action before initiating the implementation phase. Throughout the activity of caring for the older person, important concepts to bear in mind include health promotion, illness prevention, health maintenance, rehabilitation, and palliation. All of the knowledge and interpersonal and technical skills that can be mustered will be employed to make the implementation successful. As the challenges of resolving the older patients' problems become more complex, the skills of the nurse become more essential.

The acute care setting In the acute care setting, the older patient usually depends on the actions of the nursing personnel. Among these people is a registered professional nurse who is responsible for carrying out the agreed-on plans of action. Associated with the nurse are other levels of nursing personnel who assist in the caregiving activities. The nurse assigns these caregiving activities among the associated personnel; to make appropriate assignments, the nurse considers each person's level of preparation, as well as the personality traits and strengths of the multiple caregivers. Matching these traits to the needs of the older patient challenges the intellectual skills of the most able professionals: Will the nurse aide respect the frailty of an older patient? How will the patient react to the nurse aide? Many factors are considered by gerontologic nurses in hospital settings.

The nursing home setting In the nursing home the older resident is usually more familiar with the routines of care than in the acute care setting. Most residents spend a longer period of time in nursing homes than patients spend in hospitals. However, this does not reduce the challenge of matching caregiver traits to the patient, the diagnoses, and the situation. When the nurse delegates activities to other personnel, the nurse is responsible for ensuring that the goals are understood and that all activities are directed toward achieving these goals. The nurse encourages reassurance that the patient's needs are being considered and that the choices and participation of the older patient and family members are constantly being reviewed. Although the assessment and planning activities begin before implementation is initiated, assessment and planning continue during the implementation phase. New data, as they become available, are used for revising the plan; as the plan is revised, the implementation actions are reconsidered and redefined. In other words, the nurse constantly rethinks, reviews, and revises the action plan, using intellectual and interpersonal skills to ensure that the needs of the older patient are foremost in the minds of the caregivers. This is especially true in the nursing home setting.

The patient's private home setting In the patient's own home in the community, professional nurses rely on the data they obtain during assessment, the nursing diagnoses they define, the outcomes they identify, and the plans they develop, for meeting the health needs of the patient. The variable that directs the activities of the nurse is the nurse's ability to function on the patient's turf, always aware of being in the patient's environs and territory. Professionals respect the patient's privacy in all settings, but it is imperative to do so when functioning in the patient's private home.

It is crucial to establish rapport with older adults to identify expected outcomes, define plans, and determine the necessary activities that the older person, the family members, or the significant others will carry out. Although the same data are sought in this setting as in all other settings, it is important here to define the patient's needs so that care can be continued in the absence of the professional person. The teaching role of the nurse assumes major significance in the patient's private home. Mutual understanding of the expected outcomes and the goals of care, and agreement about the projected care activities are critical to achieving comfort and health for older people in their own homes.

Evaluation

Evaluation appraises the changes experienced by the patient as a result of the actions conducted during the nursing process. That is, it asks how effectively the identified outcomes were achieved. To what extent were the defined goals realized?

To initiate evaluation, the nurse reexamines the blueprint for action that was designed in the early phase of the nursing process. The patient is included in this activity to be certain that the patient's perspective is respected. If the patient believes that the goals were not achieved, this sends a clear message to the nurse, whether or not the nurse believes that the goals were met. The focus of the evaluation phase is the viewpoint of the patient and the patient's response to care. If the patient is not satisfied, and if the nursing team identifies deficits in the expected outcomes of care, the evaluation process directs the team members to reassess, replan, reimplement, and reevaluate the care as many times as

necessary until the goals are achieved. That is, the patient's needs are assessed and diagnoses are defined again, outcomes are reidentified, and a revised plan is made in terms of this reappraisal. The appropriate people implement the new plan of care, and the team then evaluates the patient's satisfaction with—and the health outcomes of—the revised care. Each of the steps is repeated in this cycle of activity as many times as necessary until satisfactory results are achieved.

Conclusion

These phases of the nursing process—assessing, diagnosing, identifying outcomes, planning, implementing, and evaluating—provide the basis of nursing care for all older adults who require a nurse's expertise in a health-related situation. To care for older adults, the nursing caregivers tailor these phases to meet the unique needs of each older person, recognizing that the care of older adults differs from the care of one who is younger.

FRAMEWORKS FOR NURSING

In addition to the elucidation of the nursing process, a second development in the 1960s was the enunciation of several theoretic frameworks for care. The writings of Florence Nightingale (published in 1859 and 1946), Hildegarde Peplau (1952), and Virginia Henderson (1966) provided valuable pronouncements about nursing and clear explanations of the goals and purposes of many professional nursing functions. Ideas such as these were being referred to as "nursing concepts" and later were called "nursing theories." These early writings stimulated discussions about professional nursing responsibilities that have continued for the past 3½ decades.

A number of these ideas have been presented in the literature and have been labeled as theories, although most of the ideas have not been validated by sufficient research. Nonetheless, many nurses are cautiously referring to these ideas as theories that aid in exploring intellectually stimulating concepts that guide nursing practice. As continuing research increasingly validates many of these nurses' ideas, the label of theory is gradually becoming justified. Meanwhile, whether labeled as theories or as ideas about nursing, these frameworks for nursing are critical to the structural formulation of what nursing is, how nurses help patients in need, and why nurses perform the activities that are called "nursing." To date, an insufficient number of research efforts have included the older population as subjects for study. This is a fertile area for exploration, offering myriad opportunities for systematic and scientific study.

Nightingale, Peplau, and Henderson had the temerity to present previously unpublished aspects of nursing, thereby stimulating others to formulate ideas that have guided major intellectual developments in nursing. For example, in the 1960s Ida Jean Orlando (1961), Ernestine Wiedenbach (1964), Myra Levine (1969), and Dorothy Johnson (1961) published their ideas about nursing. In the 1970s Martha Rogers (1970), Dorothea Orem (1971), Imogene King (1971), Joyce Travelbee (1971), Sister Callista Roy (1976), and Josephine Paterson and Loretta Zderad (1976) presented their concepts about nursing. In the 1980s Betty Neuman (1980), Jean Watson (1985), and the team of Helen Yura and Mary Walsh (1988) announced their views to their colleagues in nursing. In addition, nurses began to emphasize the applicability of these ideas to nursing practice. Thus began a greater thrust toward wholistic nursing and an emphasis on the use of frameworks to guide nursing practice.

Building on consensus developed in the 1980s regarding the "domain concepts" of nursing—person, environment, health, and nursing—nurse theorists of the 1990s remain focused on the tenor and interrelation of these concepts (Fawcett, 1984). Additionally, literature reveals continued debate regarding the type of science nursing represents—basic, applied, or practical—as well as the necessity for a practice theory separate from scientific and ethical theory (Beckstrand, 1992; Collins & Fielder, 1992; Johnson, 1991).

Despite and because of ongoing controversy regarding some basic tenets of the development and investigation of nursing knowledge, the current decade holds great promise for refinement of the scientific discipline of nursing. The wonder of the possibilities is reflected in the frameworks of contemporary nursing theorists and their application to nursing practice. Specifically, Patricia Benner, Rosemarie Parse, and Margaret Newman hold promise for further theory development, application of theory to practice, and the differentiation of nurses in their roles as health care providers.

So far, the development of theories and concepts about nursing has given little attention to the structure that can best guide the care of older adults. However, among the several frameworks for nursing that have been enunciated, the following have particular appeal for and potential applicability to the care of older people: frameworks suggested by Imogene King, Betty Neuman, Dorothea Orem, Martha Rogers, Sister Callista Roy, Jean Watson, and the team of Helen Yura and Mary Walsh. These frameworks seem to be the most constructive for guiding the care of older adults. Further research to validate these ideas in the gerontologic setting will be very important.

Gerontologic nurses are encouraged to select from the framework or frameworks with which they are most comfortable. Because some elements of several ideas may be appropriate for the care of older adults, nurses are encouraged to consider the use of an eclectic approach, which integrates the most appropriate ideas from several of the authors.

Interaction theory (Imogene King) focuses on the ways in which older adults interact both with their environment and with the nurse to set and achieve goals of health care. King defines nursing as a process of action, reaction, interaction, and transaction. She highlights the establishment of the nurse-patient relationship as the means to help the patient maintain health and to support the patient in making changes and adapting to the changes in order to improve health. The older person is perceived by King as an open system that consists of social systems (society), interpersonal systems (groups), and personal systems (individuals).

The health care systems model (Betty Neuman) views the older person as a total person who experiences stress and adversity that can affect the individual's functioning. The nurse's role in this health care systems model is to help the older person, as well as the person's family if necessary, to achieve a maximum level of wellness through purposeful interventions. Two assumptions proposed by Neuman are appropriate to the care of older adults: (1) Each person is unique and is exposed to a variety of stressors that can disturb the equilibrium of the individual. (2) Reactions to these stressors can vary, depending upon the status of each person's inherent lines of defense.

The self-care deficit theory (Dorothea Orem) encourages, supports, and empowers older adults in meeting their own needs to the extent that they are able. Orem suggests that the nurse is responsible for identifying what the person needs and then providing and managing the resources that will enable the patient to engage in self-care; assuming that these activities are continual, the outcome of these nursing endeavors will be to help the older person to sustain life and health, to recover from disease or injury, and to cope with the effects of disease or injury. The essence of Orem's ideas are the constructs of self-care, self-care deficits, and nursing systems.

Unitary man concepts (Martha Rogers) emphasize the interaction between older adults and the environment, with the goal of achieving maximal health. Rogers's beliefs that apply to the care of older adults include the concepts that each person is unique, that each human and the environment are involved in a continuous interactive process, and that all human beings are more than and different from the sum of their parts. Rogers stresses the importance of nursing

practice in multiple settings and identifies the nurse's role as helping people to prevent disease and to achieve optimal health.

Adaptation theory (Sister Callista Roy) points to the need for older people to adapt to the changes they may be experiencing. Four modes of adaptation are defined: physiologic needs, self-concept, role function, and interdependence. These constitute the framework that the nurse can use to determine how effectively older people are adapting to their life and health status. Three types of stimuli are defined in this theory: focal, contextual, and residual. These can be adjusted and/or manipulated to promote and to ensure adaptation; the patients may be the ones to manipulate these stimuli with the assistance and support of the nurse.

An interpersonal concept (Jean Watson) directs the focus of nursing to meeting the needs of the older person through a caring interpersonal relationship. The focus is a philosophy and science of caring to guide the action of the nurse. Caring is viewed as an interpersonal process that promotes health; accepts patients wherever they may be in terms of their health, their health awareness, and their health activity; and creates an environment that enables the patients to exercise choice as they consider what will be best for them. Watson views decision making as being the responsibility of the older patient. Nursing intervention is perceived as a legitimate activity that is based on a scientific-humanistic approach, using caring as a framework to direct activity. Nurses are encouraged to approach older adults in a positive manner with a wholistic outlook, liberally using faith and hope. Watson believes that without these concepts, it would not be possible to establish an interpersonal relationship. Through a positive relationship, both nurse and patient can realize teaching and learning, help and trust, and the acceptance of feelings.

Human need theory (Helen Yura and Mary Walsh) views the older person as an integrated, organized whole whose goal-directed behavior leads the person to satisfy human needs. As the nurse supports and encourages the older adults' attempts to satisfy their needs, wholistic care is practiced and the integrity of the older person is recognized. With guidance and direction from the health care professional who respects the patient's ability, it is reasonable to expect that the individual person will achieve those goals that satisfy the person's unique human needs.

A framework of *pragmatic phenomenology* is described by *Patricia Benner* and serves as a bridge between the nursing theorists of the 1980s and those of the 1990s. Her model embraces the basic domain concepts of person, environment, health, and nursing. The framework is pragmatic in that nursing is characterized as a caring association. The nurse is viewed as facilitating a relationship with the patient in which help is given and received (Benner & Wrubel, 1989). The framework is phenomenologic in that Benner's views of health, person, and situation (environment) are grounded in the works of existential phenomenologists Heidegger and Merleau-Ponty. Existential phenomenology is difficult to define; however, all existential philosophers stress individual existence, subjectivity, individual freedom, and choice. Knowing this will serve as a good basis for discerning Benner's wholistic view of nursing practice relative to the interrelationships of health, person, situation, and nursing.

Health is described as a dialectic, "the lived experience of being healthy and being ill" (Benner & Wrubel, 1989, p. 7). Benner views health as being capable of assessment and as being more than the absence of disease and illness. She further makes the distinction between illness and disease. Benner posits that people may not see themselves as ill because illness is interpreted as a "loss or dysfunction." In other words, an aging person may not recognize symptoms of congestive heart failure if those symptoms do not translate into a loss of function from the person's perspective.

Person is described as "embodied" or capable of responding to meaningful situations. "A person is a self-interpreting being" (Benner & Wrubel, 1989, p. 41), defined throughout the course of living life. Consistent with her grounding in existential phenomenology, Benner clearly views the person as being interactive with the world, a summation of mind and body, evolving over time.

Environment is described by Benner within a phenomenologic framework. Situation, rather than environment, is described in the model to emphasize meaningfulness in a full social context. This creates a comprehensive context for the concept of environment. Benner states that the unique perspectives, habits, and assigned meanings of a person enter into each situation with the person.

Benner views nursing practice as the application and study of the lived experiences of health, illness, and disease and their interrelationships framed within the caring paradigm of nursing practice. The concept of how a "person is in the situation sets up different possibilities" (Benner & Wrubel, 1989, p. 63), both for the person and for the nurse involved in the care of that person. Benner purports that "a nurse's clinical knowledge is relevant to the extent to which its manifestation in nursing skills makes a difference in patient care and patient outcomes" (Benner & Wrubel, 1989, p. 63). A thorough accounting of Benner's concepts regarding skill acquisition and nursing can be studied in her work *From Novice to Expert.* Benner resides well within the caring paradigm of nursing. Although caring is clearly a component of the application of her work with Wrubel in *Primace of Caring,* her offering is specifically related to the philosophy of caring. What remains to be articulated is the relevance and function of caring in nursing (Radsma, 1994).

Rosemarie Parse has developed a theory firmly entrenched in the domain concepts central to nursing. Although never expressly stated, this focus is understood in the process orientation of the original title of her theory: man-living-health. She further made this explicit in the coining of the term *simultaneity paradigm* to describe alternative views of the domain concepts relative to the Rogers and Parse conceptual frameworks (Parse, 1981). It is critical to point out that the language requires some work from the reader. Parse has been criticized for her difficult terminology. Holmes (1990) states the following:

> Unfortunately, [Parse's] efforts have not had the impact on nursing that might have been hoped. Their accessibility is undermined by an obscure style, a penchant for the utterly novel use of familiar words, and a large crop of ill-explained neologisms. These problems are exacerbated if the reader is not familiar with esoteric language and idiosyncratic conceptual tools of existential phenomenologists (p. 193).

That said, the reader is challenged to take up the study of this theory for all it offers.

The human becoming theory of Parse evolves from Martha Rogers's holistic interactive framework of nursing and major tenets from existential-phenomenologic works of Heidegger, Sarte, Merleau-Pongy, and Marcel (Parse, 1981). The outcome is theory rooted in the human sciences intended to guide nursing by serving as the theoretic basis of a practice and research methodology unique to nursing. The central theme is the interrelationship of the elements of the human-universe-health process described as *human becoming* (Parse, 1992). Three main principles emerge from the three central themes of meaning, rhythmicity, and cotranscendence. The three principles are as follows (Parse, 1981):

1. Structuring meaning multidimensionally is co-creating reality through the *languaging* of *valuing* and *imaging.*
2. Cocreating rhythmic patterns of relating is living the paradoxic unity of *revealing-concealing* and *enabling-limiting,* while *connecting-separating.*

3. Cotranscending with the possibles is *powering* unique ways of *originating* in the process of *transforming.*

Each principle contains three major concepts central to the understanding of Parse's theory of human becoming (as highlighted with italics).

Languaging is the communication of personal experiences through verbal and nonverbal means. Valuing is the process of living cherished beliefs while assimilating the new into a personal world view. It emerges in the human-universe process and is the human being's confirming of cherished beliefs. Imaging is the creation of perceptions of one's experiences. "What is real for each individual is structured by that individual." Revealing-concealing is the process of choosing what is to be known of one's self while simultaneously hiding other things. Connecting-separating represents the rhythm of the patterns created by making choices throughout one's life. Choosing to move toward something or someone is a simultaneous decision to move away from another. Enabling-limiting describes the paradoxic patterns that emerge when one chooses a particular path in life. Each path represents limitations, as well as possibilities. Powering is the force of human existence. It is self-affirmation in light of the possibility of nonbeing. Originating is self-differentiation through personal choices within given situations, despite uncertainty of the outcome. Transforming is defined as the changing of change. Changing unfolds as the familiar is seen in a different light, thus shifting the view and illuminating new possibilities.

Parse (1990) describes health as "a process of becoming, experienced by the person" (p. 137), whereas most others view health as a value. Parse states that "health is an unfolding that cannot be prescribed or described by societal norms, only by the person living the health. It is just the way the human is!" (Parse, 1992). She further states the following:

> Health as personal commitment, then, means that health is one's own unfolding in interconnectedness

with the world. It does not imply that one's health is an entity, lived in a vacuum without connectedness with others and environment. The belief is that one cocreates health with others and the world in mutual interrelationship and that cocreation of health is the set of choices the person with the world makes from all levels of the universe, not just from the explicit level. The person is responsible for the outcomes of choices in that the choices themselves incarnate the person's unique was, is, and will be (Parse, 1990, p. 137).

People, or human beings, are conceptualized through the simultaneity paradigm. They are thought to be a "living unity" free to choose meaning, create patterns of relating and being, assume responsibility for choices made, and move beyond the present en route to changing in the future. Consistent with these views of the human being is the broader view of human nature that depicts the human as a "creative author." This view posits that "the human creates a personal world with spirit, compassion, and honor. This view of the human shuns the idea of control, fixing, and manipulation" (Parse, 1981, 1990).

Parse refers to environment and the universe interchangeably. Her concept of environment is most clearly seen within principle #2: Cocreating rhythmic patterns of relating is living the paradoxic unity of revealing-concealing and enabling-limiting, while connecting-separating. The interrelation of man and environment is reflected in this principle. *Cocreating* meaning together, man and the environment are partners in the origination of the other (Parse, 1981).

The goal of nursing is to enhance the quality of life as perceived by the person and family. The nurse who is guided by Parse's theory in practice "seeks to participate with persons in enhancing their quality of life through being with them in true presence as they explore the meaning of personal situations and choose ways of becoming" (Cody & Mitchell, 1992). This requires a different approach to nursing. Nurses do not assume the positions of authority. They trust the individuals' commitment to the process of health and remain present with the individuals as they align their realities with those of their current or future situation. To this end Parse created a practice methodology capable of application in any given environment or nurse-client relationship (Cody & Mitchell, 1992). Dimensions and processes of this methodology are advocated: illuminating through *explication,* synchronizing rhythms through *dwelling with,* and mobilizing transcendence processes, imagine a person being allowed to explore the meaning of smoking cessation and relate it to the quality of that person's life. One way of moving beyond the current reality to future realities is to assist people in viewing their past, present, and future health with and without smoking with no imposition of the "shoulds" of a different value structure. This allows the individuals to review the meanings they have placed on smoking, its role in their lives, and possibly how those meanings have changed or will change. The first step to changing health, then, is within the context of one's own values and preferences (Parse, 1990).

The basis of *Margaret Newman's* theory of nursing is *health as expanding consciousness.* This concept describes the patterns of time, space, and movement as directly corresponding to evolving consciousness. The roots of her theory were derived from several varied disciplines: nursing, philosophy, physics, psychology, and chemistry. Flowing from the influences of Hegel's dialectic process and Rogers's model of nursing, Newman's theory concentrates on wholeness, person-environment, pattern organization, life process, and the capacity for advanced, complex process of the mind (Newman, 1979, 1986). Her major assumptions are as follows:

- Health encompasses conditions heretofore described as illness, or in medical terms, pathologic conditions.

- These "pathologic" conditions can be considered a manifestation of the total pattern of the individual.
- The pattern of the individual that eventually manifests itself as a pathologic condition is primary and exists before structural or functional changes.
- Removal of the pathologic condition in itself will not change the pattern of the individual.
- If an individual's pattern can manifest itself only through the individual's becoming "ill," then that is health for that person.

The theory of expanding consciousness is posited along a continuum from potential consciousness (freedom) to the ideal of absolute consciousness (real freedom). The continuum of consciousness is related to the dimensions of time and space. Described is a process of interrelationships among time, space, movement, and consciousness. It begins with the person coming into being in a state of potential consciousness, circumscribed in time, defined in space, and propelled toward absolute consciousness by choices made within patterns of life (movement) (Newman, 1979).

The domain concepts universal to nursing, much as in the case of Parse's theory, are not directly discussed within the theory of expanding consciousness. However, they can be inferred through examining several conceptual definitions.

Health is the focus of Newman's theory of expanding consciousness. Health is viewed as being composed of both disease and nondisease. It follows that health is "the pattern of the whole of a person"—the "undivided wholeness of the person in interaction with the environment." Newman further states that the recognition of patterns is the essence of health, thus concluding that health and evolving consciousness are one and the same (Newman, 1986, 1990).

People are defined as extensions of consciousness. They are identified and differentiated by their individual patterns. Newman describes

both implicit and explicit order in her concept of pattern and states that pattern is somehow intimately involved in energy exchange and transformation (Newman, 1986).

Newman (1986) postulates that "consciousness is coextensive in the universe and resides in all matter" (p. 33). It is through movement that one is able to control one's environment. Incorporating the concept of pattern, Newman describes the pattern of consciousness of a person as interacting with the collective consciousness of the family and/or community at large (Newman, 1986).

Newman views nursing as facilitating a relationship with the patient within the process of expanding consciousness. The nurse is capable of developing this relationship when the person is at the point of choice or movement. The task for nursing is to recognize the patterns of a person and to understand them as a unified entity, thus enabling the nurse to facilitate health within the context of person-environment (Newman, 1986).

Conclusion

A few theoretic frameworks have been summarized in this chapter. Several publications present far more comprehensive overviews of these theoreticians who have fostered a sophisticated level of intellectualization in the discussion of the practice of nursing. Readers of this text are advised to review these publications, which present the various authors' ideas in considerable detail, and which provide guidance regarding the use and value of specific frameworks in clinical practice. Students and practitioners are encouraged to consider each author's views about nursing, about people, and about how to apply these ideas in practice.

A more recent group of publications provides the scholar of theories with presentations and analyses that enable deeper thoughts about the proposed theories of nursing. A variety of nurses have accepted the challenge of describing conceptual frameworks and theories. Each

The focus of gerontology experts is on determining answers about the normal aging process rather than the diseases of old age. There has been a concerted effort during these recent years to address the changes that occur in every human cell as a person ages; hence, the emergence of biogerontology. This is a science with a vast subject area for those who are courageous enough to explore it (Hayflick, 1994).

Biogerontologists generally agree that there is enough observational data available about aging to test a number of theories about aging. Theories that are presently accepted are continuously changing as new research reports become available. The recent increase in theories about the causes of age changes can cause confusion about the validity of the multiple theories.

Strehler (1977) suggested a group of criteria that must be met before any theory is accepted. According to Strehler, the theory must explain why

1. The losses in physiologic function occur (deleterious)
2. The losses are gradual (progressive)
3. The losses cannot be corrected (intrinsic)
4. The losses occur in all members of a species (universal)

Application of these criteria allows a more precise definition of biologic aging, setting aside, for example, the effect of disease on the human cell (Strehler, 1977).

The major challenge for nurses is to determine just what areas of knowledge are important for providing the best care for older adults. The more nurses understand about the process of aging, the better they will be able to meet the needs of older people. This knowledge provides a better basis for decision making about measures to control and cope with the major problems of aging, such as incontinence, cognitive impairment, susceptibility to infection, lack of or difficulty with mobility, loneliness, changes in human needs, and a host of other difficulties that continue to grow in number and complexity as people age.

■ Psychosociologic Theories

Psychologic aging is characterized primarily by behavioral changes. Closely associated with the psychologic and biologic sciences are the sociologic changes that relate to the environmental influences that contribute to and affect aging people.

As research about aging increases, "there appears to be an openness to accept contributions from . . . adjacent sciences," as well as pressure to establish a theoretic structural framework for reporting the results of scientific study (Birren & Birren, 1990, p. 14). Each of the three disciplines (psychology, sociology, and biology) is increasingly aware of the need for research to explain the aging process, and a multidisciplinary approach is being strongly advocated.

Potential for the growth of knowledge within each discipline is phenomenal. Witness the growth in the psychologic gerontologic literature alone. Until 1945, only about 500 publications could be found in this area. In each 10-year period since 1945 the literature has doubled. The reports about research and aging in each discipline have continued to increase exponentially. Similar pronouncements can be made about the biologic and sociologic literature, which indicates the potential significance and value of the literature in guiding the study of gerontology.

Explanation for psychosocial (i.e., psychosociologic) aging are complex. Psychologists and sociologists show a marked desire to arrive at a single cause or explanation for aging. As the population of older adults increases, the complexity of this issue also grows. Each older person is an individual, and each life experience and each change in a person's environment has an effect on that person. Explaining these events and experiences, tracing the origin of each change, and describing the resulting influences on the person leads the scholar down a very convoluted trail. By isolating one experience at a time and discretely analyzing the data related to

---

BOX 3-1 PSYCHOSOCIOLOGIC THEORIES OF AGING

- Disengagement theory
- Activity theory
- Life-course theories
- Continuity theory

---

the particular experience across a variety of individuals, one can reach logical conclusions about the experience. If this process is implemented for a variety of experiences, the various conclusions about each experience can be clustered and arranged in some order that will allow inspection and application to future groups of people.

A few psychosocial theories, listed in Box 3-1, are presented in the following pages. Experts are also discussing many other valid and intriguing theories. Readers are advised to consider the theories presented here to be only a sampling among the many that will be developed in the future. Readers should critically analyze each of the theories they encounter, whether presented here or elsewhere. The developments in the theories of aging are emerging so rapidly that while new reports are being written, still-newer information is being discovered. The diligent and conscientious reader is challenged to maintain an open and inquiring mind while carefully monitoring the exciting emergence of information in this rapidly developing field.

PSYCHOSOCIAL PERSPECTIVES ON AGING

Aging is defined as the transformation of the human organism after the age of physical maturity so that the probability of survival constantly decreases, and it is accompanied by regular transformations in appearance, behavior, experience, and social roles (Birren, 1988). The underlying assumption on which all scholars of aging theory operate is that whatever is observed or described will change in some way, given time, experience, and exposure to the environment. Growth, development, and aging are characterized by change; stagnation is not a characteristic of life.

Psychosocial aging can be described as a result of the disuse of previously acquired skills; a consequence of random wear and tear; a change in adaptive capacity because of environmental variables; a loss of various internal and external resources; a result of genetic influences over the life span, which cause changes in an individual's psychosocial characteristics; and/or a consequence of the choices made by an individual and the creation of new solutions that have never been used before.

Social scientists generally agree that genetics—that is, heredity—is a major factor in determining the length of human life, although environment plays an important role in modifying the expected life span. Within the limits of heredity and despite the environmental factors that influence life, scientists recognize that genetically controlled characteristics interact with the biologic characteristics of individuals and their knowledge and attitudes about life; the resulting characteristics become known as "culture." Culture can be considered the "DNA of society"—that is, the collection of roles, beliefs, and behaviors that are handed down from one generation to another (Birren, 1988).

The psychosocial literature of gerontology contains many closely related yet different views of aging. These various perspectives agree that as people grow older, their behavior changes, their social interactions change, and the activities in which they engage change. At this point, the common views diverge into a great variety of theories, two of which focus on either the individual's social interactions (disengagement theory) or the individual's activities (activity theory—originally called implicit theory).

DISENGAGEMENT THEORY

Cumming and Henry (1961), of the University of Chicago, reported the empiric study that prompted their development of disengagement theory and activity theory. These two scholars investigated various aspects of the aging process and reported the results of their work in publications that others have relied on for more than the past 35 years. Data were gathered by observing and interviewing a sample of older people to "construct inductively a theory of aging" (Cumming & Henry, 1961). Cumming and Henry acknowledged the work of colleagues who had identified and described "outcomes of the aging process," or the end point of the aging process. However, their colleagues had not identified the actual *process* of aging. Unanswered questions were, How did the older person reach the end point? What stages were experienced by the individual in reaching the end point? Stimulated by the desire to describe what happens between adulthood and old age, these researchers observed a panel of aging people over a period of time to identify what occurs to healthy, economically stable Americans as they experience the process of aging. Based on the resulting data, they enunciated two theories of aging. Talcott Parsons presciently predicted, in the foreword to the report of their findings, that this study would serve as a focus of discussion for some time to come, and indeed it has proven to be just that.

As a result of this investigation, the disengagement theory of aging was developed. This was perceived as a commonsense theory. *Disengagement* was viewed as "an inevitable process in which many of the relationships between a person and other members of society are severed, and those remaining are altered in quality" (Cumming & Henry, 1961, p. 14). The process may be initiated by aging people themselves, or it may be initiated by others in society. When the withdrawal takes place, it may be partial or total; that is, the aging people need not withdraw from everyone around them. They might selectively withdraw from some groups of people and not from others.

The research plan was based on a social-psychologic theory, and it was suggested that the theory was a bridge between personality theory and social theory. A wide variety of hereditary and environmental factors were known to influence human behavior, and all of these factors were to be considered when studying human behavior. Cumming and Henry went on to acknowledge that development follows a pattern in which each phase of development is influenced by the phase that has preceded it. For example, older people are influenced by the experiences they have had in adulthood, which in turn have been influenced by experiences during adolescence and, still earlier, by occurrences in childhood. The major emphasis of the researchers, however, was on the experiences of old age and adulthood, with little attention given to childhood experiences. Given these assumptions, the goal of the study was to develop a theory of aging through the use of the *inductive process* (i.e., the process of deriving general ideas from a lot of specific information).

It was observed that older people are less involved with life than they were as younger adults. This is a statement of fact; no value judgments were made regarding whether older people should or should not behave in this way. It was noted that during middle age, adults usually establish an equilibrium between themselves and society; as they age, this state of equilibrium is altered and a new equilibrium is established, in which the older people experience a greater distance from society, and they develop a new kind of relationship with society. In America there is evidence that society forces withdrawal on the older people whether or not they wish it.

Although this theory has had staunch supporters over the years, it has also had strong opponents. Some suggest that this theory does not consider the large number of older people who do not withdraw from society. The rebuttal to this criticism is that the theory still holds and that those older people who do keep in touch with society are "unsuccessful adjusters to old age," or "off time" disengagers, or members of a "biological or psychological elite." Although disengagement theory has been roundly criticized and its limitations are acknowledged, even those who argue against it admit that it has stimulated important discussion and investigation and has had a lasting effect on theory development in social gerontology. It is recognized as the first formal theory that attempted to explain the process of growing older.

ACTIVITY THEORY

Disengagement theory is not the only common-sense theory that describes the psychosocial aging process. The implicit theory of aging, more recently called the activity theory of aging, looks at and considers the phenomenon of aging quite differently than does disengagement theory. Missing from the literature and from research reports were data that could provide a basis for an *explicit* theory of aging. Many assumptions about aging gave credence to an implicit theory of the aging process. The following were among the assumptions that supported the implicit theory:

- There is an abrupt beginning of old age after a specified period of time in middle age.
- The process of aging leaves the older person alone or cut off from the usual acquaintances and friends.
- People should be encouraged to remain active and to develop friendships with other people in their own age group.
- Standards and expectations of middle-aged people should be projected onto the behavior of the older person. Being successful in the aging process depends on being like a middle-aged person as much as possible.
- The aging person should be encouraged to expand and to be involved, because the more active older adult is more satisfied with life.

Activity theory emphasizes the importance of ongoing social activity; as a result of this activity, older adults develop a positive concept of self. Those who adhere to this theory suggest that a person's self-concept is related to the roles held by that person; for example, retiring from an occupational role may not be so harmful to self-concept if the person actively maintains other roles, such as familial roles, recreational roles, and volunteer and community roles. As one ages, it is expected that roles will change, but to maintain a positive sense of self, the activity theory assumes that one must substitute new roles for those roles that are lost because of age; hence well-being in later life depends on activity in newly acquired roles.

A basic assumption that underlies activity theory is that social activity, in and of itself, is beneficial for older adults and that it contributes to the achievement of life satisfaction for older adults. Also, it is assumed that older adults need and desire high levels of social activity and that older adults interpret different types of activity in exactly the same way that younger people do. Studies have reported that the relationship between activity and well-being among older adults depends on the type of activity in which they are engaged. A further component of this theory considers the preferences of the older people and their choices regarding the extent to which they wish to be active; setting aside time for quiet reflection may be as important as more active pursuits for some older people.

LIFE-COURSE THEORIES

Various scholars have placed marked emphasis on the developmental features of aging. The life span theories of the 1950s and 1960s made valuable contributions to the psychosocial literature. Their views about human development from infancy through adulthood have been a stimulus to further inquiry.

E.H. Erikson (1963) approached maturity as a process. He perceived each person as developing as a biologic organism and a social being. To illustrate this development, he defined eight distinct stages and proposed that each person progresses through these stages, from birth through maturity. Within each stage, he identified features of complete development and of incomplete development. This model cites crises that involve dilemmas that confront people as they develop. Erikson contends that each crisis can be resolved by moving forward to another stage of development or by remaining fixed at a level of incomplete development. Those who disagree with Erikson's theory acknowledge that there may be some substance to his ideas, especially regarding the early and middle years of life. However, it is felt that the model neither incorporates nor adequately defines the maturity of old age. Though the model does provide some sound ideas on which study of maturity and development can be based, the theory does not adequately address the dilemmas and crises through which older adults proceed.

Havighurst (1972) also suggested some development-related ideas and suggested that if older people (age 60 and older) are to experience satisfaction in later life, they should successfully complete the following tasks:

1. Adjustment to declining health and decreasing physical strength
2. Adjustment to the life of retirement, as well as to reduced income
3. Adjustment to the death of a spouse, of family members, and of significant others
4. Adjustment to living arrangements that differ from those to which they have been accustomed
5. Adjustment to the pleasures that accompany aging, such as increased leisure time and playing with grandchildren

In the more recent past (the 1970s and 1980s), scholars have addressed the life-course perspective, which is a conceptual development within social and behavioral analysis of aging (Passuth & Bengtson, 1988). This perspective is perceived as a "conceptual framework for con-

ducting research and interpreting data" rather than as an exact theory. Key elements of this framework are the following assumptions:

- Aging occurs from birth to death.
- Aging involves biologic, psychologic, and sociologic processes.
- Experiences during aging are shaped by historical factors.

Some who share this perspective express concern that loosely using the term *life course* in social gerontology may dilute and reduce the significance of the life-course perspective.

CONTINUITY THEORY

The central premise of continuity theory is that older adults try to preserve and maintain internal and external structures by using strategies that maintain continuity; that is, the older people may seek to use familiar strategies in familiar arenas of life. Continuity is a subjective perception, and each person must uniquely adjust to changes by forming personal links to tie the new experiences to the person's previous experiences in life (Cohler, 1982). Continuity is very much *person oriented*—that is, oriented to the individual person. Only the older person can assess the here and now because the basis for assessing is the result of the person's retrospection—the recollection of the person's remembered past. In later life, adults tend to use continuity as an adaptive strategy to deal with changes that occur during normal aging. Continuity theory has excellent potential for explaining how people adapt to their own aging. It is supported by individual preference and social approval (Atchley, 1989).

A fundamental assumption of this theory is that evolution occurs as people age and that change can be integrated into a person's historical context without causing major upheaval or disequilibrium. Change comes about as a result of the aging person's reflecting upon past experience and setting goals for the future. The aging people exercise choice over their experiences and recognize that some of the changes are occurring because of normal aging, which they may not have chosen for themselves.

Atchley (1989) defines *continuity* as "coherence or consistency of patterns over time." He refers to this as a dynamic concept of continuity and applies it to the issue of adaptation to normal aging. Change is ever present and may be perceived as such against the backdrop of the person's past, especially the person's perceived past. Thus continuity may be a general cognitive construct within which many specific changes can occur.

Continuity may be viewed more readily over a long life span than over a short one. Thus the changes that occur in human development in later life appear to be more subtle than the changes that occur earlier (Fry, 1992).

■ Biologic Theories

Theories of cellular aging have been classified as genetic and nongenetic by Brookbank (1990), with the suggestion that genetic theories seem to be the most promising in terms of arriving at answers through research. Genetic theories include those involving deoxyribonucleic acid (DNA), error and fidelity, somatic mutation, and glycation. Nongenetic theories include those involving "wear and tear," nutrient deprivation, and aging pigment accumulation, as shown in Box 3-2.

GENETIC THEORIES
Theories of molecular aging

Error and fidelity theory The error theory of aging has been extensively studied, yet it is difficult to determine exactly where an identified error might have occurred in the molecular development of the cell. The error may have occurred at the level of DNA or at the level of transcription, translation, or posttranslation. *Fidelity* is defined as the faithful reproduction of the correct proteins from the point of gene transcription and translation of the messenger ribonucleic acid (RNA) into the proteins that become components of cellular structure. As the

> ### BOX 3-2 GENETIC AND NONGENETIC THEORIES OF AGING
>
> Genetic theories
>   Theories of molecular aging
>   Error and fidelity
>   Somatic mutation
>   Glycation
>   Theories of cellular aging
>   Programmed cellular aging
>   Aging pacemaker
>   Theories of the organ system
>   Autoimmunity
>   Neuroendocrine control
> Nongenetic theories
>   Effects of temperature
>   Nutrient deprivation
>   Lipofuscin

fidelity of transcription or translation is decreased, an error occurs that results in the insertion of improper amino acids into the sequence of a particular protein. As a result of the identification of these data in scientific experiments, further studies were done to determine the relationship of this information to aging. Despite the demonstrated existence of altered proteins in aging cells, there is little evidence to support the theory of error and fidelity as a cause of aging (Brookbank, 1990).

According to Cristofalo (1988), the theory of error is an example of a *stochastic theory*—that is, a theory describing random events that occur in the organism or in the environment that may have a cumulative and predictable effect. The core of this theory recognizes that the normal process of faithfully replicating that is carried out by normal molecules of protein occasionally—at random—goes awry. The error occurs when an incorrectly replicated or synthesized protein is faithfully (fidelity) replicated over and over, which produces numerous faulty molecules in the genetic apparatus. Over a lifetime these random changes lead to a continually increasing production of erroneous protein molecules, which eventually leads to an "error catastrophe" that causes the death of the person.

Somatic mutation theory A very similar example of a stochastic theory is the somatic mutation theory. *Mutations* are those inheritable changes that occur in the cellular DNA. If there is extensive damage to DNA and it is not repaired, then there will probably be an alteration in a genetic sequence. The suggestion is that random genetic mutations caused by background radiation of various types, as well as other factors, gradually produce failure in various body systems that eventually causes death (Cristofalo, 1988). The frequency of spontaneous somatic mutation is low, and the possibility of linking the aging process to these genetic changes is not very likely. Although x-rays do increase the rate of mutation, the lesions of aging and of radiation damage differ. Radiation primarily affects the cells of the skin, of the intestinal lining, and of the bone marrow. Age effects, however, are noted primarily on the nerve and muscle cells. Scientists advise that much more research and study will be necessary before a direct link can be established between radiation-related or other mutations and aging (Brookbank, 1990).

Glycation theory Glycation theory suggests that glucose acts as a mediator of aging. *Glycation* is the nonenzymic reaction between glucose and tissue protein. Cellular studies of the effect of glycation suggest that glycated proteins show less enzyme activity, less degradation of abnormal proteins, and inappropriate *cross-linking* (i.e., they do not form appropriately parallel connections with other proteins). A number of studies conclude that glycation may have a profound cumulative effect during a person's life. The negative effects of this process on proteins may be a major contributor to age changes. In addition, the effects of this process appear to parallel the elevated glucose levels and shorter life span of diabetic patients (Masoro, et al., 1989). However, no definitive relationship between diabetes and aging has been shown, and it has not been clearly determined that glycation effects either cause aging or are caused by aging-related changes that occur in other body processes (Brookbank, 1990).

Theories of cellular aging

Programmed cellular aging theory The theory of programmed cellular aging, sometimes termed *program restriction,* suggests that aging may be the result of an impairment of the cell in translating necessary RNAs as a result of increased turnoffs of DNA. Some scientists speculate that though the essential messages may be transcribed at all ages, the translation of these messages into functional proteins may be restricted in older people. They suggest that the cell may stop exchanging genetic information, and without genetic guidance, the cell may undergo senescence.

The significance of this theory is being debated. It has been established that either some segments of DNA become depleted with advancing age, or selected cellular structures seem to change with age so that DNA transcription is restricted. However, if aging were attributable to this alteration in the program of cellular development, a more regular and more predictable sequence of organ system failures might be expected than occurs at present (Brookbank, 1990).

Aging pacemaker theory The aging pacemaker theory proposes that one cell, or one type of tissue, interferes with cell proliferation, thereby initiating the process of senescence throughout the body. Some authors have attempted to explain this process by studying the thymus as the pacemaker, or "biologic clock," that is responsible for activating and maintaining this aging activity in humans. This theory has not been definitively and universally accepted.

Conclusion Cellular aging remains a fascinating area of study. Though various authorities agree that cells have finite limits of reproduction, they continue to debate exactly what these limits are. Some doubt that the finite limit is ever reached by cells living in the body. The body cells lose their functional abilities well before they lose their ability to reproduce; hence signs of aging cannot be attributed to cell death alone.

Theories of the organ system

Autoimmune theory Many of the health problems that older people encounter can be explained by some degree of immune system dysfunction, including diseases such as cancer, mature-onset diabetes, senile dementia, and some vascular diseases. The immune system is closely linked to the neuroendocrine system, and each body system can react to changes in the other systems. It is also known that the immune system is less able to deal with foreign organisms as the body ages, and the immune system also increasingly makes mistakes by erroneously identifying autologous tissues as being foreign. The altered ability of the body to deal with alien organisms and the increase in identification errors by the immune system increase the susceptibility to disease and to abnormalities that result from autoimmune responses (Brookbank, 1990); many known causes of death relate to these problems of the immune system.

Neuroendocrine control theory The neurologic and endocrine systems are major controllers of body activity. The loss of cells from both of these systems is documented by scientists who study the brain. During the human life span there is a 10% decrease in the weight of the brain, which is accounted for by both a loss of cells and a loss of fluids in the cerebrum. Some investigators suggest that the documented age-related changes in response to hormones may be the result of changes in the receptors for hormones rather than changes in the activity of the endocrines themselves.

Conclusion General acceptance of the neuroendocrine control theory is just as elusive as is general acceptance of the autoimmune theory. As with many scientifically correlated events, it is difficult to know which one may be causing the other or whether still other factors may be causing both events. Thus the changes in the body that are ascribed to the processes described by either of these theories may simply reflect what is happening to the systems of the body as a result of the aging process (Brookbank, 1990).

NONGENETIC THEORIES
Effects-of-temperature theory

The life span of warm-blooded species is inversely proportional to their metabolic rate; observations confirm that mammals with high metabolic rates tend to be the smaller, shorter-lived species. However, this cannot explain why members of the same species die at different ages despite a similar metabolic rate. Aging among those species with a higher metabolic rate is usually explained in terms of the cells wearing out; the rationale for this is that chemical reactions in living systems are slower at lower temperatures and are accelerated at higher temperatures. Humans might live at a much slower pace if their body temperatures were just 5 degrees lower than the usual 98.6 degrees Fahrenheit. If such a reduction were attained, humans could expect to live about 20% longer than they live at present (Brookbank, 1990).

Nutrient deprivation theory

Nutrient deprivation is another perplexing correlational theory: thus far, scientists do not know whether deprivation of cellular nutrients causes aging or is caused by aging, or even whether both may be caused by some other factor. Some theorists propose that oxygen deprivation leads to senescence of deprived cells, but the pattern of such deprivation does not approximate that of normal aging, in which cells randomly disappear from tissues (Brookbank, 1990).

Lipofuscin theory

As people age, pigment accumulates, and this accumulation becomes apparent in the skin of older people. These "age spots" have been referred to as "biochemical debris" by biochemists, and it is theorized that these waste products of the metabolic processes of the cells accumulate until they reach a critical point, when they begin to interfere with cellular functioning. This is referred to by some people as the "wear and tear" theory. However, there has been no demonstrable association between the existence of these age spots and alterations in cellular function. Scientists have concluded that this pigmentation is a result of aging rather than a cause of it (Brookbank, 1990).

CURRENT THINKING AND OLD IDEAS

In the present situation of defining theories of aging, most biogerontologists believe that several mechanisms are operating simultaneously to cause aging; there probably is not one single cause of aging, but many causes. Until there is definitive data about the causes of aging, a number of ideas and efforts will be studied, read, and reported. Those presented by Brookbank are stimulating and give cause for thought and study. In the following section, equally valid ideas are presented from the studies and work done by Hayflick.

According to Hayflick (1994), current thinking about aging is influenced by some old ideas. Three of these ideas are the following:

1. The "vital substance" theory
2. The genetic mutation theory
3. The reproductive exhaustion theory

Vital substance theory

Each person is born with a specific amount of some vital substance. Aging occurs as this vital substance is consumed, or exhausted, and the person dies. Variations in individual life expectations are the result of differences in the amount of vital substance that each person has at birth. To date, there has been no evidence to support this theory.

Genetic mutation theory

Mutations are changes that occur in genes, and several kinds of changes are known to occur.

Some are harmful and some are beneficial. Because of their essential role in the diversity of life and the adaptation of animals to their environment, mutations are serious contenders for the locus of aging and longevity phenomena. Although this idea has been intriguing to scientists, there is no experimental evidence to support it as a sound theory.

Reproductive exhaustion theory

The reproductive exhaustion theory has few followers. The central idea in this theory is that there is an initial burst of reproductive activity, then a period of rapid aging followed by death. It was concluded that this does not meet the criteria for being an acceptable theory.

■ Theories Presuming a Preexisting Master Plan

Theories of aging that are worthy of consideration at present can be classified into two broad groups: those that presume a preexisting master plan and those that are based on random events.

The chief theory in the first group suggests the presence of a *biologic clock* governed by a series of chemical events. Especially significant in this idea is the secretion of hormones by the hypothalamus or the pituitary gland in the brain.

Biologists generally accept the phenomenon of *programmed cell death*. Hayflick, however, questions the relationship of massive cell death to aging. The complex molecular changes that precede cell death might cause age changes and eventual death of the person long before the cells die. The current beliefs about programmed aging make it an unpopular theory today.

The release of hormones into the human blood creates many kinds of activity in the body. Hormones can accelerate some aging processes and can slow down other processes. Modern gerontologic endocrinologists are especially concerned with hormones as possible causes of age changes rather than looking to the hormones as a means of rejuvenation. The role of the *neuroendocrine system* is significant in reproduction and in the presence and function of biologic clocks. However, despite various research efforts to define the relationship of the endocrines to aging, conclusions can only point to the fact that the neuroendocrine system has an effect on our bodies—there is no conclusive evidence that it is the origin of age changes.

Biogerontologists cannot agree about whether or not we lose nerve cells as we age. They do agree that profound changes occur in the brain as humans age, but the effect of these changes on the life of other cells in the body is not clear. At one time it was thought that the brain produced a "death hormone," allegedly made by the pituitary. The studies have not been confirmed, and researchers are not pursuing this area of research at present. Despite the tendency to rely on the neuroendocrine theory to account for age-associated deficits, there seems to be no more compelling reason to "blame" the neuroendocrine system for age changes than to select any other body system as being responsible for these changes.

■ Theories Based on Random Events

The *wear and tear theory* has been on record for many years. The idea that supports this theory is that a body tissue, as it becomes worn from use, cannot continuously renew itself. It is generally agreed that normal cells cannot divide or function forever, but this admission does not explain *why* age changes occur. In fact, this recognition may have nothing at all to do with aging causes. Although biogerontologists may be admired for their ingenuity in developing such a theory, it will not be possible to test this theory scientifically until some type of experiment is devised to determine whether the wear and tear on body parts can account for aging.

The *rate-of-living theory* is based on the premise that animals and humans are born with a limited amount of potential or physiologic capacity that is expended at various rates. Rapid expenditure of energy precipitates early aging; slow expenditure results in slower aging. This is often referred to as the "live fast, die young" theory. Life in the fast lane is also referred to as "burning the candle at both ends"; maintaining a slower lifestyle is referred to as "being laid back." Proponents of the rate-of-living theory, and of the wear and tear theory, would assume that one who lives a laid-back life will age more slowly and will live longer. Appealing as this may sound to some, there has not been any scientific evidence generated to support this idea.

The *waste product accumulation theory* suggests that a kind of cellular constipation results if cells accumulate more waste than can be disposed of efficiently. Over time, such cells will accumulate toxins that could hamper normal cell function and the cell will slowly die. Among some scientists this is called the lipofuscin theory. The most evident sign of this process is the brownish pigment that becomes apparent in the skin of people as they age. One writer calls these age pigments "the ashes of our dwindling metabolic fires." However, this theory does not meet the criterion of universality, and there is no proven evidence that the presence of age pigmentation interferes with cell functioning. Some merchants promote the use of centrophenoxine, which in laboratory animals seems to reduce the pipovuscin content of cells. When studied in humans, the drug does reduce blood sugar levels and increase oxygen consumption; however, there is no sound evidence that this pigmentation—or the centrophenoxine—plays any role in aging.

The *cross-linking theory* of aging contends that, with age, some body proteins become cross-linked and may impede metabolic processes. Advocates of this theory contend that as errors accumulate in various molecules, age changes can occur. Belief that cross-linking of molecules in the human body causes age changes is not based on experimental evidence. Even if cross-linking of the human collagen molecules does occur, there is no good evidence that it actually interferes with the metabolic processes. Perhaps this is only one of the many biochemical changes that occur over time and contribute to aspects of aging. More systematic study is needed to arrive at conclusive evidence about the significance of this phenomenon.

■ Conclusion

There are other theories about aging, and there is a great deal of speculation about what may cause this reality of life. None of the theories that have been proposed can claim sufficient evidence to account for the aging effects that are witnessed and experienced in humans. Any one of the proposals can be pursued and studied with great interest and enthusiasm. The basic truth about the explanation of the cause or causes of aging is this: we do not know why we age. Some biogerontologists believe that aging has many causes that probably include aspects of all of the extant theories. Other scientists adhere to one or a few theories and discount all the other proposals. Because gerontology is such a young science, there is not sufficient knowledge to explain why aging occurs. For the first time in the history of biology, however, there is hope that available knowledge will be made known soon because of the increase in the number of dedicated scientists who are working in the field of aging. Hayflick suggests that our thinking about aging can be reordered by rearranging the format of the question we ask; in other words, instead of asking, Why do we age? the question should be, Why do we live as long as we do? By reformulating the question, we may conclude that the body has changed over a period of time as evidenced by the fact that longevity has increased and by the possibility that the aging process has slowed. The studies of biogerontology could prove to be very exciting and revealing in the future.

The theories of aging presented in the preceding pages share one common denominator, or central theme: change. As molecules, cells, and organ systems continue to live, they change. An interesting observation about change: When considered at the beginning of life, change is referred to and talked about as *development*. Later in life, when change is considered, it is referred to as *aging*. This idea offers an interesting basis for discussion.

The following summarizes several characteristics of the complex process of aging (Cristofalo, 1988):

- There is increased mortality with increasing age.
- Changes in the chemical composition of the body occur during the aging process.
- A broad spectrum of progressive deteriorative changes occurs with aging.
- The reduced ability of the older person to adapt to environmental change is probably a major factor in aging.
- People who are aging are increasingly vulnerable to disease.

Examination of and reflection on the theories of aging are stimulating and intellectually invigorating experiences. Witness the ever-increasing research and number of publications in the biologic, psychologic, and sociologic specialties of gerontology; with these before them, scholars cannot help but wax enthusiastic and feel very positive about the future of gerontologic knowledge. On the other hand, several improvements are sorely needed:

- Experts must communicate more, building on the strengths of existing interdisciplinary collaboration and communication.
- Researchers must develop and use a more uniform, shared language, both within each discipline and across the disciplines, to enhance communication.
- Nurses must intensively analyze existing theories to develop more specific ideas and to reduce the complexity and overlap among the defined theories.
- Nurses must maintain, and increase, the emphasis on the quality of life of older adults.
- Society must develop a positive view of older adults and their potential for contributing to

society, yet at the same time, realistically recognize when their strengths may be temporarily reduced.

- Nurses must incorporate the concept of the individuality of each older person, respecting the uniqueness of the individual whose life holds valuable experiences and recollections that should be utilized.
- Nurses must recognize the physical, psychologic, and social losses experienced by all older people.
- Society must change or eliminate the existing stereotypes about older adults.

As studies about older adults continue, it is encouraging to note that there is room for many ideas and a multitude of systematic studies.

Specialists in aging predict an "endless agenda for empirical research on the social aspects of aging" (Streib & Binstock, 1990). They advocate the development of theories and models so that acquired knowledge and discoveries about aging can be organized in such a way that the interested scholars can build on data already identified (Birren & Bengtson, 1988).

The task of defining theories of aging is complex. Biology uses genetics and evolution (commonly termed *nature*) as concepts for organizing data, whereas the social sciences use concepts of culture, social structure, and socialization (commonly termed *nurture*). Each human being is a product of both domains; hence the theories that can be called "psychologic theories" will have dimensions of genetics (nature), as well as social dimensions (nurture). To develop a theory in the behavioral sciences, multiple factors must be considered, and each must be specified carefully as the theorist struggles to meet the challenge of defining the process of aging.

During the 1950s, 1960s, and 1970s older adults in the developed nations were examined and studied as a disadvantaged group with low socioeconomic status, as compared to younger people in society (Streib & Binstock, 1990). This

stereotype of older people changed in the 1980s, probably because of society's awareness of their increased numbers and the fear of their becoming an economic burden; indeed, the stereotype became the reverse as U.S. society came to believe that all older adults were "prosperous, hedonistic and selfish" (Streib & Binstock, 1990). As a result of the change in society's view of older adults, which showed a fear of the influence that older adults will wield on the nation's economy, groups of advocates for the aging have been established. It is predicted this trend will continue throughout the remaining years of the twentieth century. These issues will probably be studied by analyzing the socioeconomic status of older adults, as well as by further developing the proposed theories about aging.

There is general agreement among the gerontologic scientists that the research efforts of many scholars will be needed to adequately explore the various theories of aging. It will take a great deal of time to explore, refine, and elaborate upon the many ideas that are being proposed as explanations of the aging process. It will be important for many to participate, especially those who work with older adults in community settings, in long-term care facilities, and in acute care settings. There are rich sources of data available to the gerontologic researcher; the availability of many hands to assist in the data collection and analysis will surely be appreciated by all older adults of today and tomorrow, as well as by their families and caregivers.

REFERENCES

Atchley, R.C. (1989, April). A continuity theory of normal aging. *Gerontologist, 29*(2), 183-190.

Birren, J.E. (1988). A contribution to the theory of the psychology of aging: As a counterpart of development. In J.E. Birren & V.L. Bengtson (Eds.), *Emergent theories of aging.* New York: Springer.

Birren, J.E., & Bengtson, V.L. (Eds.). (1988). *Emergent theories of aging.* New York: Springer.

Birren, J.E., & Birren, B.A. (1990). The concepts, models, and history of the psychology of aging. In J.E. Birren &

K.W. Schaie (Eds.), *Handbook of the psychology of aging.* New York: Academic Press.

Brookbank, J.W. (1990). *The biology of aging.* New York: Harper and Row.

Cohler, B.J. (1982). Personal narrative and life course. In P.B. Baltes & O.G. Brim (Eds.), *Life-span development and behavior* (Vol. 4). New York: Academic Press.

Cristofalo, V.J. (1988). An overview of the theories of biological aging. In J.E. Birren & V.L. Bengston (Eds.), *Emergent theories of aging.* New York: Springer.

Cumming, E., & Henry, W.E. (1961). *Growing old: The process of disengagement.* New York: Basic Books.

Erikson, E.H. (1963). *Childhood and society* (2nd ed.). New York: W.W. Norton.

Fry, P.S. (1992, April). Major social theories of aging and their implications for counseling concepts and practice. *Counseling Psychologist, 30*(2), 246-329.

Havighurst, R. (1972). *Developmental tasks and education.* New York: David McKay.

Hayflick, L. (1994). *How and why we age.* New York: Ballantine Books.

Masoro, E.J., Katz, M.S., & McMahan, C.A. (1989). Evidence for the glycation hypothesis of aging from the food-restricted rodent model. *Journal of Gerontology, 44,* B20.

Passuth, P.M., & Bengtson, V.L. (1988). Sociological theories of aging: Current perspectives and future directions. In J.E. Birren & V.L. Bengtson (Eds.), *Emergent theories of aging.* New York: Springer.

Strehler, B.L. (1977). *Time, cells and aging* (2nd ed.). New York: Academic Press.

Streib, G.F., & Binstock, R.H. (1990). Aging and the social sciences: Changes in the field. In R.H. Binstock & L.K. George (Eds.), *Handbook of aging and the social sciences* (3rd ed.). New York: Academic Press.

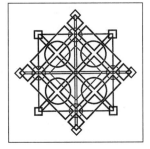

C H A P T E R   4

If I should live to a ripe old age
May I possess some bit of
individuality, charm and wit
that I may not be discarded
when I am withered, worn, and weak
But sought after and cherished
like a fine antique.

ANONYMOUS

The Transition Years

■ Learning Objectives

On completion of this chapter, the reader will be able to do the following:

1. Describe social role changes experienced by older adults in the United States.
2. Describe changing family roles experienced by older adults in the United States.
3. Discuss the patterns of late-life marriages.
4. Examine the positive and negative consequences of retirement for older adults.

Most people do not experience aging by waking each morning saying, "Well, today I am much older than yesterday." Rather, for many people the song "Sunrise, Sunset" from the musical *Fiddler on the Roof* captures their experience of growing older. Tevye, a traditional father, suddenly notices that his oldest daughter is a beautiful woman and his young neighbor has grown into a man who dearly loves her. He reveals his sense of aging by singing, "I don't remember growing older; when did they?"

Perhaps that is the way most people come to the realization of their own aging—watching their children reach adulthood, losing their parents, and realizing that they now are the oldest generation in their families.

Middle age is said to begin when a person starts to think of time in terms of the amount left to accomplish life's tasks; there is an awareness of one's mortality different from the younger person's sense of unlimited time and immortality. Taking stock of one's life is another aspect of middle age. Furthermore, as people move into their late 50s and early 60s, there is a sense, for some, of coming to terms with their own passage into the older age group. What this actually means to people is not clearly understood, especially in our youth-oriented culture.

The ambiguity surrounding the perception of growing older in the United States in the last part of the twentieth century is suggested in an interesting sociologic study. Goldstein and Heiens (1992) examined self-perceptions of aging. They asked subjects to evaluate, when compared to members of a given age group, how they looked, how they felt, and how their interests compared. The results demonstrated that older subjects overwhelmingly perceived themselves as being within younger age groups rather than within their own chronologic age boundaries, leading the investigators to conclude that perceived subjective age is less than chronologic age (Goldstein & Heiens, 1992). There is a sense of the ageless self, an identity that maintains continuity over time, that draws meaning from the past and provides courage for the future (Kaufman, 1993).

There is a creative tension in the lives of many older people as they strive to meet new role expectations, to continue to develop their gifts and talents, and to realize their ambitions and dreams for their retirement years. The tension comes from being older and living in a society that values youth, speed, productivity in terms of work, and individual independence. These attributes are difficult for older people to generate and exacting for them to maintain.

What then are the psychosocial challenges and the realities that face an older person? How does society respond to the needs of older adults? And lastly, what are the gifts, talents, and dreams of older people that have the potential to enrich the community and society while providing a sense of satisfaction and fulfillment for the older adult? While trying to address these questions, this chapter will provide a view of family and social roles available to the older person and will discuss the effects of retirement, successful aging, and the involvement of older people in overall society.

■ Social Challenges of Aging

As a result of extensive studies of today's older population, a great deal is known about the older people of today. Significant for nursing is the realization of the wide diversity of the older population and the important differences in health care needs. Because of the wide diversity, it is most difficult to generalize about appropriate health care for the individual older adult. The diversity is seen in ethnic origin, language, health, family relationships, intelligence, lifestyle, educational background, and socioeconomic status (Silverstone, 1996). The need for individualized health care is of vital importance and should be uppermost in the nurse's mind when the nurse approaches the care of older adults. The need for nursing care soars as people age because of increases in disabling illness, the occurrence of which rises sharply in the older age groups. There is an opportunity for nurses to focus on the functional level of the older person rather than on the disease or illness state. The understanding of diversity among older people will assist the nurse in bringing a realistic but wholistic perspective to the delivery of services to older people.

The social roles available to older adults are in a way reflections of their lives. Family roles many times are a result of investments made over years of being a family member. Traditions handed down through generations—celebrations of holidays, family events, celebration of family members' accomplishments, traditional gifts, vacations—are part of the glue that binds generations together through both good and bad times. There is a reciprocity in life, a mutuality of sharing, celebrating, laughing, and crying together. To live fully is to give of oneself for the joy of life's journeys. Not always, but most of the time, people make a place for the older person as they journey through life.

Today many older people are challenged to embrace the leisure time they have forfeited along their life's journey. The rewards of an older age should not be dismissed. The freedom from the competitive struggle so often typical of the workplace, the time to pursue creative talents, and the time to travel to faraway and exotic places are a few of the pleasures that are afforded to many of today's older adults.

FAMILY ROLES

Significant changes in family composition—such as declining family size with fewer children, changes caused by increasing divorce and second-marriage rates, and expanding numbers of women in the work force with dual workers, single parents, and single-person households—will lead to adjustments in the lives of older adults. Although these changes may seem overwhelming, it is appropriate to pause and realize that older adults in their 70s, 80s, and beyond have survived and adapted to depression, war, countercultures, and phenomenal changes in the use of information processes, from listening to radios on crystal sets to working with computers and the Internet. As society responds to the cultural changes, it may be that the older and wiser people will provide the continuity that will support growth and stability for family life.

The family roles depend on the composition of the family and the availability of different members to augment whatever roles are played by the older person. Family life provides many roles for older people. The connections in three-, four-, and even five-generation families lead to multiple roles. Many older people have roles that stretch from being a caregiver for a frail 80-plus-year-old parent to being a great-grandparent. Over 50% of people over 65 years of age are members of four-generation families, and 20% of women over 80 who died were great-great-grandmothers, the matriarchs of five generations (Silverstone & Hyman, 1992). Longevity and early childbearing create multiple roles for older members.

The following two situations emphasize factors that influence role attainment for an older adult:

Charles and Maria have been married for 45 years. Charles, who is 67 years old, has his 86-year-old mother living with his family; he shares expenses for her care with his two brothers. Maria's father, who has severe dementia, lives in a nursing home close to their home. Charles's eldest son, Harold, who is 45, is a new grandfather; his 22-year-old daughter, Emily, has just given birth to her first child. Charles's roles in this family include husband, son, son-in-law, brother, father, father-in-law, grandfather, and great-grandfather. Charles has made a lifetime investment in his family roles. He enjoys close relationships with his wife, his children, his siblings, his mother, his father-in-law, and his grandchildren.

Bryan is 62 years old and has been divorced once and has remarried. He was 35 years old when he first married, and his marriage lasted for 14 years. He had two sons by this marriage; they are 13 and 19 years old. Bryan remarried when he was 52. He is an only child and his parents are both deceased. He has a poor relationship with his sons and does not see them more than twice a year. His second wife's parents are also deceased. She has a sister who lives close to them and is often a visitor at their home. Bryan's family roles are husband, father, and brother-in-law. His strained relationship with his sons will probably limit his future enjoyment of not only the father role, but also the grandparent role. At present he is very satisfied with his life, but the structure of the family system may limit his ability to fulfill all available family roles.

GRANDPARENTING

Age is not an accurate predictor of family roles, although grandparenting is always projected to be the special role reserved for older adults. A favorite saying regarding grandchildren is the classic "If I had known grandchildren were such fun, I would have had them first"; or consider another statement, overheard from a retired money manager: "The children are the investment, the grandchildren the dividends."

How older adults assume the role of grandparenting varies, with interactions ranging from fun loving and game playing to a distant, formal type of interaction. One role of grandparenting that has become too common is that of caregiver or protector of grandchildren. As the scourge of drug abuse ravages some young adults, their parents are stepping in to take care of their grandchildren. Many times grandparents have gone to court to protect the grandchildren from abuse or neglect and have won custody of their grandchildren (Minkler et al., 1992).

Most grandparents are not faced with such a heavy responsibility, but enjoy the role of grandparent with a sense of continuity of family and a sense of fulfillment. The old idea of the grandparents' being aged, doddering, fragile, and dependent has been changed. Grandparents are now often hale, hearty, active, healthy, and quite independent. As the younger, middle-aged, and older generations consider grandparents of today, they think of quite a different group of people than existed a few years ago.

Because people are living longer, healthier lives, the role of the grandparent has taken on a very different style. This is the age when grandparents celebrate life and love; they love and are involved with grandchildren very intimately, quite a bit more freely than they interacted with their own brood. They celebrate their life with their spouse in a more romantic way than when they were burdened with the responsibilities of child rearing, mortgage paying, grocery shopping, meal preparing, and all the other daily tasks of working families. The grandparent couple can spend time with the grandchildren in a relaxed, fun-loving way; they can involve themselves and the children in games and activities, depending on the ages of all. They can reflect and comment on the strengths of their grandchildren, appreciate the talents and potential they observe in the children, and introduce and use humor to appreciate and talk about the mistakes and shenanigans that are experienced in the course of the days when they are together. The ease with which the children and the grandparents experience being together, for whatever purpose and period, is certainly one of the potential gifts available to the older adult.

This relationship with grandchildren affords an opportunity for the older person's own children, now parents themselves, to view their older parents in a special way. The bonds between generations may become stronger as the young parents come to appreciate not only the

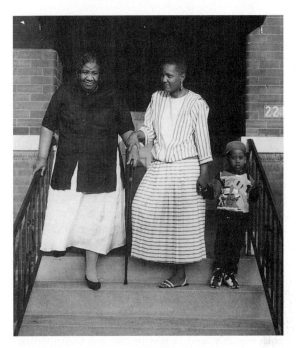

Strong intergenerational bonds are important.
Courtesy Loy Ledbetter, St. Louis.

present grandparenting, but also the parenting they received when they were young. They may now come to an increased understanding of all the trials and tribulations that are part of child-rearing experiences. There is great opportunity for intergenerational reflection and expression of love and affection through the act of active grandparenting.

■ Late-Life Marriage

The role of spouse or the role of being part of a couple is available to those who choose marriage as part of their life's journey. Silverstone and Hyman (1992) suggest that couples who grow old together live out their later years in several different patterns. With great respect for the diversity in relationships and the difficulty in categorizing people, it is helpful for nurses to look at the different patterns late-life marriage may take.

How individual partners in a marriage respond to aging influences the life of the married couple. Certainly health and illness are key factors in the couple's ability to maintain the relationship over time. Nonetheless, taking these factors into consideration, there are six patterns that typify late-life marriage: the inseparables, the collaborators, the quiet despairers, the not-so-quiet despairers, the parallel pairs, and the tie breakers (Silverstone & Hyman, 1992).

THE INSEPARABLES

The inseparable couple is a poet's dream—love forever, together forever. The partners in these couples talk for each other, always referring to themselves as "us," and their entangled identity leaves no room for individual differences. They like the same sports, vacations, movies, people, and other elements in their lives. Whether or not this type of marriage pattern makes for a healthy relationship for individuals is not for anyone to judge. The important thing for nurses to recognize with this pattern is that the partners need one another, and illness in one has the potential to leave the other incapacitated.

THE COLLABORATORS

The collaborators have developed, over time, the ability to respect individual differences, but they are emotionally connected, with mutual appreciation for each other's talents and gifts. Problem solving is their mode of operation, and this continues into their later life. They work efficiently together; at times there are disagreements and arguments, but solutions are their goals. One example of a late-life problem could be the simultaneous retirement of both members of a professional working couple. Collaborators will spend time working toward an equitable solution, which may entail different times for individual retirement. The problem-solving focus of this couple will need to be recognized and valued by any health professional who will be providing the spouses' health care.

THE QUIET DESPAIRERS

Marriage is viewed as a trap by the quiet despairers. Many spouses have gone through long years of not experiencing intimacy, support, or personal recognition for their talents or gifts. Many lead lives of quiet desperation. They stay together for a myriad of reasons that others may find incomprehensible: for the good of the children, for financial security, because of religious or social beliefs, or out of fear of being alone. These are some of the reasons health professionals may hear as individuals explain their lives together, although most suffer in silence. In fact, many times these couples go unrecognized; they seem contented and perhaps even comfortable in their relationship. The nurse, however, should always be aware that there may be despair below the surface of silent contentment.

THE NOT-SO-QUIET DESPAIRERS

For the not-so-quiet despairers, fighting is a way of life, and the partners have spent years bickering, carping, and even physically abusing one another. In fact, later years may see an increase rather than a decrease in the fighting. One or both individuals may have difficulty in accepting changes brought about by the aging process. These feelings of frustration may lead to venting of unrecognized rage that increases hostility and results in more fighting within the marriage. Because these spouses do not endear themselves to many, they become more dependent on each other as their children and their friends maintain a distance from the constant discomfort of watching or participating in the pattern of fighting.

THE PARALLEL PAIR

The parallel pair long ago decided, for reasons similar to those of the quiet despairers, that marriage was essential but not necessarily an emotional or loving involvement. Many times, either one or both of the partners have found intimacy outside of the marriage. There is either open or tacit acknowledgment of the arrangement, and these spouses live compatible but separate lives. Later years may find that this pattern does not continue, and disruption may bring forth resentment if in fact there was not mutual acceptance of extramarital behavior.

THE TIE BREAKERS

Some spouses find that the late-life transition is not one they want to share, and they realize that their goal is to escape the relationship. Late-life divorce and separation are still uncommon, but they are on the rise. Although infrequent, divorce among older couples has become such a major concern that the American Association of Retired Persons has published a guide entitled "Getting Divorced after 50" (Silverstone & Hyman, 1992).

CONCLUSION

How older adults relate to each other through their marriage is a reflection of their history together. Most marriages maintain or actually escalate their pattern of relationship. It is important for the nurse to be aware of the diversity of marriage patterns and the possible impact these relationships will have on the health of the individual partner.

■ Widowhood

Even though older couples know that they will be separated by the death of one member, most older adults experience great difficulties in adjusting to the reality. The adjustment includes coping with loss and acceptance of the role of widow or widower. Following the death of their husbands, older women are most economically vulnerable because of a loss of income and benefits.

For many older adults, widowhood is accompanied by adverse health. It is difficult to appreciate all the stresses that impinge on an older person who has suffered a severe loss such as the loss of a long-term spouse. Whether or not this type of stress is related to or a cause of illness is a moot question. The reality is that the recent widow may be at risk because of a combination of factors, such as increased age, self-neglect, stress response, and genetic makeup. The nurse must consider where the person is in the life cycle and incorporate this knowledge in the assessment process when managing the care of older adults.

On the other hand, the new role of widowhood may in time bring unforeseen joys as many older adults are able to find new companionship with new marriage partners. The gender distribution in the older population, of three women for every man over the age of 65 years, favors the remarriage of older men over that of older women (White House Conference on Aging, 1995).

■ Retirement

Retirement is defined as the withdrawal from the labor force, either voluntary or involuntary, coupled with the earned right to pension income. This is a recent sociologic development, which may not survive in its current form for future older generations. Actually, the practice of setting retirement age at 65 years was started in Germany in 1889 by Chancellor Bismarck. He arrived at the age of 65 by adding 20 years to the average life expectancy, which at that time was 45 years. Bismarck ensured that few, if any, pension benefits would be paid to workers. Even though life expectancy has increased, the age of 65 has remained the marker for retirement in Western countries.

Two historical events have influenced the American retirement process: (1) in 1908 Great Britain adopted 70 as the age of retirement, and (2) in 1935 the United States established the first nationalized pension system for adults 65 years of age. In 1967 age discrimination in places of employment was made illegal in the United States, ending a long history of age discrimination in the workplace. In 1986 the Age Discrimination in Employment Act made involuntary retirement at either 65 or 70 a thing of the past. As of then, involuntary retirement predicated on age alone was to be considered an act of discrimination and therefore illegal.

In 1900 an average man spent about 3% of his life in retirement; men and women in the late 1990s will spend from 20 to 35 years in retirement. Therefore retirement is to be considered a normative event in the third age of life, and for most people it is a welcome and widely anticipated stage of life: a time to reap the rewards of work and family life and to have an abundance of free time to pursue forestalled pleasures.

Retirement can have a major impact on the financial condition of the retiree. The economic status of older Americans has improved significantly since the 1950s, with poverty rates declining from 35% in 1959 to 12% in 1986 (McLaughlin & Jensen, 1993). Income in older age is linked to multiple interacting past and present variables such as past and current labor force participation, marital status, gender, age, educational attainment, and living arrangements. Factors that increase the possibility of a comfortable income stream during later life are high wages during the work years, higher educational attainment, being male and married, and living in an urban area.

Professional and self-employed older adults have personal investments and continued employment opportunities and are more apt to retire later rather than earlier. However, more people are retiring earlier, and the trend is thought to be accelerating because of the restructuring of the American business community. Younger retirees have lower projected Social Security benefits, fewer private pensions, and longer life expectancy. This does not bode well for their future economic well-being. (Table 4-1.)

A Canadian longitudinal study of men over the age of 65 indicated that men with higher earnings in midlife had significantly lower mortality at older ages and that mortality was associated with early retirement (Wolfson et al., 1993).

TABLE 4-1 U.S. labor force participation

Year	Age	Men (%)	Women (%)
1950	55-64	87.0	27
	65+	45.8	10
1980	55-64	72.0	42
	65+	19.0	8

From Social Security Administration (1995). *Social Security Handbook* (12 ed.). Washington D.C.: Government Printing Office.

On the other hand, many studies show a continuity of involvement and well-being among most retirees as they make the transition to retirement. A study of the short-term effects of retirement on a group of 60- to 66-year-old health maintenance organization (HMO) participants indicated no negative effects. Retired men reported less stress and were more apt to exercise regularly than those who were still working (Midanik et al., 1994). The mixed results of retirement studies demonstrate the diversity of experiences and characteristics of older adults. Retirement is a personal experience and a shared family experience.

There are large ethnic inequalities in the income of older U.S. citizens, with black and Hispanic Americans having much less in assets and private pensions than white citizens. Median income of white older men is almost twice that of black and Hispanic older men. Retirement patterns are sensitive to differences in mortality rates and to the occurrence of disability over the life course. Black men spend more time working, experience more disability, die younger than white men, and therefore spend less time in retirement (Hayward et al., 1996).

Women make up one half of the population, but they compose 75% of the poverty group of older adults. Median income of single older men is substantially higher than that of single older women. Poverty in retirement for women is a result of past discrimination in the workplace coupled with lifetime low salaries. Eighty percent of all working women can be found in 20 of the 420 jobs listed by the Department of Labor. Women are most frequently found in clerical and sales and service jobs. They occupy a limited number of professional jobs including teacher, nurse, librarian, and dental assistant—certainly not the highest-paying jobs in America. Poverty of postretirement women affects social, psychologic, and physical well-being (Perkins, 1993). Noncash factors that benefit all older adults are tax treatment, reduced family size, Medicare, and Medicaid.

The inequality in the distribution of wealth is mitigated, though not resolved, in the United States through our social program known as

BOX 4-1 POTENTIAL RETIREMENT ISSUES

LOSSES
Psychologic

1. Loss of valued self-identity
2. Loss of prestige

3. Loss of companionship
4. Loss of satisfaction

Social

1. Loss of income
2. Loss of valued role

3. Loss of benefits

Physical

1. Loss of physical routine
2. Loss of health

GAINS

1. Gain in companionship of family members
2. Increase in involvement in community affairs as volunteer
3. Increase in control of own time

1. Acceptance of new roles
2. Increase in value to family for grandparenting skills

1. Increase in time to exercise
2. Increase in attention to health behaviors
3. Decrease in stress

Social Security. Thirty-five percent of income for older persons comes from the Social Security system, and nine out of ten people over 65 receive benefits (Social Security Administration 1995). Interesting is the fact that after a lifetime of work, only 29% of Americans over 65 years of age receive a private pension.

Issues that surround retirement reflect the complexity of the human condition, which becomes more extreme as people age. When assessing a person's response to retirement, the nurse should consider that that response may have psychologic, social, and physical aspects (Box 4-1).

How retired people spend their time is of interest to the nurse because social interaction is considered a fundamental element of a healthy lifestyle. However, it must be remembered that individuals differ greatly in their approach to life. Furthermore, the diversity of the older population is a major premise of this chapter, and it calls for great respect for the patterns of social interaction that older adults have chosen for their

third age. It is of interest to note that 22.6 million people over the age of 55 provide direct help for their children or grandchildren. Seventy percent report membership in churches or synagogues, and 60% attend religious activities once a week. Another important aspect of life for people who have retired from the work force is volunteerism. Over 6 million older Americans volunteer through organizations and add their contributions to maintaining community structures. The services of older volunteers influence the nation's political system and support much of the country's system of social programs. For a summary of leisure activities of older adults, see Table 4-2 (White House Conference on Aging, 1995).

In spite of the potential losses associated with retirement, there are certainly significant gains for many retired people, including more leisure time, relief from monotonous work patterns, more control over daily living patterns, ability to pursue interests, time to renew relationships, and time to travel. Retirement has become

TABLE 4-2 Leisure activities of older adults

Activity	Percentage participating
Travel	50
Handcrafts	43
Photography	30
Playing musical instruments	18
Singing in choir	18
Painting	15
Writing	12

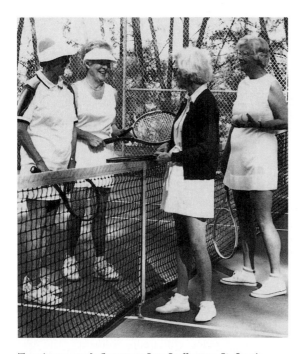

Tennis anyone? *Courtesy Loy Ledbetter, St. Louis.*

an acceptable and anticipated role in modern society. Studies have shown that men and women look forward to retirement and suffer few if any adverse effects that can be attributed solely to retirement from the organized work force.

The nurse must be cognizant of the social roles that older adults carry out in their daily lives. The older person's response to social roles of later life and to retirement may fall anywhere within a wide range—the changes may result in almost no difference in daily life, or they may constitute the best or worst event that the couple or individual has had to face. The event may be a life crisis or the reason for unending joy. But the nurse will always consider social roles and response to retirement—both psychosocial and economic aspects—when doing any assessment of an older adult.

REFERENCES

Goldstein, R., & Heiens, R. (1992). Subjective age: A test of five hypotheses. *Gerontologist, 32*(3), 312-317.

Hayward, M., Friedman, S., & Chen, H. (1996). Race inequities in men's retirement. *Journal of Gerontology, 51B*(1), S1-S10.

Kaufman, S. (1993). Reflections on the "ageless self." *Generations, 17*(2), 13-16.

McLaughlin, D., & Jensen, L. (1993). Poverty among older Americans: The plight of the nonmetropolitan elders. *Journal of Gerontology, 48*(2), S44-S54.

Midanik, et al. (1994). Retirement and health behaviors. *Journal of Gerontology: Social Sciences, 50*(1), S59-S61.

Minkler, M., Roe, K., & Price, M. (1992). The physical and emotional health of grandmothers raising grandchildren in the crack cocaine epidemic. *Gerontologist, 32*(6), 752-762.

Perkins, K. (1993). Recycling poverty: From the workplace to retirement. *Journal of Women and Aging, 5*(1), 5-23.

Silverstone, B. (1996). Older people of tomorrow: A psychosocial profile. *Gerontologist, 36*(1), 27-32.

Silverstone & Hyman. (1992). *Growing older together.* New York: Pantheon Books.

Social Security Administration. (1995). *Social Security handbook* (12th ed.). Washington, DC: U.S. Government Printing Office.

White House Conference on Aging. (1995, May). Background papers. Meeting held in Washington, DC.

Wolfson, M., et al. (1993). Career earnings and death: A longitudinal analysis of older Canadian men. *Journal of Gerontology: Social Sciences, 48*(4), S167-S179.

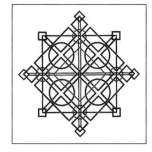

C H A P T E R 5

In spite of illness, in spite even of the archenemy sorrow, one can *remain alive long past the usual date of disintegration if one is unafraid of change, insatiable in intellectual curiosity, interested in big things, and happy in small ways.*

EDITH WHARTON

Drug Therapy in Older Adults

■ Learning Objectives

On completion of this chapter, the reader will be able to do the following:

1. Discuss physiologic-age-related changes that affect the pharmacologic dynamics of the older person.
2. Identify signs and symptoms of adverse drug reactions common in older adults.
3. Recognize high-risk drugs and their potential for harm and benefit to older adults.
4. Identify drug-drug interactions in older adults.
5. Recognize the risks and benefits of the use of over-the-counter (OTC) drugs in older adults.
6. Discuss methods to increase older adults' ability to understand and to follow medication prescriptions.

Appropriate drug prescribing in older adults is an important component of both the day-to-day primary care evaluation and comprehensive assessment of an older patient. The basic concepts of appropriate drug prescribing in older adults differ significantly from those used in other age groups because the effects of a drug on an older patient may be magnified by certain changes that occur during the aging process. This may be secondary to either an alteration of absorption, metabolism, or excretion of the drug; structural and physiologic changes of aging organ systems; or blunting of immune defenses (Hazzard et al., 1994).

Because of these changes and because older patients in general have significantly more ill-nesses, they take more prescription and over-the-counter-drugs, and in many instances, inappropriately, than do members of other age groups. This syndrome, referred to as polypharmacy, is defined as the use or administration of many medications; it differs according to subgroup within the older population. The average older American takes 4.5 prescription and 3.5 over-the-counter medications at any given time. That same individual may refill about 15 prescriptions per year. As would be expected, the highest incidence of polypharmacy occurs in the nursing home population burdened with advanced age and chronic disease, averaging eight medications per patient. The least incidence occurs in the community-dwelling older adult population (Beck, 1991-1992).

Older adults are at greater risk for and experience the greatest severity of adverse drug reactions (ADRs). An adverse drug reaction is "the development of unwanted symptoms, signs, changes in laboratory values, or death directly related to the use of a medication" (Beck, 1991-1992). In addition to those instances secondary to alterations in drug absorption, metabolism, or elimination, ADRs may also occur in the form of drug-drug or drug-disease interactions (Gurwitz & Avorn, 1991; Lesage, 1991; Lindley et al., 1992). This increased risk is not independently related to age, however.

Older adults are also at greater risk for both polypharmacy and adverse drug reactions because they tend to be referred to or to visit more specialist physicians. Therefore they may visit more pharmacies, both in frequency and in numbers of sites, possibly because their regular pharmacy may not have the drug "in stock" and they perceive an urgent need to take the drug as soon as possible. Also, various family members serving as caregivers for an older loved one may use their own respective pharmacies, when refilling the drug, adding to the confusion and the number of "pill" bottles. Older patients may not be aware that they are taking several different forms of aspirin or acetaminophen because they are not aware of some of the basic ingredients of OTC drugs.

■ Physiologic-Age-Related Changes

Older adults, especially the advanced elderly (those over 85 years of age), have blunted immune defense systems to fight infection, leading to a greater risk of pneumonia and influenza, and less chance of recovery because of inadequate antibody production (Hazzard et al., 1994). Manifestations of this blunted response may be seen in the gastrointestinal system (at the junction of the esophagus and the stomach-cardiac sphincter of the stomach) and genitourinary system (at the junction of the urinary sphincter and urethra), in which bacteria may have a tendency to reflux

beyond otherwise "sterile" areas close to these sphincters, leading to a greater risk of aspiration pneumonia or bladder infection in the presence of disease (Beck, 1991-1992). Therefore these patients lose the "margin of reserve" that allows the human body to fight off stresses, whether physiologic, psychologic, or physical. In the presence of various disease processes, this loss of reserve plays a significant role. An example is precipitation of congestive heart failure (CHF) in a patient with angina and cardiomegaly when the system is challenged with intake of a "few" grams of extra dietary salt, failure to take a morning dose of fluid medication or digoxin, a mild upper respiratory tract infection, or slight excesses of physical exertion (Beck, 1991-1992).

Normal changes of aging include reduction in total body water and muscle mass, and increase in total body fat (Beck, 1991-1992). These changes may translate into a greater risk of adverse drug reactions. Water-soluble drugs, such as digoxin and theophylline, and alcohol are distributed in a smaller compartment in older adults and may accumulate at toxic levels at the same dose that would be safe in other age groups. Fat-soluble, long-acting benzodiazepine minor tranquilizers accumulate in body fat to a greater extent, leading to excess sedation, lethargy, and risk of falls, whereas these problems do not tend to occur in younger patients with less body fat (Calkins et al., 1992). Reduction in muscle mass with "normal" aging translates into reductions in renal clearance, especially in the advanced elderly and for drugs dependent on renal clearance, including digoxin, H_2 blocking agents, fluoroquinolones, penicillins, and aminoglycosides (Calkins et al., 1992).

The normal aging process is accompanied by a reduction of the total number of receptors in the nervous system. In some older adults there is a reduction in the number of functioning receptors in the pancreas; in the responsiveness to stimuli of organ-specific receptors and specific organ systems; in blood supply to the liver; and in the size of organs such as the kidneys, liver, and brain (Beck, 1991-1992; Calkins et al., 1992). Examples of reduction of responsiveness of a specific organ (central nervous system) to stimuli are increased refractory time between responses and inability to learn new material with advancing age. An example of reduction of organ-specific receptors' responsiveness to a stimulus is reduced maximum heart rate, or "blunted" heart rate increase, initiated by the carotid baroreceptors, sensing an acute change in blood pressure when the patient is standing or sitting from a supine position. Normally the expected increase in heart rate would neutralize the negative effects of any transient reduction in blood pressure and prevent any symptoms of "dizziness" or lightheadedness. The blunted process may precipitate postural hypotension in an otherwise normal older patient in 10% to 15% of instances. Postural hypotension is a reduction in systolic blood pressure of 15 mm Hg or more when the patient stands or sits from the supine position (Calkins et al., 1992). The presence of various disease processes and drugs may potentiate these responses. Examples of drug-induced exaggeration of normal aging responses include development of cognitive dysfunction secondary to usage of alcohol and other drugs, including centrally acting antihypertensive agents; psychotropics in high doses or with high anticholinergic activity; long-acting minor tranquilizers; anticholinergic agents; high doses of certain antibiotics—aminoglycosides, fluoroquinolones, and penicillins; high doses of H_2 blocking agents; and non-steroidal anti-inflammatory drugs (NSAIDs). These agents might cause reduction in responsiveness to stimuli, leading to confusion, sedation, or lethargy. An example of drug-induced exaggeration of reduced responsiveness of an organ-specific receptor to a stimulus is the heart block that might be caused by the use of cardiovascular agents—including digoxin, antiarrhythmic drugs, and calcium channel blocker drugs—at high doses in older adults.

"*Five body systems*" deserve mention in a discussion of the absorption, metabolism, and excretion of drugs in older adults and the development of adverse drug reactions. The least important system is the "*integumentary system.*" In the outer layers of the skin, 7-dehydrocholesterol is converted by ultraviolet light of the sun to vitamin D_3 (Hazzard et al., 1994). Though the sun is not the only source of vitamin D production, institutionalized older patients with chronic renal or liver failure who do not get regular exercise may develop vitamin D deficiency, leading to the development of osteomalacia, because the metabolically active form of vitamin D requires metabolism in the liver and the kidney (Hazzard et al., 1994). (See Table 5-1 for a summary of the effects of drugs on body systems.)

The "*central nervous system*" plays an important role in the development of adverse drug reactions in older adults primarily because of normal structural and physiologic changes; in addition, Alzheimer's and related diseases may cause the patient to be more susceptible to acute confusion (delirium) and chronic confusion (cognitive dysfunction). The development of confusion syndromes is thought to be related to an anticholinergic hypothesis (Hazzard et al., 1994; Mach et al., 1995). Use of drugs with significant anticholinergic or muscarinic activity (e.g., antihistamines, antispasmodics, tricyclic antidepressants, phenothiazines, and narcotics) should be minimized or avoided in older patients.

The second least important system involves the "*gastrointestinal tract.*" In the normal older adult, physiologic changes include a reduction in acid secretion and motility, an increase in transit time, and a greater tendency for constipation (Hazzard et al., 1994). These changes do not usually translate into clinically significant disease. Certain drugs dependent on an acid medium in the stomach may be absorbed to a greater or lesser degree (Calkins et al., 1992). Albumin decreases slightly with normal aging, which is of no clinical significance. However, in the presence of gastrointestinal tract disease (previous gastrectomy, Crohn's disease, ulcerative colitis, or sprue), older patients may develop malabsorption syndromes leading to hypoproteinemia and hypoalbuminemia. Albumin and total protein levels may also decrease in older adults secondary to one or a combination of three other possible

TABLE 5-1 Classes of drugs associated with frequent adverse drug reactions by mechanism and body system

Body system	Drug class	Mechanism of ADR	ADR
Cardiovascular system	Diuretics	Fluid contraction, hypokalemia, hyponatremia	Lethargy; inappropriate antidiuretic syndrome; postural hypotension, falls, hip and other fracture
	Alpha-blocker drugs	Arterial vasodilation	Presyncopal lightheadedness and falls, especially with high doses
	Beta-blocker drugs	Nonselective blockade of beta-receptors	Precipitation or exaggeration of congestive heart failure, masking of hypoglycemia, postural hypotension, masking of symptoms of endocrine disease, reduction in exercise capacity, exacerbation of chronic lung disease or bronchospasm, memory loss, depression, arthropathy
Central nervous system	Anticholinergic agents (antihistamines, antispasmodics, phenothiazine and tricyclic antidepressants)	Stimulation of parasympathetic nervous system, central anticholinergic disruption	Sedation, cognitive dysfunction, lethargy, acute confusion; postural hypotension, falls, hip fracture; constipation, fecal impaction; worsening of glaucoma; urinary retention; dry mouth
	Benzodiazepine tranquilizers, barbiturates, hypnotics	Depression of central nervous system	Sedation, cognitive dysfunction, lethargy, acute confusion; postural hypotension, falls, hip and other fracture
	Centrally acting antihypertensive agents (methyldopa, reserpine, clonidine)	Depression of central nervous system	Sedation, cognitive dysfunction, lethargy, acute confusion; postural hypotension
	Nonsteroidal anti-inflammatory drugs	—	Sedation, cognitive dysfunction, lethargy, acute confusion

TABLE 5-1 Classes of drugs associated with frequent adverse drug reactions by mechanism and body system—cont'd

Body system	Drug class	Mechanism of ADR	ADR
Gastrointestinal system	H$_2$ blocking agents, sucralfate	Reduction in acid secretion leading to achlorhydria	Increased risk of aspiration pneumonia in the presence of swallowing dysfunction in bed-bound patients
	Nonsteroidal anti-inflammatory drugs	Direct irritation of gastric and duodenal mucosa (inhibition of surface prostaglandin)	Gastrointestinal bleeding
	Antacids, iron preparations, tetracyclines	Binding between agents	Diarrhea or constipation; malabsorption
Liver	Anticoagulant (warfarin) and antiseizure medications (carbamazepine [Tegretol], phenytoin [Dilantin], barbiturates, meperidine)	Increased bleeding time (warfarin); sedation, lethargy, acute confusion, cognitive dysfunction (phenytoin, carbamazepine, barbiturates, meperidine); ataxia and incoordination (phenytoin)	—
	Barbiturates, meperidine, diphenhydramine, lidocaine, theophylline, ibuprofen, tolbutamide, salicylates, long-acting benzodiazepine tranquilizers (diazepam, chlordiazepoxide, flurazepam)	Increased risk of gastrointestinal or other bleeding (salicylates, ibuprofen)	Sedation, lethargy, acute confusion, cognitive dysfunction, postural hypotension, falls, hip fracture
Kidney	H$_2$ blocker drugs, antibiotics (penicillins, aminoglycosides, fluoroquinolones)	Reduction in creatinine clearance	Confusion, irritability, drowsiness, lethargy, dizziness
	Digoxin	Reduction in creatinine clearance	Anorexia, decreased appetite, nausea, cardiac conduction problems, confusion, irritability, anxiety
	Nonsteroidal anti-inflammatory drugs	Inhibition of prostaglandin-mediated renal vasodilation	Fluid retention, worsening hypertension, aggravation of CHF
Integumentary system	Tetracyclines	Photosensitivity	Dermatitis

mechanisms: decreased metabolism secondary to liver diseases such as cirrhosis; increased catabolism secondary to malignancy; or decreased intake secondary to socioeconomic issues or the anorexia associated with dementia or depression. Certain drugs are highly bound to protein or albumin in the inactive (ineffective) state. A reduction in total protein or albumin level may lead to a greater fraction of free drug that is bioavailable, leading to toxicity. Examples include phenytoin, meperidine, digoxin, and warfarin (Calkins et al., 1992). Reduction of the dosage of these drugs may be necessary to prevent confusion and ataxia secondary to the use of phenytoin; lethargy, drowsiness, falls, or cognitive dysfunction secondary to the use of meperidine; confusion, anorexia, and nausea secondary to the use of digoxin; and bleeding secondary to the use of warfarin. Specific formulas are available that allow dose-specific adjustments according to protein and albumin levels (Winter, 1988). The use of anticholinergic drugs or sucralfate may predispose the older patient to constipation or gastric reflux (by relaxation of the sphincter of the stomach) and aspiration risk. In addition, the use of H_2 blocking drugs to reduce acid secretion in the stomach of an older patient with peptic ulcer disease or hiatal hernia theoretically might seem a logical step in the treatment process; however, the use of such drugs could lead to further reduction in acid secretion and a neutral or basic medium that would be an appropriate environment for bacteria refluxing from the stomach cavity to the lower esophagus. The problem is compounded when the patient develops swallowing problems from a stroke, Parkinson's disease, or other esophageal disorder and becomes bed bound, becoming further predisposed to aspiration risk (Beck, 1991-1992; Cook et al., 1994).

The second most important system regarding the development of adverse drug reactions in older adults is the *"liver."* The liver is the most important organ system for metabolism of various drugs. This metabolism involves two processes. The first one, phase I metabolism, undergoes significant reduction in activity with age. Drugs metabolized in this phase are either oxidized, reduced, or hydrolyzed, and their half-lives are prolonged because of this phase. This includes drugs such as diazepam, chlordiazepoxide, flurazepam, barbiturates, meperidine, phenytoin, propranolol, quinidine, warfarin, theophylline, tolbutamide, salicylates, nortriptyline, diphenhydramine, lidocaine, and ibuprofen. Phase II metabolism, conjugation or deactivation, is not altered with age. Drugs metabolized by phase II include the short-acting benzodiazepines (lorazepam, oxazepam, temazepam, and triazolam) with relatively short half-lives (Calkins et al., 1992). This correlation of metabolism phase to half-life is reflected clinically by studies indicating a difference in hip fracture risk between patients using long-acting and short-acting benzodiazepines, with the long-acting drugs causing a greater risk (Berggren et al., 1987; Cummings et al., 1995).

The most important organ system involved in the elimination of drugs dependent on renal blood flow is the *"kidney,"* because kidneys are dependent on creatinine clearance, which decreases with advancing age even in the presence of normal blood urea nitrogen and serum creatinine levels. Examples of these drugs are digoxin, penicillins, aminoglycosides, H_2 blocking agents, and fluoroquinolones (Calkins et al., 1992). Significant reduction in the dose of these drugs is necessary with reduced creatinine clearance to avoid adverse drug reactions, which may manifest themselves with acute changes in mental status, cognitive dysfunction, dizziness, falls, or syncope. A formula useful for estimating creatinine clearance is as follows: creatinine clearance (CrCl) equals 140 minus the age of the patient times the weight of the patient in kilograms divided by the serum creatinine value (values less than 1 rounded to 1) times 72. In the case of women, the creatinine clearance should be multiplied by 0.85 (Calkins et al., 1992). A useful rule of thumb to remember is that if the serum blood urea nitrogen or serum creatinine is elevated above the normal range, the creatinine clearance will be below at least 50 ml/min and the dosage of these drugs should be reduced by one half.

■ High-Risk Drugs

Certain categories of drugs that present high risk of adverse drug reactions to the older patient warrant special consideration and discussion. This list includes the nonsteroidal anti-inflammatory drugs, H_2 blocking drugs, beta-blocking drugs, diuretics, psychotropics, centrally acting alpha-blocker drugs, ganglionic antihypertensive drugs, anticholinergic drugs, antibiotics, antiarrhythmic drugs, drugs for dementia, and other miscellaneous drugs.

Recent studies show a correlation between advancing age, peptic ulcer disease, and the presence of helicobacter pylori, a gram-negative bacterium that colonizes the lining of the stomach, especially in the presence of chronic disease (Graham et al., 1991). Excluding alcoholic and nonsteroidal anti-inflammatory drug–induced causes, one study of 49 older patients with gastritis showed a high correlation with helicobacter pylori (O'Riordan et al., 1991). In such cases, "H_2 blocker drugs" have been shown to be inadequate for healing stomach and duodenal ulcers, with a greater chance of recurrence than with a combination of 2 weeks of antibiotics, metronidazole, and milk of bismuth (Graham et al., 1992; Hentschel et al., 1993). Because of this increasingly popular concept about the etiology of gastrointestinal disease, this regimen appears to be gaining momentum as an ideal alternative in the presence of a positive helicobacter stomach biopsy, urea breath test, or serum antibody level (Culter et al., 1995; Peura, 1995). Both H_2 blocker drugs and sucralfate have been used nonspecifically as prophylaxes to prevent stomach ulceration—in older patients with or without a history of gastrointestinal disease and in patients placed on salicylates or nonsteroidal anti-inflammatory drugs to prevent ulceration. This regimen is not an accepted indication for use of these drugs (*Physicians Desk Reference*,

1995). A study of over 700 nursing home patients revealed that 41% were taking H_2 blocker drugs per indications that had not been substantiated by clinical studies (Gurwitz et al., 1992). Another common protocol is for critically ill patients in the intensive care unit setting to receive one of these agents to prevent stress-related gastrointestinal bleeding. Another study, however, indicated only two conditions that warranted use of these agents in this setting to prevent this complication: respiratory failure or coagulopathy (Cook et al., 1994).

Omeprazole and lansoprazole are proton pump inhibitors, a new class of drugs useful for the treatment of duodenal ulcer and gastroesophageal reflux disease. They have been shown to be more effective than conventional therapy with H_2 blocker drugs in the short-term (2- to 4-week) healing of duodenal ulcer disease. They should not be used for longer than 8 weeks because they may produce achlorhydria and hypergastrinemia; prolonged use has been associated with a dose-related increase in the production of gastric carcinoid tumors in rats (*Physicians Desk Reference*, 1995). These drugs should be reserved for treating intractable symptoms after conventional therapy has failed or for severe disease.

Metoclopramide and cisapride are drugs commonly used to increase gastric emptying and cause contraction of the lower esophageal (cardiac) sphincter. Indications for metoclopramide use are for the treatment of gastroesophageal reflux, diabetic gastroparesis, prevention of nausea and vomiting secondary to chemotherapy and postoperatively, and before implementation procedures. Common side effects include restlessness, drowsiness, confusion, fatigue, extrapyramidal symptoms, and diarrhea. Because cisapride has less affinity for crossing the blood-brain barrier than does metoclopramide, central nervous system symptoms are negligible. Cisapride is the preferred agent for treating gastroesophageal reflux in older adults but is not currently indicated for the other conditions. Both drugs are frequently used nonspecifically to increase gastric emptying in older patients with feeding tubes to prevent aspiration. However, they are not approved for this use (*Physicians Desk Reference,* 1995).

In addition to their effects on cognitive status, other common side effects of *anticholinergic drugs* include dry mouth, constipation, dry eyes, difficulty with urination, blurred vision, drying of bronchial secretions, and prevention of sweating. Medical diseases such as glaucoma, benign prostatic hyperplasia, Sjögren's syndrome (dry eyes and dry mouth), constipation, chronic bronchitis, and peripheral vascular disease may be aggravated by these drugs, predisposing the older patient to the development of fecal impaction, worsening glaucoma, urinary retention, hypothermia and hyperthermia, and exacerbation of chronic bronchitis secondary to mucous plugging (Beck, 1991-1992; Cahill et al., 1994; *Physicians Desk Reference,* 1995).

Nonsteroidal anti-inflammatory drugs, known as NSAIDs, are a particularly hazardous category of drugs that should be avoided in older adults, if at all possible, because of their potential for causing adverse drug reactions by three different mechanisms: precipitating confusion, gastrointestinal bleeding, and renal insufficiency or failure. In one study, NSAID use was found to have caused or exacerbated medical conditions in 86% of the 500 emergency admissions to a general hospital ward (Jones et al., 1992). In high doses, all of these drugs may cause acute or cognitive dysfunction. Indomethacin, because of its high affinity for penetrating the blood-brain barrier, causes the greatest risk of central nervous system side effects such as confusion, dizziness, lethargy, restlessness, and depression (*Physicians Desk Reference,* 1995), and thus is inappropriate for use in older adults (Willcox et al., 1994). NSAIDs also cause direct irritation of the gastric and duodenal mucosa leading to gastritis, peptic ulcer, and esophagitis after first-time or sustained use. Often, a patient may develop bleeding from an undiagnosed, asymptomatic hiatal hernia or reflux that was precipitated by the use of these drugs. Several studies indicate

that all NSAIDs, in high enough doses, may cause gastrointestinal bleeding, with the least risk being from low doses of ibuprofen (200 to 400 mg) (Griffin et al., 1991; Langman et al., 1994).

The third mechanism by which NSAIDs cause adverse drug reactions in older adults is by prostaglandin-mediated renal vasodilation leading to fluid retention and subsequent renal injury via several mechanisms, renal failure, and glomerulopathy (Shankel et al., 1992). By causing fluid retention, NSAIDs may be responsible for worsening of hypertension or inability to control existing hypertension adequately, or for precipitating or aggravating existing congestive heart failure. Discontinuance of NSAIDs in an older patient with hypertension may result in a statistically significant reduction in mean blood pressure (Gottlief et al., 1992; Gurwitz et al., 1994).

The use of NSAIDs also is associated with acute liver injury and a hepatitis-like syndrome (Garcia Rodriquez et al., 1992). A recent study comparing acetaminophen (4000 mg) to high (2400 mg/day) and low doses of ibuprofen (1200 mg/day) for osteoarthritis of the knee indicated no difference in relief of symptoms (Bradley et al., 1991). However, for acute flare-ups of inflammation (swollen, warm, tender joints), for which a nonsteroidal agent may be beneficial, some practical guidelines include the following: (1) using the agent as needed, alternating it with acetaminophen; (2) using the agent in the lowest possible dose; and (3) using the agent for 5 to 7 days and then discontinuing use. Occasionally, persistent patients will demand that they be prescribed an NSAID for continuous use. In such cases, patients should be advised of the potential side effects and should agree to routine monitoring of the blood urea nitrogen for early signs of renal insufficiency, and a hemogram to monitor for early gastrointestinal bleeding. In these cases, misoprostol, a cytoprotective agent given 4 times daily, may provide some protection of the mucosa from gastrointestinal problems (Levine, 1995). Disadvantages of the drug include high cost, the need to be administered 4 times daily, and the common side effect of diarrhea. NSAIDs should not be used concomitantly with aspirin or warfarin because of the higher risk of causing bleeding complications (*The Complete Drug Reference,* 1992).

"*Beta-blocker drugs*" should be used with caution in older adults, particularly propranolol, which is often an inappropriate drug because of its side effects. These include the precipitation or exacerbation of congestive heart failure, masking of hypoglycemia, development of postural hypotension, masking of symptoms of endocrine disease such as hypothyroidism, reduction in exercise capacity, exacerbation of chronic lung disease or bronchospasm, depression, memory loss, and production of arthropathy (Cahill et al., 1994; Newbern, 1991; Thiessen et al., 1990). However, some studies indicate that propranolol may be beneficial for the treatment of anxiety in demented patients and tremor disorders in older adults (Colenda, 1991). The drug was also used to prove efficacy of treatment of systolic hypertension (systolic blood pressure greater than 160) for the prevention of stroke and death (Systolic Hypertension in the Elderly Program [SHEP] Cooperative Research Group, 1991). Use of the drug should be based on a risk-benefit ratio for the particular patient, including an evaluation of the patient's medical conditions.

Beta-blocker drugs may also produce adverse effects on lipid metabolism (*Physicians Desk Reference,* 1995). Pragmatically, the use of beta-blocker drugs in older adults would seem illogical because of the low incidence of high-renin, high-aldosterone hypertension in this group and because renin and aldosterone levels decrease with normal aging (Beck, 1991-1992). However, beta-blocker drugs may be used as first-line agents for the older hypertensive patient with a history of angina or myocardial infarction because they can reduce overall mortality by as much as 76% in this population (Park et al., 1995). Beta selective blocking drugs such as atenolol or metoprolol have fewer side effects and also have the advantage of once- or twice-

daily dosing and therefore increased compliance. They also may be particularly appropriate for the older patient for treatment of dual conditions of atrial arrhythmias and hypertension. Beta-blocker drugs used selectively in patients with good left ventricular function have been shown to decrease the risk of congestive heart failure and death over a 2-year period (Lichstein et al., 1990).

"*Diuretics*" constitute another class of high-risk drugs that should be used with caution in older adults because of the reduction in total body water with normal aging and other factors. Side effects include hypokalemia, possibly linked to sudden death; worsening renal function, left ventricular hypertrophy; and increase in total cholesterol and triglycerides. Diuretics also may cause a contraction alkalosis. In addition, they may precipitate an exaggerated postural hypotensive response leading to lightheadedness, falling, and further morbidity or death from a hip or other fracture (Beck, 1991-1992; *Physicians Desk Reference,* 1995; Weinberger, 1992). Extreme caution is advised in administering thiazides to older patients with dementia or depression because of the tendency of these patients to drink less or even to forget to drink fluids because of the associated memory loss. Frail older adults and those over 85 years of age are also at high risk because of their greater tendency to develop postural hypotension. Older patients taking diuretics should be advised to drink lots of isotonic fluids during the summer months, especially during times of exercise and sweating. Diuretics may actually be harmful in hypertensive diabetic patients. A recent study indicated that such patients treated with diuretics had higher cardiovascular and total mortality than untreated patients (Warram et al., 1991).

Thiazides are generally not effective in the presence of renal insufficiency. Loop diuretics (metolazone, furosemide, bumetanide) are popular drugs used to treat dependent leg edema in older adults but also have the potential of exaggerating the postural hypotension caused by chronic venous insufficiency and stasis, further increasing the risk of inducing lightheadedness, dizziness, falls, and fracture or other morbidity (Beck, 1991-1992). These agents should be reserved for severe edema that is refractory to leg elevation, stockings, and exercise, or for patients with renal insufficiency or congestive heart failure, to mobilize fluid and promote brisk diuresis. By causing calciuria, they may serve a useful purpose in the initial treatment of hypercalcemia (Beck, 1991-1992). Both loop and thiazide diuretics may be a significant cause of urinary incontinence. Removing or minimizing the dose or changing the time of day for administration from the afternoon to midmorning may alleviate the problem in many cases (Beck, 1991-1992).

Advantages of using thiazide diuretics in older adults for treating mild hypertension include low cost and once-per-day dosing. The systolic hypertension in the elderly program, or SHEP, trial, using a first-line drug of chlorthalidone, a long-acting diuretic, showed that reduction in systolic blood pressure below 160 mm Hg reduced significantly the incidence of stroke and cardiovascular disease and, to a lesser extent, cardiovascular deaths and total mortality (SHEP Cooperative Research Group, 1991). Recent case control studies indicate that older women with hypertension using thiazides as compared to those not using thiazides have a significantly lower risk of hip fracture, possibly secondary to reduced excretion of calcium in the urine and resulting retardation of osteoporosis (Heidrich et al., 1991). Doses of more than 50 mg are generally not effective in achieving blood pressure control. African-American patients seem to benefit more from thiazides than do Caucasian patients. For stepwise treatment of hypertension, diuretics used in combination with other agents may potentiate the effect of other drugs but also have the disadvantage of being more expensive.

Centrally acting and "*alpha-blocker antihypertensives*" represent another group of high-risk drugs. Centrally acting drugs such as clonidine, reserpine, and methyldopa can cause significant central nervous system side effects in older adults, including headache, irritability, sedation, cognitive dysfunction, and depressive symptoms (*Physicians Desk Reference,* 1995). Alphamethyldopa is an old drug that must be given 4 times per day because of its short half-life. It may also cause drug-induced lupus syndrome, a rare hemolytic anemia, and hepatitis syndrome in a small percentage of cases (*Physicians Desk Reference,* 1995). Reserpine offers the advantage of once-per-day dosing and is inexpensive, but may produce other bothersome side effects including postural hypotension, dry mouth, constipation, bradycardia, bronchospasm, and hypersecretion of the digestive tract. It causes a hypertensive crisis when used in conjunction with food and drugs containing MAO inhibitor. Thus the use of methyldopa and reserpine is inappropriate in older adults (Willcox et al., 1994). Alpha-blocker drugs such as prazosin, terazosin, and doxazosin reduce blood pressure by causing vasodilation (*Physicians Desk Reference,* 1995). They have become popular because of their recent promotion as first-line agents for treating hypertension in the older patient with benign prostatic hyperplasia with associated signs and symptoms of urgency, frequency, or hesitancy. They have the added advantage of once- or twice-daily dosing. However, to achieve the dual effect of blood pressure and prostatic symptom control, dosages of 7 to 10 mg are often necessary, which also increase the risk of postural hypotension. This risk can be minimized by giving the drug before bedtime (Guthrie, 1994).

Apresoline is an old drug that has traditionally been used for treating hypertension. Its mechanism of action involves vasodilation, especially of the renal arteries. Side effects of the drug include negative effects on the cardiac muscle and increase in heart rate, which subsequently increase the work load of the heart and, in some cases, contribute to the development of congestive heart failure, especially in patients with impaired left ventricular function (*Physicians Desk Reference,* 1995). Disadvantages of the drug include short half-life and 4-times-per-day dosage. The drug can also cause a lupus-like syndrome. The dual-acting alpha- and beta-blocking drugs are newer agents that combine the advantages of beta-blockers with the vasodilating effects of alpha-blockers without increasing heart rate; they can be used for treating heart failure (Lessem & Weber, 1993). However, these combination drugs tend to be more expensive than other classes of drugs in general. Other classes of drugs appropriate for the treatment of hypertension in older adults include the angiotensin-converting enzyme (ACE) inhibitor and calcium channel blocker drugs.

The *angiotensin-converting enzyme, or ACE inhibitors* are a popular group of drugs used to treat hypertension. They have been shown in numerous studies to improve cardiac function in cases of acute congestive heart failure secondary to diastolic dysfunction and to increase survival in patients with chronic severe congestive heart failure, with one study showing a reduction in mortality in cases of mild to moderate congestive heart failure at 41 months using enalapril (Braunwald, 1991; Cohn et al., 1991). Captopril, the first of these agents, has been shown to reverse the reduction in renal blood flow that occurs with normal aging in healthy normotensive older adults by causing significant renal vasodilation (Hollenberg & Moore, 1994). It also has been shown to limit myocardial infarction expansion if given within 24 hours (Oldroyd et al., 1991), and to limit short-term mortality at 5 weeks (ISIS-4 Collaborative Group, 1995). This drug may also slow the progression of renal disease, reduce mortality, and alleviate the need for transplantation or dialysis as opposed to placebo when followed for 3 years (Lewis et al., 1993). Enalapril has also been shown to slow the progression of renal disease, proteinuria, and albuminuria when taken for hypertension, as compared to the effects of using metoprolol, when followed for 3 years (Bjorck et al., 1992). Furthermore, use of enalapril, as compared to beta-blocker drugs, resulted in a significant reduction in proteinuria at 6 months and significant reduction in end-stage renal failure when followed for 3 years in patients with nondiabetic renal insufficiency (Hannedouche et al., 1994). Other positive effects of ACE inhibitor drugs include slower rates of renal function decline and significant reductions in albuminuria using lisinopril, as opposed to using furosemide and atenolol, in hypertensive patients with moderate diabetic renal insufficiency when followed for 18 months (Slataper et al., 1993). In most cases, ACE inhibitor drugs offer the added advantage of once- or twice-daily dosing. ACE inhibitor drugs are contraindicated in the presence of renal artery stenosis. Frequent side effects of these drugs include cough and angioedema (*Physicians Desk Reference,* 1995). Potassium levels should be monitored in patients given ACE inhibitors because of the tendency for these patients to develop hyperkalemia.

Calcium channel blocker drugs are another popular group of drugs used to treat older hypertensive patients by producing vasodilation and promoting loss of sodium and water. Side effects include flushing, headache, dependent edema, and constipation, depending on the specific drug. Calcium channel blocker drugs also offer the advantage of once- or twice-daily dosing, although they are more expensive than diuretics or beta-blocker drugs (Weinberger, 1992). However, a recent case control study suggests increased mortality in hypertensive patients treated with these agents, with the risk increasing with increasing dose, particularly of short-acting agents. Because of the possible limitations and criticisms of the study, a clinical trial is ongoing to prove or disprove these findings, but the results are not expected until 2002. Because these findings relate mostly to the short-acting agents, until there are further findings, long-acting agents are the preferred agents for treating hypertension according to recommendations of the National Heart, Lung, and Blood Institute (Buring et al., 1995; Furberg et al., 1995; Pinkowish, 1995).

PSYCHOTROPIC DRUGS

Another group of high-risk drugs is the *psychotropic drugs* that include minor tranquilizers, major tranquilizers, antidepressants, barbiturates, and hypnotics. Adverse effects of these drugs in general include cognitive dysfunction, sedation, drowsiness, lethargy, and functional decline. In inappropriately high doses for the older patient, they may produce or exaggerate postural hypotension leading to lightheadedness on standing or sitting from a supine position, leading to falls, fracture, and other morbidity (Beck, 1991-1992; Cummings et al., 1995; Grisso et al., 1991; Ray et al., 1991). Because of their side effect profile and their traditional overuse in institutional settings for such nonspecific conditions as insomnia, general agitation, anxiety, and dementia syndromes, OBRA 1987, a federal law, limits use of psychotropics in these settings to specific indications only and in a time-limited fashion. Proper documentation in the medical record is also required. Major and minor tranquilizers are only indicated for psychotic behavior, for hallucinations or delusions that are potentially harmful to the patient or to his or her surroundings, or for the prevention of aggressive, hostile, or combative behavior. Antidepressants should only be used for depressive symptoms. Antianxiety drugs should only be used to alleviate these symptoms in a patient with anxiety that is potentially harmful to the patient's medical or social condition. Barbiturates should only be used for prevention of specific seizures. Hypnotics should only be used for occasional inducing of sleep and not on a daily basis. The first component of the law involving the use of major tranquilizers was implemented in 1994. As a result, the use of these agents has decreased significantly (Rovner et al., 1990).

The "*major tranquilizers*," commonly known as the phenothiazines, can also cause a drug-induced Parkinsonian syndrome consisting of bradykinesia, resting tremor, and cogwheel rigidity of the extremities (Beck, 1991-1992). It has been traditional that they be prescribed prophy-lactically with an anticholinergic drug (diphenhy-dramine, benztropine, trihexyphenidyl) to prevent these side effects. However, the older patient with this syndrome may not have the associated tremor, alleviating the need for these agents, especially with their additional troublesome side effects mentioned previously. In many cases, older patients are inappropriately treated for presumed Parkinson's disease instead of having their dose of phenothiazine eliminated or lowered (Kalish et al., 1995). The phenothiazines have a particularly disturbing and, in many cases, nonreversible side effect of tardive dyskinesia, characterized by abnormal, involuntary, repetitious muscle movements. Increasing the drug dosage may temporarily suppress the involuntary movements with subsequent "breakthrough" and worsening of the involuntary movements. Discontinuance of the drug may help to alleviate the movement disorder, but there is no predictable pattern to the syndrome. Anticholinergic drugs used to treat the parkinsonian side effects of phenothiazine major tranquilizers usually are of no benefit for this condition. The antipsychotic clozapine may be effective in treating severe cases, but can cause agranulocytosis in 1% of cases. Patients treated with this drug should have a hemogram performed monthly to monitor for this side effect. The risk of tardive dyskinesia in older adults may be as high as 6 times that for younger patients using the phenothiazine drugs (Saltz, 1992; Saltz et al., 1991; Yassa & Nair, 1992). The newest agent available for the treatment of psychotic disorders in older adults is risperidone, a serotonin and dopamine antagonist. Because it is not a phenothiazine derivative, it has a safer side effect profile, especially as related to dyskinesia (*Physicians Desk Reference,* 1995).

The choice of a major tranquilizer (phenothiazine) used in the older patient depends on the side effect of the agent and the patient's signs and symptoms. All of the phenothiazine major tranquilizers cause tardive dyskinesia, postural hypotension, anticholinergic side effects, and sedation, and have differing potency. For instance, an older patient with sleep-wake cycle problems secondary to sundowning from Alzheimer's disease may benefit from the sedative properties of chlorpromazine (10 to 25 mg) or thioridazine (25 mg at bedtime) to produce sleep; a dose sufficient to induce postural hypotension or cause significant anticholinergic disruption, leading to the development of delirium, worsening cognitive dysfunction, or other anticholinergic or parkinsonian side effects, is not warranted. On the other hand, haloperidol in a dose of 0.5 to 1 mg may be an ideal drug to treat aggressive, hostile, combative, or psychotic behavior in an agitated demented patient during the day because it is the least sedating, is the least hypotensive, and has the least anticholinergic side effects of these agents, yet is the most potent. However, the use of haloperidol at night for sleep would be counterproductive. The use of these agents, especially in high doses, may reduce the older demented patient's self-care activities, as a result of cognitive dysfunction secondary to the drug. This may lead to the development of functional decline manifested by reduction in independent mobility, bathing, feeding, dressing, eating, and toileting, leading to fecal and urinary incontinence and subsequent hygiene problems (Beck, 1991-1992).

The "*tricyclic antidepressants*" should be used with caution because of their side effect profile, similar to that of the phenothiazines, including postural hypotension, anticholinergic side effects (dry mouth, blurred vision, tachycardia, constipation, urinary retention), sedation, and cognitive dysfunction, and because of their differing potency (Beck, 1991-1992; Calkins et al., 1992; *Physicians Desk Reference,* 1995; Sheikh, 1995). They nonselectively block the reuptake of various neurotransmitters, including norepinephrine, serotonin, and dopamine. In low doses these agents promote a "quieting" or quinidine-like effect on the myocardium, and they produce an arrhythmogenic effect when used in high doses. These drugs can cause significant risk to older adults because of their high rate of successful suicide. Suicide risk related to anti-depressants in general is not related to the specific class, but rather to the dose used, with higher doses associated with increased risk (Jick et al., 1995). Tricyclic drugs with the least anticholinergic properties should be used over those with high-anticholinergic side effects to limit the risk of precipitating acute confusion or precipitating or worsening cognitive dysfunction, especially at high doses. Desipramine and nortriptyline should be given during the morning because of their nonsedating properties. They also offer the safest profile, whereas imipramine and amitriptyline offer the worst. The latter, considered an inappropriate drug for older adults in a majority of cases (Willcox et al., 1994), should not be given during the day because of the associated high risk of sedation and postural hypotension, and it should be avoided in doses exceeding 25 mg. Few current indications exist for its use, except to treat chronic pain syndromes associated with depressed mood, or depression associated with both insomnia and anorexia, because of its ability to stimulate appetite. It should be used with caution in patients with Alzheimer's disease.

The newest and most popular class of agents useful for the treatment of depression in older adults includes the "*serotonin selective reuptake inhibitors (SSRIs).*" These have the same efficacy as the tricyclic agents, but may be tolerated better because of their selectivity (Sheikh, 1995). Recent studies indicate that depression may be caused primarily by a deficiency of serotonin, among other chemical agents in the brain. These agents offer an advantage over the traditional tricyclic antidepressants because of their lack of significant anticholinergic side effects. Theoretically, their use in patients with Alzheimer's disease would seem appropriate to avoid worsening the anticholinergic disruption that typically occurs in these patients structurally as the disease process worsens (Hazzard et al., 1994; Mach et al., 1995). This is an especially important concept because Alzheimer's disease accounts for 93% of cases of dementia, either in the pure form

(51%) or combined with vascular causes (42%) (Calkins et al., 1992). However, side effects of SSRIs include insomnia, agitation, decreased appetite, and nausea (Sheikh, 1995). Fluoxetine, the first of these agents, has a half-life of several days and is less selective in its side effect profile. Other, newer agents such as sertraline and paroxytyline, with half-lives approximating 24 hours and more selectivity for serotonin receptors, are more appropriate for the older patient (*Physicians Desk Reference,* 1995). The SSRIs are strong inhibitors of the cytochrome P-450 system, which is involved in the metabolism of many medications. When used with other agents such as the tricyclic agents, antihistamines, theophylline, erythromycin, benzodiazepines, and steroids, they can double or triple the levels of these agents, leading to a greater risk of adverse drug reactions (Sheikh, 1995). Fluoxetine has been shown to be an independent factor related to higher suicide risk, probably because of its multiple antidepressant use (Jick et al., 1995). Caution should be exercised when using SSRIs to treat depressive symptoms with or without dementia and in the malnourished patient, because the drug may magnify the symptoms of weight loss, nausea, and anorexia related to the disease process itself. This class of drugs also has the advantages of once-daily dosing and rapid onset of action—in 2 to 4 weeks, as compared to the tricyclic antidepressants, which require 6 to 8 weeks. These drugs should be administered in the morning because of their side effect profile. Because of its direct serotonergic effects, trazodone, in an initial dose of 25 to 50 mg at bedtime, provides an excellent option for the dual purpose of treating dementia and/or depression along with insomnia or sundowning. Side effects include postural hypotension and—rarely, if the drug is given in much higher doses than normally used in older adults (150 to 300 mg)—priapism (Beck, 1991-1992). The SSRIs are also used in combination with trazodone for treating depression. Patients given such a combination should be monitored for signs and symptoms of

the so-called serotonin syndrome, associated with restlessness and increased anxiety (Hazzard et al., 1994).

Atypical antidepressants include venlafaxine and bupropion. Venlafaxine has a broader spectrum of neurotransmitter reuptake in addition to that of serotonin, but it does not inhibit the cytochrome P-450 system, which results in less risk of adverse drug reactions when it is used in combination with other drugs (Sheikh, 1995). Bupropion is a relatively safe drug with low anticholinergic and antiadrenergic side effects used for the treatment of depression. However, it should be used with caution in patients with a history of seizure disorder because it lowers the seizure threshold (Beck, 1991-1992).

Lithium is a drug used to treat bipolar (manic depressive) disorder. Regular monitoring of serum levels is recommended because of the frequency of adverse side effects associated with this drug, especially when used with other agents. Because the drug is distributed in the total body water content, excretion is dependent on adequate renal function. Dosages should be reduced for renal insufficiency. Levels of the drug may be increased in patients taking ACE inhibitor and nonsteroidal anti-inflammatory drugs. Other agents such as acetazolamide, urea, xanthine preparations (theophylline), and alkalinizing agents may decrease serum levels. Lithium may interfere with blood monitoring for thyroid disease. Use with calcium channel blocker drugs can increase the risk of nervous system toxicity. Use of lithium with diuretics or in patients with restricted sodium diets for treatment of congestive heart failure or hypertension decreases sodium reabsorption by the renal tubules, leading to an increased risk of hyponatremia and lithium toxicity (*Physicians Desk Reference,* 1995). Other agents that may interfere with lithium metabolism include antipsychotics and medications containing iodine. Early symptoms of toxicity include diarrhea, drowsiness, loss of appetite, muscle weakness, nausea or vomiting, slurred speech, and trembling. Late symptoms include confusion, unsteadiness or blurred vision, convulsions, dizziness, and increased urination. Less common side effects include postural hypotension, weight gain, bradycardia, cardiac arrhythmias, and heart block (*The Complete Drug Reference*, 1992).

The "*benzodiazepine minor tranquilizers*" are useful agents for the treatment of agitation, anxiety, and insomnia in older adults. In this category, short-acting drugs such as lorazepam (0.5 to 1 mg) and oxazepam (15 mg) are the drugs of choice to prevent worrisome side effects encountered with the long-acting agents (Beck, 1991-1992; *Physicians Desk Reference*, 1995). Flurazepam, chlordiazepoxide, and diazepam are inappropriate for use in older adults (Willcox et al., 1994). Although requiring metabolism by the liver, alprazolam, a short-acting benzodiazepine, has minor antidepressant effects in addition to its antianxiety effect if used in a low dose (0.25 mg) 2 or 3 times daily (*Physicians Desk Reference*, 1995). Other relatively short-acting benzodiazepines (triazolam and temazepam) serve a useful purpose for the occasional treatment of insomnia. Triazolam, having a half-life of 4 to 6 hours, is useful for inducing sleep, whereas temazepam will maintain sleep. Triazolam, in doses higher than 0.125 mg and when used on a regular basis, has been implicated as a cause of delayed recall of tasks in older patients. For this reason it should be used in a dose of 0.125 mg only on an occasional basis (Bixler et al., 1991; Greenblatt et al., 1991). The benzodiazepines in general are known to cause short-term memory impairment, although the long-term effect is unknown (Rummans et al., 1993). Meprobamate is an older drug used for the treatment of anxiety. However, its use in older adults is inappropriate because of its risk of causing sedation, confusion, and lethargy (*The Complete Drug Reference*, 1992; Willcox et al., 1994). Buspirone is a useful agent for the treatment of chronic anxiety, but must be given on a regular basis to be effective. Because onset of action requires 7 to 10 days, use of a short-acting benzodiazepine for this period may be necessary (*Physicians Desk Reference*, 1995).

Zolpidem tartrate is a new, short-acting non-benzodiazepine hypnotic with a chemical structure unrelated to the benzodiazepines, barbiturates, or other hypnotic drugs. Because it interacts with GABA receptor sites, it shares some of the properties of the benzodiazepines, including the potential to depress the central nervous system and impair motor and cognitive performance in older adults. It also has been associated with signs and symptoms of other central nervous system depressant drugs with abrupt withdrawal. It is indicated for the occasional treatment of insomnia, but because it is a new drug, experience in older adults is limited (*Physicians Desk Reference*, 1995).

Agents useful in the treatment of agitation and anxiety associated with dementia syndromes include trazodone and buspirone (Colenda, 1991). Carbamazepine has also recently become a popular agent for the treatment of agitation and aggressive, hostile, and combative behavior in such cases—in lower doses traditionally used to treat seizure disorder (100 to 200 mg twice daily). It offers a safer side effect profile than the traditional psychotropic agents, with little toxicity (Tariot et al., 1994, 1995).

"*Drug therapy for dementia*" has shown little to no progress in ameliorating the symptomatology of the disease. Various agents have been recommended in the past for the treatment of Alzheimer's disease, because of the recognition that lecithin deficiency and acetylcholine deficiency may play a role in its development. These various agents include lecithin-containing health foods and megadoses of other vitamins. Even though popularly used, clinical trials do not prove their efficacy. Hydergine, an old drug, has been used in the past for the treatment of dementia but has shown no clinically significant effects (Beck, 1991-1992). Cerebral vasodilators were once a popular group of drugs for the treatment of organic brain syndrome, Alzheimer's disease, or vascular dementia. The theory behind the use of these agents was that vascular and oxygen supply to the brain should be increased. These drugs are contraindicated because of their risk of causing postural hypotension, falls, fracture, and other morbidity (Willcox et al., 1994). Pentoxifylline, a drug approved for use in treating peripheral vascular insufficiency, has been shown to slow the cognitive deterioration in patients with multiinfarct dementia, but with little effect on memory (Black et al., 1992).

Tacrine, an acetylcholinesterase inhibitor, is the first of a new class of drugs approved for Alzheimer's disease. Studies prove its effectiveness for mild cases of the disease and only for short-term benefit (up to 30 weeks); long-term studies are not available. In addition to cost, disadvantages include the need for regular blood monitoring because the drug causes asymptomatic elevation of the liver function tests. This toxicity is usually associated with higher doses of the drug, and discontinuance of the drug will usually resolve the problem. Another disadvantage is a high frequency of other side effects, including diarrhea and nausea, occurring in up to 74% of patients, with 59% of patients stopping the drug (Knapp et al., 1994; Maltby et al., 1994).

ANTIBIOTICS

Because of their risk of causing confusion, sedation, and lethargy, classes of antibiotics for which the dosage should be reduced in older adults consistent with creatinine clearance (as mentioned earlier) include the orally and parenterally administered penicillins and fluoroquinolones (Beck, 1991-1992; Calkins et al., 1992). Aminoglycosides, used in high doses, may cause hearing loss. In addition, appropriate use of antibiotics in older adults is important to prevent the development of resistant strains of bacteria, which appears to be an increasing and alarming concern among health care providers and public health officials. Appropriate general indications for the use of antibiotics include a productive-colored sputum, evidence of bacteria and leukocytes in the urine, evidence of cellulitis or sus-

pected osteomyelitis or bacterial meningitis, and abscess formation. The indiscriminate use of these agents can lead to diarrhea secondary to *clostridium difficile*, and related morbidity and death from pseudomembranous colitis, if not treated appropriately (Beck, 1991-1992). Mild cases should be treated with oral metronidazole (250 mg 3 times daily for 10 days), whereas moderate to severe cases with systemic symptoms of fever and leukocytosis should be treated with intravenous vancomycin (Beck, 1991-1992; *The Complete Drug Reference,* 1992). The fluoroquinolone group of antibiotics should be given 4 hours before or 2 hours after administration of antacids or sucralfate, because these agents may interfere with antacid's effectiveness (*The Complete Drug Reference,* 1992).

A frequent misperception among health care professionals is that the presence of bacteria or leukocytes in the urine of a patient with an indwelling urinary catheter or the presence of foul-smelling or pustular drainage from a pressure ulcer requires antibiotic administration. Patients with indwelling catheters and pressure ulcers will commonly develop colonization of the urinary tract or ulcer site, respectively. The use of oral antibiotics in such cases is not only ineffective, but will also promote resistance. Indications for the administration of parenteral antibiotics are the presence of fever greater than 102° as determined rectally, elevation of the serum leukocyte count above 15,000 with a shift to granulocytosis, and/or other signs of systemic sepsis including hypotension, change in mental status, central pallor, peripheral cyanosis, diaphoresis, and/or tachycardia (Beck, 1991-1992).

Acyclovir is an antiviral agent used for the treatment of herpes zoster (shingles). Initially approved for the treatment of herpes type II infections, this agent should be given for zoster at a much higher dose of 800 mg every 4 hours 5 times per day for 7 to 10 days. If given within 48 hours of infection, it has been shown to reduce the duration and severity of symptoms. The dosage and/or frequency of administration of the drug should be lowered in patients with creatinine clearance below 25 ml/min to prevent neurologic side effects from high doses, including confusion, dizziness, hallucinations, paresthesia, and lethargy (*Physicians Desk Reference,* 1995). Other side effects include skin rash, itching, myalgia, diarrhea, nausea, fever, headache, peripheral edema, lymphadenopathy, and leukopenia. When acyclovir is taken concomitantly with cobenemid, levels may become elevated. The drug can be administered intravenously in severe cases of infection associated with systemic involvement (ocular) or when infection is associated with immune deficiency states (*Physicians Desk Reference,* 1995). Famciclovir is a newer antiviral agent for acute zoster infection with the advantage of less frequent dosing (3 times per day) and a safer side effect profile. Dosage should be reduced for renal insufficiency (*Physicians Desk Reference,* 1995).

AGENTS FOR DIZZINESS

It is common practice among practitioners to prescribe meclizine for a patient who complains of dizziness, especially in a hurried office visit. Older patients with such a complaint may be exhibiting one or a combination of three different syndromes: "true" dizziness, presyncopal lightheadedness, or disequilibrium. True dizziness implies a vertical or horizontal spinning of the surroundings, which may or may not be associated with sensory or neurologic signs or symptoms. It can be secondary to a multitude of causes related to the inner ear or the central nervous system. Disequilibrium usually implies unsteadiness on the feet, usually on walking or turning. Disequilibrium may be secondary to a host of other disease processes as well. Presyncopal lightheadedness implies a "feeling of being faint," usually on standing or sitting from the supine position, and lasting 1 to 2 minutes in most cases. Various disease states and drugs previously mentioned in other sections may cause this syndrome. Appropriate evaluation of the type of dizziness, as well as the associated signs

and symptoms, time frame, and circumstance, is necessary before prescribing meclizine, because the treatments for these three syndromes are different. In addition, meclizine is an anticholinergic drug and should be used in as low a dose as possible, preferably 12.5 mg, to prevent side effects (Baloh, 1992).

CARDIAC DRUGS

There are only a few current indications for the use of digoxin—for systolic dysfunction of the myocardium and for the treatment of atrial arrhythmias. This drug should be avoided if possible in older adults because it is excreted 90% unchanged in the urine and is highly dependent on renal clearance, which in the absence of disease declines steadily with age. Inappropriately high doses of digoxin may cause confusion, agitation, anxiety, nausea, vomiting, heart block, arrhythmias, and the visual perception of yellow or green colors. An early sign of digitalis toxicity is usually anorexia. When used concomitantly with other cardiac drugs such as quinidine, verapamil, or amiodarone, the dosage of digoxin should be monitored closely and reduced accordingly because of the potentiating effects of these drugs. Digoxin is contraindicated in certain cardiac disease states such as incomplete heart block, pericarditis, aortic stenosis, and hypertrophic cardiomyopathy. The drug may also worsen myocardial ischemia with acute pulmonary edema (Luchi et al., 1991).

Quinidine is an old drug traditionally used to treat ventricular and atrial arrhythmias including atrial fibrillation. A recent meta-analysis of controlled trials using quinidine to control normal heart rhythm after conversion indicates that use increases mortality rate (Coplen et al., 1990). Common side effects of quinidine include ringing in the ears, diarrhea, flushing of the skin, bitter taste, nausea, stomach pain or cramping, headache, dizziness, lightheadedness, blurred vision, skin rash, and wheezing. Rare side effects include confusion, fatigue, increased bleeding, and hemolytic anemia (*The Complete Drug Reference,*

1992). Other more recent and more potent anti-arrhythmic agents such as flecainide and encainide have also been shown to increase mortality in patients with ventricular arrhythmias after acute myocardial infarction, with age being an independent risk factor (Akiyama et al., 1992). Amiodarone is an agent used for treatment and prophylaxis of frequently occurring (refractory) ventricular fibrillation and unstable ventricular tachycardia. Hypotension is a major side effect. Procainamide has been shown to decrease short-term survival after cardiac arrest and resuscitation outside the hospital (Hallstrom et al., 1991). Side effects include diarrhea and, less commonly, fever, chills, joint pains, skin rash, confusion, depression, dizziness, and lightheadedness (*The Complete Drug Reference*, 1992). Procainamide can also cause a lupus syndrome. Because of the limited benefit-to-risk ratio for these drugs, they should be prescribed only under the close supervision and monitoring of a cardiologist. Nitroglycerin preparations (nitrates), both administered orally and applied to the skin for treatment of ischemic heart disease and angina, may predispose the older patient to the development of lightheadedness, postural hypotension, syncope, and falls, especially when used in increasing doses. Other common side effects include headache, faint or rapid heartbeat, nausea, and vomiting. Rare side effects include blurred vision, dry mouth, skin rash occurring at the site of administration for topical preparations, and—with very high doses—seizures (*The Complete Drug Reference,* 1992). Patients using patch preparations should remove the patch for 4 to 6 hours per day to prevent the development of tolerance to the drug.

■ Hypolipidemic Agents

Hypocholesterolemic agents should be used with discretion in older adults because a recent meta-analysis of 35 randomized trials of cholesterol-lowering treatments questions the value of intensive treatment of hypercholesterolemia; this treatment is likely to benefit only people with significant risk factors for coronary heart disease, including the presence of smoking, hypertension, sedentary activity, previous stroke or myocardial infarction, and/or family history of risk factors (Smith et al., 1993). Two recent studies indicate that serum lipid levels (elevated levels of cholesterol and low levels of high-density lipoprotein [HDL] cholesterol) are poor predictors of coronary risk (for coronary heart disease mortality or hospitalization for myocardial infarction or unstable angina) and all cause death in *older adults* between the ages of 60 and 79 years and after age 70, respectively (Grover et al., 1994; Krumholz et al., 1994). A recent meta-analysis of clinical trials involving cholesterol reduction has also failed to show any correlation with stroke risk (Hebert et al., 1995). In fact, since serum cholesterol screening in healthy postmenopausal women has not been shown to change serum cholesterol levels significantly over the long term (7 to 10 years), a serum cholesterol performed every 5 to 10 years in older women without cardiovascular risk factors is sufficient (Hteland et al., 1992). Lastly, cholesterol-lowering agents used for patients with a total cholesterol level of over 309 mg/100 ml in the general population have not been shown to be cost-effective, costing $190,000 per extra year of life saved as opposed to population-based promotion of better eating habits at a cost of $20 per extra year of life saved (Kristiansen et al., 1991).

Normal aging is accompanied by dulling of taste and smell sensations (Beck, 1991-1992). Certain older patients are predisposed to the development of malnutritional states, including patients with anorexia secondary to dementia, depression, or malignancy; patients with visual or oral sensory deficits; and patients living alone, with low income and lack of transportation, or living in an institutional setting (Beck, 1991-1992). Inappropriate dietary cholesterol restriction in these patients is unnecessary because it may worsen the process, leading to further anorexia, weight loss, and death. Liberalization of salt, carbohydrate, protein, and cholesterol restrictions in these patients may be one of the few quality-of-life measures that may make life worth living. Hypocholesterolemia (4 mmol/L) has been linked to increased mortality in older adults, probably secondary to chronic inflammatory processes producing a catabolic state (Verdery & Goldberg, 1991). Restricted diets found in a majority of malnourished nursing home patients can contribute to the situation (Buckler, et al., 1994).

For those patients with cardiovascular risk factors and a higher-than-normal low-density lipoprotein (LDL) cholesterol level, the statin (HMG-CoA reductase inhibitor) drugs are very effective in lowering the LDL and total cholesterol, with the disadvantage of higher cost and need for regular monitoring of liver function tests because of the development of rare hepatitis (*The Complete Drug Reference,* 1992; Verdery & Goldberg, 1991). These agents should not be used in combination with cyclosporine, gemfibrozil, or niacin, because renal failure may result (*The Complete Drug Reference,* 1992). Nicotinic acid lowers total cholesterol to some extent but significantly elevates the HDL cholesterol (Vega & Grundy, 1994). Gemfibrozil reduces total cholesterol and elevates HDL cholesterol to a lesser extent than do nicotinic acid and the statin drugs (Vega & Grundy, 1994). Niacin and gemfibrozil also reduce serum triglyceride levels. When used to treat serum triglyceride levels, niacin and gemfibrozil should be used after an adequate trial of diet has failed, and for levels between 1000 and 2000 mg/100 ml, and for patients who have a history of pancreatitis or of recurrent abdominal pain resembling pancreatitis (*Physicians Desk Reference,* 1995). Frequent bothersome side effects of niacin include pruritus, flushing, tingling, headache, and diarrhea, especially when given in high doses of several grams per day (*The Complete Drug Reference,* 1992). Concomitant administration with aspirin can prevent cutaneous side effects (Whelan et al., 1992). Common side effects of gemfibrozil include stomach pain, gas, and heartburn. Less frequent side effects

include diarrhea, low back pain, cough, fever or chills, nausea or vomiting, and muscle pain. This agent should not be used concomitantly with anticoagulants because it may increase the risk of bleeding. Use of the drug may increase the severity of gallstones and, in the presence of liver disease, may increase levels of the drug, subsequently increasing chances of side effects (*The Complete Drug Reference,* 1992).

Probucol is a drug used to lower LDL cholesterol and, to a lesser extent, triglycerides. Probucol is not the preferred agent for use in older adults because, in addition to causing gastrointestinal side effects, it carries the risk of worsening cardiac conduction problems, as evidenced in many instances by prolongation of the QT interval on the electrocardiogram (*The Complete Drug Reference,* 1992; *Physicians Desk Reference,* 1995). Clofibrate is a drug that causes modest reduction in cholesterol with a somewhat greater reduction in triglyceride level. The use of this drug is associated with potentially bothersome gastrointestinal side effects including diarrhea and nausea. It is relatively weak as compared to other agents. It may potentiate the effect of anticoagulants when used concomitantly with them. It also has been shown to increase the incidence of cholelithiasis and subsequent morbidity and death from surgery (*Complete Drug Reference,* 1992; *Physicians Desk Reference,* 1995). Regular isotonic exercise (walking, running, swimming, bicycling) for 20 to 30 minutes 3 times per week is a very effective way of raising the high-density cholesterol and can be effective in causing slow, progressive weight loss (Schuler et al., 1992). Moderate alcohol intake (one or more drinks per day) has been shown to be effective in elevating HDL cholesterol, and in achieving a reduction in the subsequent risk of stroke, myocardial infarction, and total cardiovascular mortality (Scherr et al., 1992).

The most potent cholesterol-lowering agent is estrogen, which increases HDL, reduces LDL, and lowers total cholesterol (Scherr et al., 1992;

Stampfer et al., 1991). Recent studies indicate that it improves word recall, increases quality of life, retards osteoporosis, and reduces fracture risk at all bone sites (Daly et al., 1993; Fogelman, 1991; Robinson et al., 1994). Other positive effects of estrogen include reduced risk for myocardial infarction, less intimal thickening of the carotid arteries, and reduced stroke risk in postmenopausal women as seen in a follow-up of less than 2 years (Finucane et al., 1993; Manolio et al., 1993; Psaty et al., 1994). In the older woman who has had a hysterectomy, in the presence of cardiovascular risk factors and an elevated total cholesterol level, low HDL component, and high LDL component, estrogen may offer a substantial advantage over the conventional cholesterol-lowering agents. In the nonhysterectomized patient, estrogen should be used sequentially or in combination with progesterone to reduce the risk of endometrial cancer caused by taking unopposed estrogen (Voight et al., 1991). New formulations that combine estrogen and progesterone are currently under review by the Food and Drug Administration. Relative contraindications to the use of estrogen include fibrocystic disease and a history of migraine headaches. Absolute contraindications include a history or family history of breast cancer and previous pelvic cancer (Colditz et al., 1995; *Physicians Desk Reference,* 1995). There is also a slight risk of breast cancer with consecutive use of estrogen (Colditz et al., 1995). Progesterone has also recently been shown to reduce the risk of osteoporosis (Prince, 1991). The effect of estrogen in regard to osteoporosis can be enhanced by the concomitant use of calcium (in a dose of at least 1000 mg daily) and Vitamin D (400 IU) (Hazzard et al., 1994).

■ Drugs for the Prevention of Osteoporosis

The question of whether to use hormone replacement therapy (estrogen and progesterone) in a woman involves the presence or absence of four factors: older age, osteoporosis risk factors,

cardiovascular risk factors, and status of the uterus and ovaries. The effect of estrogen for the prevention of osteoporosis is thought to be dependent on a "window of opportunity" during which maximum effect can be achieved. The sooner hormone replacement therapy is started after surgical or natural menopause, the greater the effect, with maximum effect achieved from therapy initiated within 3 to 5 years afterward. The usefulness of hormone replacement therapy after age 62 solely for prevention of osteoporosis is thought to be minimal, though specifics are unknown and studies are ongoing (Hazzard et al., 1994). The presence of osteoporosis risk factors after menopause may strengthen the argument for use of hormone replacement therapy for osteoporosis, although this therapy by itself will have little impact for an older woman unless cardiovascular risk factors are present, because the benefit for the latter has been shown to be short-term. The use of hormone replacement therapy for prevention of cardiovascular risk is beneficial at any age. For the older woman with osteoporosis risk factors and no cardiovascular risk factors, modification of osteoporosis risk factors may be all that is necessary, including cessation of smoking and drinking, consumption of extra calcium and vitamin D, and regular exercise. The presence of a uterus when hormone replacement therapy is used necessitates an understanding of the risk of endometrial cancer; the need for follow-up if prolonged, unexpected, or heavier than usual bleeding occurs; and the fact that the patient may have a regular period.

Other drugs that may be beneficial in the treatment of osteoporosis for the patient who has relative or absolute contraindications to hormone replacement therapy include calcitonin, sodium fluoride, and biphosphonates (Beck, 1991-1992; Hazzard et al., 1994). Calcitonin has to be given parenterally (subcutaneously) 3 times per week, and has the added disadvantage of being expensive. Sodium fluoride, considered an experimental agent, has been shown to increase bone formation, but with increased risk of fracture because the bone that is formed is more brittle. Etidronate, a biphosphonate, has been shown to be effective for the prevention of recurrent vertebral compression fractures in older women with osteoporosis when used cyclically in combination with calcium (*The Complete Drug Reference,* 1992). Disadvantages include cost and side effects, including, most commonly, diarrhea and nausea (*The Complete Drug Reference,* 1992). Sodium alendronate has recently been approved for primary prevention of postmenopausal osteoporosis. It has been shown to significantly decrease the risk of vertebral and other fractures when used over a 3-year period. Common side effects include abdominal and musculoskeletal pain, acid reflux, dyspepsia, esophageal ulcer, vomiting, abdominal distention, and gastritis in 1% to 3% of patients.

■ Drugs That Cause Anorexia

In the evaluation of causes of anorexia in older adults, review of the patient's drug list with prompt removal of the suspected offending agent is a simple but expedient method of resolving the problem before instituting a potentially unnecessary extensive workup to rule out organic causes such as malignancy, dementia, and depression. Drugs known to cause anorexia include digoxin, procainamide, thyroxin, theophylline, nitrofurantoin, and the selective serotonin reuptake inhibitors (Thompson & Morris, 1991).

Inappropriately high doses of thyroxin may also cause agitation, insomnia, unexpected weight loss, tachycardia, arrhythmias, and premature osteoporosis (*The Complete Drug Reference,* 1992; *Physicians Desk Reference,* 1995). Theophylline may also precipitate anxiety, arrhythmias, postural hypotension, nausea, insomnia, and even seizures (*The Complete Drug Reference,* 1992; Hazzard et al., 1994). Because of these side effects, higher incidence of comorbid disease, and concomitant use of other drugs, theophylline is more difficult to use in older patients. The use of theophylline and fluoroqui-

nolones together can cause a severe adverse drug reaction that includes seizures, agitation, confusion, nausea, and vomiting, because of possible doubling of the theophylline concentration (Grasela & Dreis, 1992). For these reasons, if theophylline is to be used at all, a dose in the lower therapeutic range is appropriate (Hazzard et al., 1994). It is also prudent to use theophylline for selected instances of wheezing and for the treatment of asthma; the beta-agonist drugs, oral or inhaled, are the first line of treatment for chronic lung disease (Hazzard et al., 1994).

Drugs such as cotrimoxazole, tetracyclines, and nitrofurantoin should be avoided in the advanced elderly and in patients with renal dysfunction, and used with caution in older patients in general because of these drugs' dependence on renal excretion (Sanderson, 1990). Long-term administration of tetracyclines may cause staining of the teeth and skin, photosensitivity of the skin, diarrhea, or stomach cramping. Tetracyclines also will chelate with other drugs taken orally—including antacids, iron preparations, laxatives, and calcium supplements—preventing absorption (*The Complete Drug Reference,* 1992).

■ Drugs for Health Maintenance, Disease Prevention, and General Prophylaxis, Minerals, Vitamins, and Antioxidants

Because of the greater risk of malnutrition secondary to multiple diseases, limited income, social isolation, or dental problems, patients 62 years of age or older should be prescribed a general multiple vitamin. Recent advertisements on television, on the radio, and in newspapers and periodicals encourage megadoses of specific vitamins—A, C, and E—to prevent premature aging, especially with case control studies indicating that vitamins A and C may reduce the incidence of heart disease and stroke (Gale et al., 1995; Riemersma et al., 1991). A popular theory of aging involves the production of free ionizing and chemical radical formation, which causes damage to the DNA and RNA responsible for the production of proteins and enzymes and for cell function (Kristal & Yu, 1992). These vitamins may function as scavengers against free radicals, or antioxidants, preventing the aging process, and have been shown to increase cell-mediated immunity in older adults (Penn et al., 1991). Although popular among older adults, the use of specific vitamin and health food supplements should be discouraged until the results of clinical trials prove their effectiveness. Rather than a deficiency of vitamins, a more common problem among community-dwelling older adults is hypervitaminosis (Beck, 1991-1992). The fat-soluble vitamins, A, D, E, and K, accumulate in fat tissue with continued use, leading to vague and nonspecific but toxic symptoms that may be difficult to recognize. Specifically, megadoses of vitamin C can cause gastrointestinal irritability, a false negative result on fecal occult testing, renal stones, and rebound scurvy. Megadoses of vitamin A can cause malaise, liver dysfunction, headache, hypercalcemia, and leukopenia (Beck, 1991-1992). Specific indications include the following: vitamin B_{12} for dementia, pernicious anemia, or malabsorption syndromes; vitamin C for pressure ulcers and for skin healing from incisions; vitamin D and calcium for osteomalacia and osteoporosis; vitamin K for bleeding problems; thiamine for chronic alcohol abuse; and folic acid supplementation for patients on phenytoin (phenytoin inhibits the production of folic acid) (Hazzard et al., 1994; Yao et al., 1992).

The need for supplemental iron therapy in older patients for nonspecific chronic anemia should be thoroughly investigated before use. Older adults, in general, tend to have a greater frequency of normal or increased tissue iron stores because of the high frequency of chronic diseases that cause iron-deficient erythropoiesis (Beck, 1991-1992). Side effects of oral iron therapy include constipation, black stools, hemosiderosis, and browning of the skin and teeth (*The Complete Drug Reference*, 1992). The diagnosis of a microcytic hypochromic anemia re-

lated to iron deficiency in older adults should always be distinguished from the diagnosis of this anemia related to other common causes such as malignancies and acute or chronic inflammatory diseases, both of which also manifest themselves with a microcytic hypochromic anemia. Blood studies such as those measuring serum iron, ferritin level, transferrin level, and total iron binding capacity can easily distinguish between anemia secondary to iron deficiency and that secondary to other disease states (Damon, 1992).

Erythropoietin is one of the first of the new biotechnology drugs being used to treat anemias secondary to chronic disease. By stimulating the production of erythropoietin, the drug has been shown to increase mean hemoglobin levels and improve quality of life. It is indicated in patients with chronic renal failure and for rheumatoid arthritis; it also has been used to treat patients with chronic anemia secondary to human immunodeficiency virus (HIV) disease. It is a relatively safe drug, with little associated risk of anaphylactic reactions. There are no contraindications to its use in older adults. Because of its tendency to cause volume expansion, and to worsen blood control, it should be monitored in patients with high blood pressure or chronic renal insufficiency (Damon, 1992). When the drug is used, an adequate substrate of iron supplementation should be given for the production of red blood cells.

Aspirin in a dose of 75 mg has been shown to be effective in significantly reducing the incidence of cerebral infarction, fatal myocardial infarction, subsequent risk of stroke, subsequent transient ischemic attack, and death in older patients (average age 66) during a follow-up period of 32 months. These results occurred with an associated nonsignificant increase in hemorrhagic stroke in older patients with a history of transient ischemia attacks, as compared to those given a placebo (Swedish Aspirin Low-Dose Trial [SALT] Collaborative Group, 1991). Aspirin also has been shown to reduce signifi-

cantly the risk of severe angina, myocardial infarction, and death at 6 and 12 months in older
patients (younger than age 70) with non–Q-wave
myocardial infarction or unstable angina (Wallentin et al., 1991). Because of its relative safety, a
baby aspirin should be a part of every older
patient's medication regimen unless contraindicated by active gastrointestinal bleeding, a history of bleeding diathesis or other blood disorder, or a history of allergy to aspirin. Higher
doses of aspirin (325 mg) have been shown to be
as effective as warfarin in preventing stroke in
patients younger than 75 years of age with a
history of nonrheumatic atrial fibrillation, except
in patients with risk factors such as a history of
hypertension, thromboembolism, or heart failure
(Stroke Prevention in Atrial Fibrillation Investigators, 1994). Aspirin has also been shown in a case
control study to reduce the risk of colon cancer
(Thun et al., 1991).

Heparin, in a low dosage (5000 units twice
daily), may be more effective than aspirin in
preventing deep venous thrombosis and subsequent fetal or nonfetal pulmonary embolus and
death in older patients who are temporarily immobile for an acute illness, for a history of deep
venous thrombosis or pulmonary embolus, for
obesity, for a history of congestive heart failure,
or for chronic venous insufficiency (Beck, 1991-
1992). This regimen is also recommended for
general postoperative prophylaxis other than for
patients undergoing surgery for malignancies,
repair of femoral or hip fracture, or lower extremity joint replacement. In these instances, a
regimen of subcutaneous heparin 3 times daily
or, preferably, low-dose warfarin (coumadin)
starting on the day of surgery and continuing for
up to 10 weeks postoperatively is recommended,
because these patients are at greater risk for deep
venous thrombosis and embolization. However,
to prevent significant bleeding, the prothrombin
bleeding time (INR) should be adjusted to between 1.2 and 1.5. A newer regimen using enox-
aparin, a low–molecular weight heparin, twice

daily in a dose of 5000 units is equally effective
for the prevention of deep vein thrombosis after
hip replacement (*Physicians Desk Reference,*
1995).

Whether to use warfarin or aspirin in an
older patient is often a difficult question. Issues
that should be factored into decision making
include compliance, risk of falling, associated
medical conditions, economic issues, and cognitive dysfunction, weighing overall risk against
benefit to the individual patient. A patient with
significant cognitive dysfunction may not be an
ideal candidate for warfarin because the patient
may ultimately take too much in a single dose,
which might lead to either increased risk of
bleeding or insufficient amount in a subsequent
dose to achieve a desired effect. The availability
of a willing and able caregiver or interested party
to administer the medication on a regular basis
can resolve this issue. Pill administration vehicles
may also be of benefit. In addition, communication and understanding of the need for regular
monitoring of the bleeding time, physician and
laboratory costs involved, availability of transportation, and distance of the patient from the
medical facility are essential components in the
decision. The wrong value for any of these
factors will make the use of warfarin impractical.
Associated medical conditions such as liver disease, malabsorption syndrome, cognitive dysfunction, and malignancy may predispose the
patient to a greater risk of adverse drug (disease-
drug) reactions when using warfarin because of
its protein-binding properties. The presence of
other chronic medical conditions necessitating
the use of other medications may increase the
risk of drug-drug reactions. Finally, a patient at
increased risk for falls secondary to mobility
problems, arthritis, neurologic disease, or specific drug therapy may be a less than optimal
candidate for warfarin because of the increased
risk of bleeding secondary to trauma.

Ticlopidine is a platelet aggregation inhibitor.
It is indicated for the prevention of thrombotic

stroke in patients with a history of transient ischemic attack who have not responded to aspirin therapy or who are intolerant to aspirin (allergy or previous bleeding). In patients with reductions in creatinine clearance (50 to 80 ml/min), there has been no significant difference in clinical effects of the drug. The drug has the potential for causing neutropenia, which is usually reversible but can be life threatening in severe cases, in less than 2% of patients. Because of this, patients who are candidates for ticlopidine therapy should have a neutrophil count taken before starting treatment, and every 2 weeks for the first 3 months of therapy. Ticlopidine becomes 50% effective within 4 days of starting treatment and 60% to 70% effective in 10 to 11 days. It is contraindicated in patients who are hypersensitive to it, or in patients with a history of hematopoietic disorders, severe liver impairment, or active intracranial or peptic ulcer (*Physicians Desk Reference,* 1995).

Influenza vaccine should be given yearly, usually between October and December, to all older adults except for those with a history of egg allergy, because 90% of deaths caused by influenza epidemics occur in patients over the age of 64. If influenza develops in a long-term care institution, patients who have not been vaccinated or those allergic to the vaccine may be prophylactically treated with amantadine in a dose of 100 mg per day until the infection resolves. When the vaccine is given in high doses, common side effects include confusion, irritability, headache, rash, lethargy, nausea, and fluid retention; rare side effects include seizures (*The Complete Drug Reference,* 1992). The drug can shorten the duration and lessen the severity of influenza type A if started early in the course of the infection, but is not effective against influenza type B (Beck, 1991-1992). Pneumonia vaccine should be administered to all older patients at least once, and some geriatricians advocate a repeat vaccination after 6 years for those at high risk for pneumococcal pneumonia, such as asplenic patients (Beck, 1991-1992). Patients

who have received the older 18 polyvalent strain do not need a repeat injection. Even though older patients have the greatest need for these vaccinations, studies indicate that they often develop an inadequate antibody response to these agents because of their blunted immune responses. Diphtheria tetanus prophylaxis is often ignored in older adults, but recent studies indicate that only about 20% of older adults have adequate antibody levels. Patients especially at risk include diabetic patients with chronic foot ulcers and nursing home or homebound older adults with chronic pressure ulcers. Many older adults were not exposed to childhood tetanus vaccinations because this program had not yet been initiated in their youth. Any older patient who has not had a vaccination should receive three separate injections of diphtheria tetanus vaccination—initially, at 6 weeks, and then at 1 year from the time of the initial vaccine (Beck, 1991-1992; Gergen et al., 1995; Holt, 1992).

Older patients with a recent conversion to positive tuberculin skin testing should be treated with isoniazid—300 mg per day for 6 months—because studies of the drug indicate that it provides a high degree of protection (69%) against conversion from tuberculous infection to disease. Patients with a history of positive skin testing of unknown duration should not be treated with this drug because of the risk of morbidity and subsequent death in older patients who develop isoniazid-induced hepatitis. Patients taking the drug should have liver function tests performed monthly to monitor for the development of this adverse reaction (*Core Curriculum on Tuberculosis,* 1994). The drug should be administered with vitamin B_6 (pyridoxine), because the drug interferes with the metabolism of this vitamin.

STEROIDS

Oral corticosteroid use in the older patient population should be a last resort for specific indications and after conventional therapy has failed, because of the side effects that occur after prolonged use. These include dependence, weight gain, masking of infection, fluid retention, worsening or precipitation of hypertension, diabetes, cataracts, and osteoporosis. Steroids serve no purpose for the treatment of uncomplicated osteoarthritis and should be reserved for severe cases of rheumatoid arthritis. Steroids may be very beneficial for the treatment of asthma resistant to conventional therapy, and for initial treatment of certain dermatoses, polymyalgia rheumatica, and temporal arteritis (Beck, 1991-1992). Inhaled steroids are as effective as oral steroids for the treatment of chronic lung conditions without producing the systemic side effects seen with oral administration (Beck, 1991-1992).

LAXATIVES

The long-term use of stimulant laxatives (cascara, bisacodyl, senna) should be discouraged in older adults because of these drugs' tendency to produce a chemical deinnervation of the autonomic nerves as they detach from the mucosa of the large colon after many years of frequent use (Cefalu & Pike, 1981). This may subsequently lead to the development of a chronic, nondilating megacolon syndrome, resulting in worsening constipation and even fecal impaction when the patient becomes immobile. Non–systemically acting and bulk laxative agents (stool softener, psyllium) are the preferred agents for the treatment of constipation (*The Complete Drug Reference*, 1992). Prune juice serves an excellent purpose as a natural mild cathartic without long-term sequelae. Additional measures that should be used in conjunction with these agents include regular exercise, added fiber in the diet in the form of bran, fruits, and vegetables, and extra fluid intake (Beck, 1991-1992). An excellent laxative regimen for the patient with gastrointestinal symptoms of hyperacidity could include an inexpensive antacid containing liquid magnesium. Because these agents tend to cause diarrhea, patients should be advised that the frequency of bowel movements depends on a variety of factors, including associated medical conditions.

What may be "abnormal" for one patient may be "normal" for another. In addition to discouraging frequent laxative use, drugs known to cause constipation, including narcotics, anticholinergic agents, antispasmodics, antihistamines, and major tranquilizers, should be identified and discontinued if possible (Cefalu & Pike, 1981).

MISCELLANEOUS DRUGS

Certain groups of drugs deserve special mention as being inappropriate and in some instances having no specific indications. Dipyridamole is an old drug that has been popular for the treatment of vascular problems by decreasing platelet "stickiness" and preventing stroke or myocardial infarction. It has not been shown to be superior to aspirin alone for the treatment of cerebral or coronary artery disease, nor in maintaining the patency of autologous grafts. It is an inappropriate drug for use in older adults (Willcox et al., 1994).

Muscle relaxers can cause sedation, lethargy, confusion, and cognitive dysfunction and should be avoided in older adults if possible (Willcox et al., 1994). The need for a "short-acting" muscle relaxer can best be served by the use of a short-acting benzodiazepine such as lorazepam, administered in a dosage of 0.5 to 1 mg every 8 hours, and used in a time-limited fashion.

Chlorpropamide, a long-acting agent used for treatment of type II diabetes, is very potent and has been popular in the past. However, this agent has a half-life of 48 to 72 hours in some cases, and carries a high risk of causing prolonged hypoglycemia, especially in patients with reduced appetite or cognitive dysfunction. It is generally considered an inappropriate drug for use in older adults and should be reserved for cases of diabetes complicated with diabetes insipidus (Willcox et al., 1994).

Oxybutin, an older drug with smooth muscle and anticholinergic properties, has traditionally been used to treat detrusa hyperreflexia associated with temporary or chronic urge incontinence in older patients. A recent study, however, indicates that it is only effective in selected patients who have not responded to prompted voiding (Ouslander et al., 1995). Phenazopyridine is an old drug that may be useful for treating the uncomfortable symptoms of urinary tract infection initially (48 to 72 hours), until the antibiotic can become effective. It stains the urine a dark orange (*The Complete Drug Reference*, 1992).

Quinine is another old drug that has been used traditionally for the treatment of nonspecific, nocturnal leg cramps. A recent meta-analysis of five clinical trials using doses from 200 to 500 mg indicated that quinine reduces the frequency but not the severity or duration of leg cramps (Man-Sons-Hing & Wells, 1995).

Older patients may have intractable anorexia and weight loss, especially in association with a worsening dementia process or cancer. Cyproheptadine is a serotonin- and histamine-blocking agent that may be effective in these patients by stimulating central appetite centers (Beck, 1991-1992).

■ "Cold" and OTC Pain Medications

Older patients frequently seek advice about prescription and over-the-counter cold and cough medications. These agents will usually have an antihistamine and/or decongestant component. In general they should be avoided, especially in the presence of any medical illness that might contraindicate their use. Decongestants relieve nasal stuffiness, whereas antihistamines "dry up" bothersome watery secretions. Decongestants should be avoided for conditions such as anxiety and panic disorder, arrhythmias, and congestive heart failure. Recent studies indicate, however, that these agents do not interfere with blood pressure control in patients with hypertension (Coates et al., 1995). In addition, though studies in older patients are lacking, the use of OTC decongestant-antihistamine preparations has not been shown to improve symptoms in children (Hutton et al., 1991). Patients with chronic nasal or allergic rhinitis or stuffiness should be in-

structed to use simple, normal saline nasal spray 3 to 4 times daily to loosen secretions. If this remedy is insufficient, and if infection has been treated, topical steroid sprays combined with normal saltwater sprays are available by prescription to relieve symptoms, as a safer alternative to decongestants or antihistamines.

Many older patients take over-the-counter analgesics for pain relief. These drugs often contain caffeine, which may be responsible for chronic symptoms of insomnia, especially if the drug is taken before bedtime (Brown et al., 1995).

■ Chronic Pain Control

Chronic pain is often the rule rather than the exception in older patients burdened by multiple chronic diseases, especially secondary to arthritis and malignancy. For these patients, the intensity and chronicity of perceived pain may produce or aggravate depressive symptoms. The latter can be a common symptom complex in older patients because of the loss of independence that occurs secondary to mobility problems; multiple sensory deficits in hearing, vision, taste, and smell; social isolation; institutionalization; and other losses including family, friends, money, and personal possessions (Parmelee et al., 1991).

Relieving chronic pain for an older patient in a pharmacologically safe and effective manner requires that certain principles be followed. These include (1) avoiding high-risk drug administration that may increase the risk of adverse drug reactions and side effects; (2) avoiding use of "as needed" medications for pain relief; (3) using the oral route of administration and reserving parenteral treatment for patients with alimentary dysfunction; (4) remembering that dependence should not be a concern and tolerance is a minimal problem; (5) starting with the simplest and safest drug available and switching to other categories as necessary; (6) always providing support for the patient in the form of counseling, both informally from family, friends, and clergy, and formally from social workers and psychologists as necessary; (7) never abandoning the patient so that he or she feels alone or isolated; and (8) providing pharmacologic support for symptoms of depression (Patt, 1992; Rhymes, 1991).

Regarding specific drug therapy: Acetaminophen given around the clock starting in a dose of 5 to 10 grains every 4 to 6 hours is often effective initially in providing pain relief secondary to arthritis. Patients with chronic pain and associated depressive symptoms will often have associated insomnia and anorexia (Parmelee et al., 1991). In these cases, 25 to 50 mg of amitriptyline may be effective because of its sedating side effects and appetite stimulation properties. Trazodone, starting in a dose of 25 to 50 mg at bedtime, is an alternative antidepressant for the patient with Alzheimer's dementia that avoids the anticholinergic side effects of amitriptyline. If acetaminophen is not effective, propoxyphene and acetaminophen (*The Complete Drug Reference,* 1992), a narcotic antagonist, may be more effective without the side effect profile of nonsteroidal anti-inflammatory drugs or narcotics.

For patients with the chronic pain of bone metastasis from a terminal malignancy, nonsteroidal anti-inflammatory drugs are particularly useful, but increasing the dose creates a "ceiling effect" after which the patient gets no further relief from pain (Rhymes, 1991). Steroids may also be effective for the relief of this type of pain (Rhymes, 1991). The around-the-clock use of a narcotic such as codeine, with judicial use of laxatives, stool softeners, and phenothiazines to alleviate the side effects and potentiate the effect of the narcotic, including relief of nausea, is the next step in relieving this type of pain. If this regimen is not effective, fentanyl patches with half-lives of 72 hours or morphine infusion pumps delivering a constant infusion with steady serum levels provide better relief (Patt, 1992; Rhymes, 1991). Meperidine and meperidine-like preparations, given orally or parenterally, with their short half-lives, have the disadvantage of causing breakthrough pain and provide no added benefit over the use of morphine derivatives (*The*

Complete Drug Reference, 1992). If meperidine is used for acute pain, a dose of no more than 25 mg, used in combination with an equal dose of a phenothiazine antiemetic (promethazine), may be effective. Higher doses may induce anticholinergic delirium.

■ Drug Compliance

Compliance with drug regimens is a significant problem in older adults, more so than in other age groups, because of a host of factors including the following: (1) multiplicity of disease requiring multiple medications, often obtained through multiple pharmacies, all of which may cause confusion for the patient; (2) cognitive dysfunction with associated memory loss and subsequent failure to take medication appropriately, leading to exacerbation of disease (too low a dose) or to excessive medication in some instances (too high a dose), leading to toxicity; (3) restricted income and inability to pay for medication, leading to exacerbation of disease; (4) difficulty with complying with office or hospital visits or with obtaining medication from the pharmacist promptly—or at all, in some cases—because of mobility problems or transportation problems for the patient; (5) visual problems that may increase the frequency of inappropriate medication or dosing, leading to adverse drug reactions; and (6) medical diseases—such as stroke, Parkinson's disease, cervical stenosis, dementia, and arthritis—that may interfere with fine and gross coordination of the upper extremities necessary for medication administration.

For the older patient, the nurse can enhance drug compliance in the following general ways: (1) educating the patient and/or family about the purpose of the medication and potential side effects; (2) educating the patient and/or family about the disease process and signs or symptoms of worsening disease; (3) asking the patient and/or family to bring all prescription and over-the-counter medications for each clinic or hospital visit for reevaluation; (4) assigning key family members or friends to assist the patient in securing needed medication from the pharmacy and clinic in a timely fashion; (5) asking family or friends, when available, to assist in or monitor medication administration for the older patient with visual, coordination, or cognitive problems; (6) using pill administration boxes that can be refilled weekly by the patient, family, or friends; and (7) referring the patient and/or family to social service agencies, home health agencies, senior citizen centers, and volunteer agencies for securing financial and transportation assistance.

■ Conclusion

Appropriate drug prescribing in older adults requires an understanding of normal changes that occur during the aging process, including reduction of immune defenses, blunting and reduction of receptor sites, loss of physiologic reserve, and physiologic and structural changes in organ systems. These systems include the integumentary system, gastrointestinal system, liver, kidney, and central nervous system. Advancing age is associated with the development of chronic disease, in many cases in multiple fashion, with the need to take more over-the-counter and prescription medications. All of these factors increase the risk of adverse drug reactions. The high incidence of sensory deficits, cognitive dysfunction, mobility problems, transportation difficulty, socioeconomic concerns, and arthritis necessitates extreme caution, and attention to compliance issues as well. All of these points make the topic of drug therapy in older adults much different from that of drug therapy in the general adult population. Table 5-2 summarizes the effects of drug therapy on older adults.

TABLE 5-2 Appropriate and inappropriate drug therapy in older adults

Drug	Appropriate use	Inappropriate use	Special consideration
Antiarrhythmic agents (quinidine, procainamide, flecainide, encainide)	For treatment of complicated arrhythmias	For treatment of routine arrhythmias	Use recommended for complicated cases under cardiologist supervision only
Antibiotics	For systemic symptoms of infected pressure ulcer or indwelling urinary catheter; fever; leukocytosis; hypotension; cellulitis; osteomyelitis; colored sputum	For surface exudate of pressure ulcers; bacteruria and pyuria associated with indwelling urinary catheter; uncomplicated upper respiratory tract infection (viral)	May cause pseudomembranous colitis or promote resistance to antibiotics; adjust doses of penicillins, aminoglycosides, and fluoroquinolones to be consistent with creatinine clearance
Anticholinergic agents (antihistamines, tricyclic antidepressants, phenothiazine tranquilizers, narcotics)	—	—	Minimize or avoid use in patients with benign prostatic hyperplasia, glaucoma, chronic constipation, peripheral vascular disease, chronic bronchitis, or Alzheimer's dementia, or in advanced elderly
Antidizziness agents (meclizine)	For true dizziness	For disequilibrium or presyncopal lightheadedness	Use in low doses; anticholinergic effects may cause or worsen cognitive dysfunction
ANTIHYPERTENSIVE AGENTS			
Alpha-blocker drugs	For hypertension	High doses—may cause postural hypotension or syncope	Dual indication for hypertension and benign prostatic hyperplasia
Beta-blocker drugs	Shorter-acting selective agents—atenolol or metoprolol	Propranolol	For dual indications—angina and high blood pressure or atrial arrhythmias; after myocardial infarction or angina to reduce cardiovascular mortality

Continued

TABLE 5-2 Appropriate and inappropriate drug therapy in older adults—cont'd

Drug	Appropriate use	Inappropriate use	Special consideration
CENTRALLY ACTING DRUGS			
Cold and OTC analgesic agents	See Antihistamines and Decongestants	See Antihistamines and Decongestants	Antihistamine-decongestant combination agents not found to be clinically effective in children
Antihistamines	For drying of excessive secretions	For Alzheimer's patients	See Anticholinergic Agents
Decongestants	For relief of nasal stuffiness	For patients with congestive heart failure, arrhythmias, anxiety disorders	Not found to significantly affect mean blood pressure control in patients with hypertension
Analgesic agents	For pain relief	For patients with anxiety disorders or insomnia	Caffeine a frequent ingredient
DEMENTIA DRUGS			
Hydergine	—	—	Not significantly effective
Tacrine	For mild impairment (Alzheimer's type) for up to 30 weeks	For moderate to severe Alzheimer's disease	Monitor liver function tests monthly while patient is taking drug because of potential liver toxicity
Pentoxifylline	For multi-infarct dementia?	—	Slows cognitive deterioration but not memory loss
Vasodilators	—	Not effective	May cause postural hypotension
DIGOXIN	For congestive heart failure secondary to systolic dysfunction, atrial arrhythmias	Nonspecifically for other cardiac conditions	May cause anorexia, nausea, agitation, confusion; reduce dose according to creatinine clearance

130

TABLE 5-2 Appropriate and inappropriate drug therapy in older adults—cont'd

Drug	Appropriate use	Inappropriate use	Special consideration
DIURETICS			
Loop diuretics	For treatment of fluid retention secondary to congestive heart failure or renal insufficiency; refractory and severe leg edema secondary to venous stasis or chronic venous insufficiency	For routine treatment of dependent edema or venous stasis secondary to chronic venous insufficiency; for treatment of hypercalcemia; to be used with caution in advanced elderly or older patients with dementia or depression; for treatment of uncomplicated hypertension	May cause contraction alkalosis, postural hypotension, hypokalemia, arrhythmias, increased mortality; causes hypercalciuria
Thiazides	For treatment of mild hypertension alone or in combination with other agents	For routine treatment of dependent edema or venous stasis secondary to chronic venous insufficiency; to be used with caution in advanced elderly or older patients with dementia or depression; doses greater than 50 mg ineffective for hypertension	May cause contraction alkalosis, postural hypotension, hypokalemia, arrhythmias, increased mortality; prevents loss of calcium in urine; may have secondary benefit in retarding osteoporosis
GASTROINTESTINAL AGENTS			
H₂ blocker drugs	For treatment or prevention of peptic ulcer disease or gastroesophageal reflux	Prophylactically to prevent NSAID-induced gastric or duodenal bleeding; as prophylaxis to prevent bleeding secondary to stress-induced gastritis in intensive care unit patients	Increases risk of aspiration pneumonia in bed-bound patients with swallowing abnormalities; indicated for prophylaxis against stress-induced gastritis for intensive care unit patients with a history of respiratory failure or bleeding disorders
Proton pump inhibitors (omeprazole, lansoprazole)	For severe or intractable gastrointestinal reflux disease	For treatment of uncomplicated peptic ulcer disease	Expensive; approved for short-term (4- to 8-week) use only

Continued

TABLE 5-2 Appropriate and inappropriate drug therapy in older adults—cont'd

Drug	Appropriate use	Inappropriate use	Special consideration
Smooth muscle relaxers (metoclopramide, cisapride)	For gastrointestinal reflux disease—for diabetic gastroparesis, prevention of nausea and vomiting postoperatively or secondary to chemotherapy, and (metoclopramide only) implementation procedures	For gastric emptying for gastrostomy patients	Less central nervous system sedation with cisapride
Sucralfate	For treatment or prevention of peptic ulcer disease	Prophylactically to prevent NSAID-induced gastric or duodenal bleeding; as prophylaxis to prevent bleeding secondary to stress-induced gastritis in intensive care unit patients	Increases risk of aspiration pneumonia in bed-bound patients with swallowing abnormalities, indicated for prophylaxis against stress-induced gastritis for intensive care unit patients with a history of respiratory failure or bleeding disorders
HYPOLIPIDEMIC AGENTS			
Hypocholesterolemic drugs	For patients with significant history of heart disease or cardiovascular risk factors	For population-based treatment of hypercholesterolemia to prevent cardiovascular mortality	HMG-CoA reductase agents used with niacin, gemfibrozil, or cyclosporine may cause rhabdomyolysis and renal failure; need to monitor liver function tests when using HMG-CoA reductase (statin) agents; HMG-CoA agents more expensive; probucol can worsen cardiac conduction abnormalities; clofibrate may increase the incidence of cholelithiasis, subsequent morbidity, and death from surgery; gemfibrozil and clofibrate may increase risk of bleeding when used with anticoagulants

TABLE 5-2 Appropriate and inappropriate drug therapy in older adults—cont'd

Drug	Appropriate use	Inappropriate use	Special consideration
Hypotriglyceridemic drugs	For patients in whom diet has failed; triglyceride levels between 1000 and 2000 mg/100 ml; pancreatitis, recurrent abdominal pain resembling pancreatitis	—	See Hypocholesterolemic Drugs
MISCELLANEOUS DRUGS			
Chlorpropamide	—	Long-acting (half-life 48 to 72 hours), potent chlorpropamide	Use only in patients with diabetes mellitus and diabetes insipidus
Dipyridamole	—	—	Not shown to be superior to aspirin for vascular disease or for autologous grafts
Meperidine	For acute pain—in low doses (25 mg)	For chronic pain	Short half-life
Muscle relaxers	—	—	May cause sedation, lethargy, cognitive dysfunction, postural hypotension, falls
Oxybutin	—	—	Only effective in selected patients who have not responded to prompted voiding
Quinine	For leg cramps—meta-analysis indicates it reduces the frequency but not the duration or severity	—	—

Continued

TABLE 5-2 Appropriate and inappropriate drug therapy in older adults—cont'd

Drug	Appropriate use	Inappropriate use	Special consideration
Nonsteroidal anti-inflammatory drugs	As needed, in lowest possible dose, for acute "flare-ups of arthritis" for 5 to 7 days	Indomethacin; frequent use of NSAIDs; for active bleeding	May cause or worsen hypertension, congestive heart failure, renal insufficiency, hepatitis; high doses associated with acute confusion and cognitive dysfunction, especially indomethacin; monitor hemogram and renal function with frequent use; acetaminophen as effective for osteoarthritis
PSYCHOTROPIC DRUGS			
Antidepressants	For treatment of depressive symptoms	For nonspecific treatment of insomnia or agitation; amitriptyline, in most cases	SSRIs can worsen appetite, insomnia, anxiety, and weight loss in frail older patients or patients with dementia or depression; high doses of tricyclic agents can cause or worsen cognitive dysfunction, precipitate postural hypotension and falls; properly document need for drug; reduce dose of drug when possible
Hypnotics	Occasional use for sleep	Regular use for sleep	Can cause sedation, cognitive dysfunction, falls
Major (phenothiazine) tranquilizers	For psychotic behavior; hallucinations or delusions that are troublesome for patient; aggressive, hostile, combative behavior in dementia patients	For nonspecific diagnosis of dementia	May cause or worsen cognitive dysfunction, functional decline, postural hypotension, falls; parkinsonian side effects and risk of tardive dyskinesia; reduce dose and discontinue drug when possible; properly document need for drug

TABLE 5-2 Appropriate and inappropriate drug therapy in older adults—cont'd

Drug	Appropriate use	Inappropriate use	Special consideration
Minor (benzodiazepine) tranquilizers	For anxiety that is troublesome for patients	Nonspecific use for sleep	Reduce dose and discontinue when possible; avoid as-needed use; properly document need for drug
Barbiturates	For seizure disorder	For nonspecific treatment of insomnia or anxiety	Monitor drug levels; properly document need for drug; may cause or worsen cognitive dysfunction, postural hypotension, falls
Theophylline	For acute wheezing or a diagnosis of asthma	For routine treatment of chronic obstructive lung disease	Can cause postural hypotension, nausea, anorexia, weight loss, arrhythmias, anxiety, insomnia
VITAMINS AND PROPHYLACTIC AGENTS			
Aspirin (75 mg)	Daily for all patients older than 62 years	For active gastrointestinal bleeding or history of bleeding diathesis or other blood disorders, allergy to aspirin	—
Aspirin (325 mg)	For patients with a history of stroke	For active gastrointestinal bleeding or history of bleeding diathesis or other blood disorders, allergy to aspirin	—
Iron supplements	For proven iron deficiency	For nonspecific treatment of microcytic hypochromic anemia	—
Vitamins (antioxidant)	For deficiency states only	For prophylaxis against premature aging	—
Vitamins (multiple)	For all patients older than 62 years		—

REFERENCES

Akiyama, T., et al. (1992). Effects of advancing age on the efficacy and side-effects of antiarrhythmic drugs in post-myocardial infarction patients with ventricular arrhythmias. *Journal of the American Geriatrics Society, 40,* 666-672.

Baloh, R.W. (1992). Dizziness in older people. *Journal of the American Geriatrics Society, 40,* 713-721.

Beck, J.C. (1991-1992). *Geriatric review syllabus—A core curriculum in geriatric medicine.* New York: American Geriatrics Society.

Berggren, D., et al. (1987). Postoperative confusion after anesthesia in elderly patients with femoral neck fractures. *Anesthesia and Analgesia, 66,* 497.

Bixler, E.O., et al. (1991). Next-day memory impairment with triazolam use. *Lancet, 337,* 827-831.

Bjorck, S., et al. (1992). Renal protective effect of enalapril in diabetic nephropathy. *British Medical Journal, 304,* 339-343.

Black, R.S., et al. (1992). Pentoxifylline in cerebrovascular dementia. *Journal of the American Geriatrics Society, 40,* 237-244.

Bradley, J.D., et al. (1991). Comparison of an anti-inflammatory dose of ibuprofen, an analgesic dose of ibuprofen, and acetaminophen in the treatment of patients with osteoarthritis of the knee. *New England Journal of Medicine, 325,* 87-91.

Braunwald, E. (1991). Ace inhibitors—A cornerstone of the treatment of heart failure. *New England Journal of Medicine, 325,* 351-353.

Brown, et al. (1995). Occult caffeine as a source of sleep problems in an older population. *Journal of the American Geriatrics Society, 43,* 860-864.

Buckler, D.A., Kelber, S.T., & Goodwin, J.S. (1994). The use of dietary restrictions in malnourished nursing home patients. *Journal of the American Geriatrics Society, 42,* 1100-1102.

Buring, J.E., et al. (1995). Calcium channel blockers and myocardial infarction: A hypothesis formulated but not yet tested. *Journal of the American Medical Association, 274,* 654-655.

Cahill, L., et al. (1994). Beta-adrenergic activation and memory for emotional events. *Nature, 371,* 702-704.

Calkins, E., Ford, A.B., & Katz, P.R. (1992). *Practice of geriatrics* (2nd ed.). Philadelphia: W.B. Saunders.

Cefalu, C.A., & Pike, J. (1981, May). Fecal impaction—A practical approach to the problem. *Geriatrics,* 143-145.

Coates, M.L., et al. (1995). Does pseudoephedrine increase blood pressure in patients with controlled hypertension? *Journal of Family Practice, 40,* 22-26.

Cohn, J.N., et al. (1991). A comparison of enalapril with hydralazine-isosorbide dinitrate in the treatment of chronic congestive heart failure. *New England Journal of Medicine, 325,* 303-310.

Colditz, G.A., et al. (1995). The use of estrogens and progestins and the risk of breast cancer in postmenopausal women. *New England Journal of Medicine, 332,* 1589-1593.

Colenda, C.C. (1991). Drug treatment of behavior problems in elderly patients with dementia: Part I. *Drug Therapy,* 15-20.

The Complete Drug Reference, (1992). New York: United States Pharmacopeia.

Cook, D.J., et al. (1994). Risk factors for gastrointestinal bleeding in critically ill patients. *New England Journal of Medicine, 10*(330), 377-381.

Coplen, et al. (1990). Efficacy and safety of quinidine therapy for maintenance of sinus rhythm after cardioversion. *Circulation, 82,* 1106-1116.

Core curriculum on tuberculosis—What the clinician should know (3rd ed.). (1994). U.S. Department of Health and Human Services.

Culter, A.F., et al. (1995). Accuracy of invasive and non-invasive tests to diagnose helicobacter pylori infection. *Gastroenterology, 109,* 136-141.

Cummings, S.R., et al. (1995). Risk factors for hip fracture in white women. *New England Journal of Medicine, 23* (332), 767-773.

Daly, E., et al. (1993). Measuring the impact of menopausal symptoms on quality of life. *British Medical Journal, 307,* 836-840.

Damon, L.E. (1992). Anemias of chronic disease in the aged: Diagnosis and treatment. *Geriatrics, 47,* 47-57.

Finucane, F.F., et al. (1993). Decreased risk of stroke among postmenopausal hormone users: Results from a national cohort. *Archives of Internal Medicine, 153,* 73-79.

Fogelman, L. (1991). Viewpoint: Oestrogen, the prevention of bone loss and osteoporosis. *British Journal of Rheumatology, 30,* 276-281.

Furberg, C.D., et al. (1995). Nifedipine: Dose-related increase in mortality in patients with coronary heart disease. *Circulation, 92,* 1326-1331.

Gale, C.R., et al. (1995). Vitamin C and risk of death from stroke and coronary heart disease in cohort of elderly people. *British Medical Journal, 310,* 1563-1566.

Garcia Rodriquez, et al. (1992). The role of non-steroidal anti-inflammatory drugs in acute liver injury. *British Medical Journal, 305,* 865-868.

Gergen, P.J., et al. (1995). A population-based serologic survey of immunity to tetanus in the United States. *New England Journal of Medicine, 332,* 761-766.

Gottlief, S.S., et al. (1992). Renal response to indomethacin in congestive heart failure secondary to ischemic or idiopathic dilated cardiomyopathy. *American Journal of Cardiology, 70,* 890-893.

Graham, D.Y., et al. (1991). Epidemiology of helicobacter pylori in an asymptomatic population in the United States: Effects of age, race, and socio-economic status. *Gastroenterology, 100,* 1495-1501.

Graham, D.Y., et al. (1992). Effect of treatment of helicobacter pylori infection on the long-term recurrence rate of gastric or duodenal ulcer. *Annals of Internal Medicine, 116,* 705-708.

Grasela, T.H., & Dreis, M.W. (1992). An evaluation of the quinolone-theophylline interaction using the Food and Drug Administration spontaneous reporting system. *Archives of Internal Medicine, 152,* 617-621.

Greenblatt, D.J., et al. (1991). Sensitivity to triazolam in the elderly. *New England Journal of Medicine, 324,* 1691-1698.

Griffin, M.R., et al. (1991). Nonsteroidal anti-inflammatory drug use and the increased risk for peptic ulcer disease in elderly persons. *Annals of Internal Medicine, 114,* 257-262.

Grisso, J.A., et al. (1991). Risk factors for falls as a cause of hip fracture in women. *New England Journal of Medicine, 324,* 1326-1331.

Grover, S.A., et al. (1994). Serum lipid screening to identify high-risk individuals for coronary death. *Archives of Internal Medicine, 154,* 679-684.

Gurwitz, J.H., & Avorn, J. (1991, June). The ambiguous relation between aging and adverse reactions. *Annals of Internal Medicine, 114,* 956-966.

Gurwitz, J.H., et al. (1992). Reducing the use of H_2-receptor antagonists in the long-term-care setting. *Journal of the American Geriatrics Society, 40,* 359-364.

Gurwitz, J.H., et al. (1994). Initiation of antihypertensive treatment during non-steroidal anti-inflammatory drug therapy. *Journal of the American Medical Association, 272,* 781-786.

Guthrie, R. (1994). Terazosin in the treatment of hypertension and symptomatic benign prostatic hyperplasia: A primary care trial. *Journal of Family Practice, 39,* 129-133.

Hallstrom, A.P., et al. (1991). An antiarrhythmic drug experience in 941 patients resuscitated from an initial cardiac arrest between 1970 and 1985. *American Journal of Cardiology, 68,* 1025-1031.

Hannedouche, T., et al. (1994). Randomized controlled trial of enalapril and B blockers in non-diabetic chronic renal failure. *British Medical Journal, 309,* 833-837.

Hazzard, W.R., et al. (1994). *Principles of geriatric medicine and gerontology* (3rd ed.). New York: McGraw-Hill.

Hebert, P.R., et al. (1995). An overview of trials of cholesterol lowering and risk of stroke. *Archives of Internal Medicine, 155,* 50-55.

Heidrich, F.E., et al. (1991). Diuretic drug use and the risk for hip fracture. *Annals of Internal Medicine, 115,* 1-6.

Hentschel, E., et al. (1993). Effect of ranitidine and amoxicillin plus metronidazole on the eradication of helicobacter pylori and the recurrence of duodenal ulcer. *New England Journal of Medicine, 328,* 308-312.

Hollenberg, N.K., & Moore, T.J. (1994). Age and the renal blood supply: Renal vascular responses to angiotensin converting enzyme inhibition in healthy humans. *Journal of the American Geriatrics Society, 42,* 805-808.

Holt, D.M. (1992). Recommendations, usage and efficacy of immunizations for the elderly. *Nurse Practitioner, 17,* 51-59.

Hteland, M.L., et al. (1992). One measurement of serum total cholesterol is enough to predict future levels in healthy postmenopausal women. *American Journal of Medicine, 92,* 25-28.

Hutton, N., et al. (1991). Effectiveness of an antihistamine-decongestant combination for young children with the common cold: A randomized, controlled clinical trial. *Journal of Pediatrics, 118,* 125-130.

ISIS-4 Collaborative Group. (1995). ISIS-4: A randomized factorial trial assessing early oral captopril, oral mononitrate, and intravenous magnesium sulphate in 58, 050 patients with suspected acute myocardial infarction. *Lancet, 345,* 669-685.

Jick, S.S., et al. (1995). Antidepressants and suicide. *British Medical Journal, 310,* 215-218.

Jones, A.C., Berman, P., & Doherty, M. (1992). Nonsteroidal anti-inflammatory drug usage and requirement in elderly acute hospital admissions. *British Journal of Rheumatology, 31,* 45-48.

Kalish, S.C., et al. (1995). Antipsychotic prescribing patterns and the treatment of extrapyramidal symptoms in older people. *Journal of the American Geriatrics Society, 43,* 967-973.

Knapp, M.J., et al. (1994). A 30-week randomized controlled trial of high-dose tacrine in patients with Alzheimer's disease. *Journal of the American Medical Association, 271,* 992-998.

Kristal, B.S., & Yu, B.P. (1992). An emerging hypothesis: Synergistic induction of aging by free radical and maillard reactions. *Journal of Gerontology: Biological Science, 47,* B107-B114.

Kristiansen, I.S., et al. (1991). Cost-effectiveness of incremental programmes for lowering serum cholesterol concentration: Is individual intervention worth while? *British Medical Journal, 302,* 1119-1122.

Krumholz, H.M., et al. (1994). Lack of association between cholesterol and coronary heart disease mortality and morbidity and all-cause mortality in persons older than 70 years. *Journal of the American Medical Association, 272,* 1335-1340.

Langman, M.J.S., et al. (1994). Risks of bleeding peptic ulcer associated with individual non-steroidal anti-inflammatory drugs. *Lancet, 343,* 1075-1078.

Lesage, J. (1991, June). Polypharmacy in geriatric patients. *Nursing Clinics of North America, 26,* 273-289.

Lessem, J.N., & Weber, M.A. (1993). Antihypertensive treatment with a dual-acting beta-blocker in the elderly. *Journal of Hypertension, 11,* S29-S36.

Levine, J.S. (1995). Misoprostol and non-steroidal anti-inflammatory drugs: A tale of effects, outcomes, and costs. *Annals of Internal Medicine, 123,* 309-310.

Lewis, E.J., et al. (1993). The effect of angiotensin-converting-enzyme inhibition on diabetic nephropathy. *New England Journal of Medicine, 329,* 1456-1462.

Lichstein, E., et al. (1990). Relation between beta-adrenergic blocker use, various correlates of left ventricular function and the chance of developing congestive heart failure. *Journal of the American College of Cardiology, 16,* 1327-1332.

Lindley, C.M., et al. (1992, July). Inappropriate medication is a major cause of adverse drug reactions in elderly patients. *Age and Ageing, 21,* 294-300.

Luchi, R.J., Taffet, G.E., & Teasdale, T.A. (1991). Congestive heart failure in the elderly. *Journal of the American Geriatrics Society, 39,* 810-825.

Mach, J.R., et al. (1995). Serum anticholinergic activity in hospitalized older persons with delirium: A preliminary study. *Journal of the American Geriatrics Society, 43,* 491-495.

Maltby, N., et al. (1994). Efficacy of tacrine and lecithin in mild to moderate Alzheimer's disease: Double blind trial. *British Medical Journal, 308,* 879-883.

Manolio, T.A., et al. (1993). Associations of postmenopausal estrogen use with cardiovascular disease and stroke risk factors in older women. *Circulation, 88,* 2163, 2171.

Man-Sons-Hing, M., & Wells, G. (1995). Meta-analysis of efficacy of quinine for treatment of nocturnal leg cramps in elderly people. *British Medical Journal, 310,* 13-17.

Newbern, V.B. (1991). Cautionary tales on using beta blockers. *Geriatric Nursing,* 119-122.

Oldroyd, K.G., et al. (1991). Effects of early captopril administration on infarct expansion, left ventricular remodeling and exercise capacity after acute myocardial infarction. *American Journal of Cardiology, 68,* 713-718.

O'Riordan, T.G., Tobin, A., & O'Morain, C. (1991). Helicobacter pylori infection in elderly dyspeptic patients. *Age and Ageing, 20,* 189-192.

Ouslander, J.G., et al. (1995). Does oxybutynin add to the effectiveness of prompted voiding for urinary incontinence among nursing home residents? A placebo-controlled trial. *Journal of the American Geriatrics Society, 43,* 610-617.

Park, K.C., Forman, D.E., & Wei, J.Y. (1995). Utility of beta-blockade treatment for older postinfarction patients. *Journal of the American Geriatrics Society, 43,* 751-755.

Parmelee, P.A., Katz, I.R., & Lawton, M.P. (1991). The relation of pain to depression among institutionalized aged. *Journal of Gerontology: Psychological Sciences, 46,* P15-P21.

Patt, R.B. (1992). PCA: Prescribing analgesia for home management of severe pain. *Geriatrics, 47,* 69-84.

Penn, N.D., et al. (1991). The effects of dietary supplementation with vitamins A, C, and E on cell-mediated immune functions in elderly, long-stay patients. *Age and Ageing, 20,* 169-174.

Peura, D.A. (1995). Helicobacter pylori: A diagnostic dilemma and a dilemma of diagnosis. *Gastroenterology, 109,* 313-315.

Physicians Desk Reference. (1995). Montvale, NJ: Medical Economics Data Production.

Pinkowish, M.D. (1995, October). Practical briefings—Clinical news you can put into practice now. *Patient Care,* 16-21.

Prince, R.L. (1991). Prevention of post-menopausal osteoporosis—A comparative study of exercise, calcium supplementation, and hormone-replacement therapy. *New England Journal of Medicine, 325,* 1189-1195.

Psaty, B.M., et al. (1994). The risk of myocardial infarction associated with the combined use of estrogens and progestins in postmenopausal women. *Archives of Internal Medicine, 154,* 1333-1339.

Ray, W.A., et al. (1991). Cyclic antidepressants and the risk of hip fracture. *Archives of Internal Medicine, 151,* 754-756.

Rhymes, J.A. (1991). Clinical management of the terminally ill. *Geriatrics, 46,* 57-67.

Riemersma, R.A., et al. (1991). Risk of angina pectoris and plasma concentrations of vitamins A, C, and E and carotene. *Lancet, 337,* 1-5.

Robinson, D., et al. (1994). Estrogen replacement therapy and memory in older women. *Journal of the American Geriatrics Society, 42,* 919-922.

Rovner, B.W., et al. (1990). Research and reviews—The prevalence and management of dementia and other psychiatric disorders in nursing homes. *International Psychogeriatrics, 2*(13), 22.

Rummans, R.A., et al. (1993). Learning and memory impairment in older, detoxified, benzodiazepine-dependent patients. *Mayo Clinic Proceedings, 68,* 731-737.

Saltz, B.L. (1992). Tardive dyskinesia in the elderly patient. *Hospital Practice, 27,* 167-184.

Saltz, B.L., et al. (1991). Prospective study of tardive dyskinesia incidence in the elderly. *Journal of the American Medical Association, 266,* 2402-2406.

Sanderson, P. (1990). Antibiotics and the elderly. *Practitioner, 234,* 1064-1066.

Scherr, P.A., et al. (1992). Light to moderate alcohol consumption and mortality in the elderly. *Journal of the American Geriatrics Society, 40,* 651-657.

Schuler, G., et al. (1992). Regular physical exercise and low-fat diet: Effects on progression of coronary artery disease. *Circulation, 86,* 1-11.

Shankel, S.W., et al. (1992). Acute renal failure and glomerulopathy caused by non-steroidal anti-inflammatory drugs. *Archives of Internal Medicine, 152,* 986-990.

Sheikh, J. (1995, October). The pharmacological treatment of depression in older patients. *1995 Annual Meeting—Symposia Highlights—American Geriatrics Society, 6.*

Slataper, R., et al. (1993). Comparative effects of different antihypertensive treatments on progression of diabetic renal disease. *Archives of Internal Medicine, 153,* 973-980.

Smith, G.D., et al. (1993). Cholesterol lowering and mortality: The importance of considering initial level of risk. *British Medical Journal, 306,* 1367-1373.

Stampfer, M.J., et al. (1991). Postmenopausal estrogen therapy and cardiovascular disease: Ten year follow-up from the Nurse's Health Study. *New England Journal of Medicine, 325,* 756-762.

Stroke Prevention in Atrial Fibrillation Investigators. (1994). Warfarin versus aspirin for prevention of thromboembolism in atrial fibrillation: Stroke prevention in atrial fibrillation II study. *Lancet, 343,* 687-691.

Swedish Aspirin Low-Dose Trial Collaborative Group. (1991). Swedish aspirin low-dose trial (SALT) of 75 mg aspirin as secondary prophylaxis after cerebrovascular ischemic events. *Lancet, 338,* 1345-1349.

Systolic Hypertension in the Elderly Program Cooperative Research Group. (1991). Prevention of stroke by antihypertensive drug treatment in older persons with isolated systolic hypertension: Final results of the systolic hypertension in the elderly program (SHEP). *Journal of the American Medical Association, 265,* 3255-3264.

Tariot, P.N., et al. (1994). Carbamazepine treatment of agitation in nursing home patients with dementia: A preliminary study. *Journal of the American Geriatrics Society, 42,* 1160-1166.

Tariot, P.N., et al. (1995). Lack of carbamazepine toxicity in frail nursing home patients: A controlled study. *Journal of the American Geriatrics Society, 43,* 1026-1029.

Thiessen, B.Q., et al. (1990). Increased prescribing of antidepressants subsequent to beta-blocker therapy. *Archives of Internal Medicine, 150,* 2286-2290.

Thompson, M.P., & Morris, L.K. (1991). Unexplained weight loss in the ambulatory elderly. *Journal of the American Geriatrics Society, 39,* 497-500.

Thun, M.J., et al. (1991). Aspirin use and reduced risk of fatal colon cancer. *New England Journal of Medicine, 325,* 1593-1596.

Vega, G.L., & Grundy, S.M. (1994). Lipoprotein responses to treatment with lovastatin, gemfibrozil, and nicotinic acid in normolipidemic patients with hypoalphalipoproteinemia. *Archives of Internal Medicine, 154,* 73-82.

Verdery, R.B., & Goldberg, A.P. (1991). Hypocholesterolemia as a predictor of death: A prospective study of 224 nursing home residents. *Journal of Gerontology: Medical Sciences, 46,* M84-M90.

Voight, L.F., et al. (1991). Progesterone supplementation of exogenous estrogens and risk of endometrial cancer. *Lancet, 338,* 274-277.

Wallentin, L.C., et al. (1991). Aspirin (75 mg/day) after an episode of unstable coronary artery disease: Long-term effects on the risk for myocardial infarction, occurrence of severe angina and the need for revascularization. *Journal of the American College of Cardiology, 18,* 1587-1593.

Warram, J.H., et al. (1991). Excess mortality associated with diuretic therapy in diabetes mellitus. *Archives of Internal Medicine, 151,* 1350-1356.

Weinberger, M.H. (1992). Hypertension in the elderly. *Hospital Practice, 27,* 103-120.

Whelan, A.M., et al. (1992). The effect of aspirin on niacin-induced cutaneous reactions. *Journal of Family Practice, 34,* 165-168.

Willcox, S.M., et al. (1994). Inappropriate drug prescribing for the community-dwelling elderly. *Journal of the American Medical Association, 272*(4), 292-295.

Winter, M. (1988). *Basic clinical pharmaco-kinetics* (2nd ed., pp. 13-21). Vancouver, WA: Applied Therapeutics.

Yao, Y., et al. (1992). Prevalence of vitamin B_{12} deficiency among geriatric outpatients. *Journal of Family Practice, 35,* 524-528.

Yassa, R., & Nair, N.P. (1992). A 10 year follow-up study of tardive dyskinesia. *Acta Psychiatrica Scandinavica, 86,* 262-2.

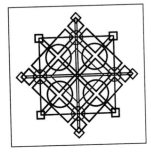

C H A P T E R 6

Age is opportunity no less
Than youth itself, though in another dress.
And as the evening twilight fades away
The sky is filled with stars, invisible by day.

HENRY WADSWORTH LONGFELLOW

Sexuality

■ Learning Objectives

On completion of this chapter, the reader will be able to do the following:

1. Describe sexuality as an integral component of the older adult's personality.
2. Identify age-related changes and health deviations that affect sexual function in older adults.
3. Describe demographic, physiologic, and social factors that affect the sexual function of older adults.
4. Discuss older adults' needs for closeness, touch, warmth, and sharing.
5. Conduct a sexual health assessment and formulate nursing diagnoses related to sexual function and sexual integrity of older adults.
6. Identify intervention strategies implemented by nurses to foster older patients' sexual function and sexual integrity.

Sexuality is a complex human characteristic that pervades the whole of an individual's life from birth to death. Every person has sexual feelings, attitudes, and beliefs; yet each person's experience of sexuality is unique because it is realized through a personal perspective.

■ Normal Function

Adult sexual feelings, behavior, and attitudes are influenced by learning and experiences of early childhood. What people learn about physical closeness and touching, and how they come to feel about themselves and others are major determinants of adult sexuality. Thus expression as a sexual being is manifested in many ways and is the result of ongoing life experiences. Although it is reasonable to expect considerable continuity over the adult life span in the expression of sexuality, new meanings may emerge as one's life situation changes.

Sexuality encompasses the biologic, psychologic, social, cultural, and spiritual aspects of sexual feelings and expression. It designates one's identity as a sexual being: the experience of maleness or femaleness; the way a person dresses, moves, speaks, and relates to others. It includes

10% of diabetic men, but the desire for sex is usually unaffected (Korenman, 1994). Diabetic women may experience orgasmic dysfunction and reduced sexual desire and/or decreased vaginal lubrication. Neuropathy is the primary cause of these changes in the sexual response. Unfortunately, the sexual problems tend to be permanent and untreatable. Some men do regain erectile ability; this is seemingly related to how well they accept their diagnosis and how they view the quality of their intimate relationship or relationships. Both men and women with good disease acceptance seem to be at lower risk for sexual dysfunction.

MALIGNANCIES

The diagnosis and treatment of cancer may have adverse effects on body image, sexual response, and sex roles. Alteration or removal of body parts, changes in their function, and psychologic responses to these changes such as anxiety, depression, or guilt may result in sexual dysfunction. Many sexual problems experienced after cancer treatment are temporary, but some are permanent. When cancer is far advanced, a person's needs for affection, sharing of feelings, and touch may be heightened.

PENILE IMPLANTS

When illness causes complete inability to have erections, sexual function can be partially restored by use of a mechanical device surgically implanted in the penis. These devices can provide erections that last long enough for intercourse to take place, but they cannot restore sensation to the penis or cause ejaculation (Masters et al., 1988). For some men, penile implants can restore a sense of masculinity and may provide some restoration of sexual function. Mechanical difficulties and infection are common problems occurring in 40% of patients who have penile implants. These problems require removal of the device or additional surgery to correct the problem (Masters et al., 1988).

■ Social Changes That Affect Sexual Function: Demographics and Gender

Demographics have a limiting impact on sexual fulfillment of older adults. It seems to be the biologic fate of many women to outlive men; consequently, older women outnumber older men. The ratio of women to men varies dramatically with age. In the under-20 age group, men outnumber women; at 30 to 34 years the age group is evenly balanced; for the 65 plus age group, women exceed men three to two. This disparity becomes more marked in the upper age ranges because women have a 7-year longer life expectancy than men (U.S. Department of Health and Human Services, 1993). There are 74 men between the ages of 70 and 74 for every 100 women, and among those 85 and over, there are only 40 men for every 100 women (Table 6-3).

The implications of these facts for older adults is that the surviving man has the opportunity to expand his sexual choices, whereas the older woman is restricted by the male-female imbalance.

Older adults' marital status and living arrangements vary tremendously by sex. Most men spend their older years married and in family settings, whereas most older women spend their later years as widows outside of family settings. Men who lose a spouse through divorce or death

TABLE 6-3 Number of men per 100 women by older age group: 1986

Age	Men per 100 women
65-69	83
70-74	74
75-79	64
80-84	53
85+	40

From U.S. Bureau of the Census. (1987). *Estimates of the population of the United States by age, sex, and race: 1980-1986* (Current Population Reports, Series P-25, No. 1000). Washington, DC: U.S. Government Printing Office.

are more likely to remarry than are women in the same situation. More often than not, older men marry or remarry women younger than themselves. Men remarry sooner (in about 3 years), whereas those widows who remarry do so in about 7 years (Corby & Solnick, 1980). Older widowed men have remarriage rates over 8 times higher than those of women (U.S. Bureau of the Census, 1987).

■ Sexual Function and Aging

Over the past 25 years the impact of aging on sexual response and function has received increased attention from investigators. Research has tended, though, to focus rather narrowly on the frequency of older adults' genital sexual activities and has underemphasized the relational and emotional content of sexuality.

Throughout adulthood women and men develop distinctively different sexual styles. Men are more sexually active than women throughout life, with the exception of the very old age groups (85 years and older), in which there is no difference. Women report lower orgasmic frequency than men throughout the life span. Although orgasmic frequency in women reaches a peak in middle age and remains constant into the 60s, it falls steadily among men in this age group. Women may be more likely than men to report increased sexual interest and activity with increasing age. In general, for both sexes, the greater the interest in sexual activity when young, the greater the interest and activity when old.

Society has differing views concerning appropriate sexual behavior for older men and women. The sexual activity of an older man is more likely to be sanctioned than that of an older woman. Older men continue to be perceived as sexually attractive, whereas older women are not. Older men usually marry younger women; society perceives this as acceptable. In contrast, sexual interest by an older woman in a younger man is less likely to be condoned. For older women, single, divorced, or widowed, the only socially sanctioned partner is an older man. Thus the population imbalance of the sexes and societal expectations combine to make the unavailability of a partner a significant factor in the sexual fulfillment of older women. For both women and men a marked change in sexual activity in old age is most frequently attributed to a new partner (an affair or remarriage) or the end of a sexual relationship through death or divorce (Turner & Adams, 1983).

Research refutes the pervasive cultural myth that the old are not interested in sex. According to Janus and Janus (1993), approximately 93% of older men and 50% of older women often or always have orgasms when they have sex. Fifty-three percent of older men and 41% of older women report sexual frequency of a few times a week (Janus & Janus, 1993).

The best predictor of sexual activity for men in old age is sexual activity and interest at a younger age, whereas for older women marital status is the best predictor. Unavailability of a partner is the primary reason in both sexes for discontinuation of sexual expression. Starr and Weiner (1981) studied 800 persons between 60 and 91 years of age and found that 36% said that sex was better for them at the time of the study than when they were younger. Of this group, about 80% were sexually active, and most had experienced an increase in spontaneity of sexual expression as they grew older. Being able to spend a long time in sexual encounters whenever they wanted was seen as a major advantage of age. Bretschneider and McCoy (1988) studied 202 healthy retirement home residents, age 80 to 102. Eighty-eight percent of the men and 72% of the women fantasized or daydreamed about being sexually intimate. The most frequently reported sexual activity was touching and caressing without intercourse. Sixty-two percent of the men and 38% of the women experienced intercourse; 72% of the men and 40% of the women experienced sexual pleasure through self-stimulation. Masturbation, or sexual self-stimulation, among older people has tended to be a highly personal topic and is surrounded by taboos. Recent research reports that only 23% of older men and 35% of older women *never* masturbate (Janus & Janus, 1993). Nurses need to accept the normalcy of this behavior in both sexes and assume the responsibility of educating other health care workers about privacy needs.

Some women who were thought to be single have in fact been in discreet lifelong relationships with other women that for reasons of public opinion had to be kept secret. Some women, after years as wives and mothers, turn to a lesbian relationship (Doress & Siegal, 1987). It is estimated that gays and lesbians make up about 10% of the U.S. population; approximately the same proportion of the older adult population can be assumed to be homosexual (Butler & Lewis, 1991). The increasing information available in recent years about sexuality and aging has served to dispel many of the myths about this stage of life. However, many people, young and old, including nurses, physicians, clergy, and family members, are astonished at the idea of people in their 70s, 80s, and 90s having sexual feelings, needs, and experiences with their own sex.

Although young and middle-aged adults have become more sexually permissive in regard to their own generations, they may have difficulty accepting an older person who has continuing sexual interest. This negative opinion may stem from a feeling that sex for most older people is unimportant, negative, distasteful, or taboo (Butler & Lewis, 1991). See Box 6-2 for myths regarding sexuality and aging.

NEED FOR TOUCH

People use their sense of touch to communicate with others. To say that one is touched by a warm thought or touched by a beautiful painting or the sound of a familiar melody is an example of the use of the word *touch* to connote positive emotions. How powerful then is the actual physical experience of touch, the act of reaching out to touch the body and spirit of another in the human expression of love and caring. Intimacy needs persist to the end of life no matter what a

> ### BOX 6-2 MYTHS OF AGING AND SEXUALITY
>
> 1. Intercourse is debilitating and will tend to hasten old age and death.
> 2. Masturbation by an older person is a sign of serious emotional disturbance.
> 3. Coital satisfaction decreases after menopause.
> 4. Older men lose their ability and desire to have sex.
> 5. Older women who still enjoy sex were probably nymphomaniacs when they were young.
> 6. Older men are subject to sexual deviations such as child molesting.
>
> Adapted from Gibson, H.B. (1992). *The emotional and sexual lives of older people: A manual for professionals.* London: Chapman and Hall.

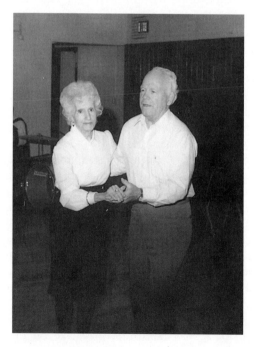

Older adults sharing a special togetherness. *Courtesy Loy Ledbetter, St. Louis.*

person's physical or cognitive abilities are. Especially important are the needs for closeness, touch, and being valued as a man or a woman. In old age, people begin to touch less and are touched less. Many older people who are frail may experience sensory deprivation because they are so seldom touched and have decreasing opportunities to touch. Touch has the potential to be a therapeutic tool to maintain contact and reduce anxiety for many older adults.

Expression of sexual feelings by older adults may add pleasure to their lives and provide relief from anxiety. Nurses have the opportunity to provide many older people with positive affirmation of their sense of self as a viable sexual person. A positive comment about a good-looking tie or a well-done hairstyle and the reaching out to touch a hand—these small acts may affirm an older man's or an older woman's sexuality.

INSTITUTIONALIZATION AND SEXUALITY

Sexuality is important to the lives of older adults who reside in institutions. Frail older adults in institutions such as hospitals or nursing homes have a capacity for sexual pleasure, which includes the need to touch and be touched and to feel warmth and caring. The gerontology literature supports the regrettable reality that nursing home staff pay little attention to the sexual needs of residents (McCartney et al., 1987). Yet certain sexual behaviors manifested by older patients in acute care units or in nursing home settings are considered by staff to be a disturbing management problem. This may be an indication of the taboo against sexual expression by older adults and a measure of staff members' lack of knowledge about sexuality. Sexual behaviors may be perceived by staff as harmful and disruptive when in fact the behavior is normal and harmless and is an expression of the older person's need for intimacy or closeness. In the absence of opportunity for direct sexual gratification, the need for sexual expression may take on many forms. Older adults may resort to clinging to possessions that can be handled or that evoke memories of lost contact with loved ones as spouse and

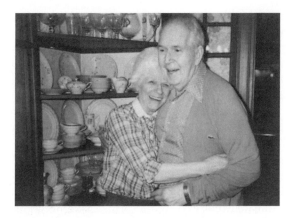

Touching or hugging has a therapeutic effect on both the young and the old alike.

friends die and children move away (Ebersole & Hess, 1994). Or they may use sexual jokes as a way of drawing attention to themselves as sexual beings. The sexual behaviors most frequently labeled as "problems" by staff are sexual talk—describing past or present sexual experiences; requesting staff to enter into some form of sexual activity; sexual acts—exposing genitalia, touching, or grabbing staff inappropriately; and implied sexual behavior—removing clothes, masturbating publicly, or making suggestive comments. Sexual behaviors that staff consider acceptable are limited physical contact between staff and residents such as hugging, hand holding, and kissing on the cheek or forehead, and perhaps masturbation in private.

Nursing home staff should have opportunities to participate in classes that discuss the sexual needs of older residents. It is helpful for staff to understand that sexual interest in old age is a reflection of prior levels of activity and interest. If this expression has been a significant method of coping in the past, it is likely to remain so.

■ Nursing Process

ASSESSMENT

Sexual function and integrity of older adults should be a concern for nurses and can be first approached by conducting a sexual assessment.

The purpose of an assessment is to determine the individual's degree of satisfaction or dissatisfaction in fulfilling sexual needs. Early discussion of patient concerns assures the patient that sexual health is an important and an acceptable topic to discuss. Some older people are willing to talk about sexuality with a nurse if the nurse projects ease and openness. Other patients will be reluctant to initiate discussion about a sexual concern with a nurse or any health professional. Instead, they may express generalized somatic complaints such as back pain, fatigue, headache, or pelvic and abdominal pain (Sheahan, 1989). When individuals feel ill or are in pain, they usually are not interested in discussing sexual matters. However, sexual difficulties can be concerns that lead to physical depletion and emotional pain. The professional nurse must be willing to become knowledgeable about and to take responsibility for dealing with the sexual aspects of the patient's illness experience. The nurse must be aware of the unique and specific sexual problems caused by various chronic illnesses.

The scope of sexual assessment will be dictated by the nurse's preparation and experience, as well as by the patient's health problems. Sexual health assessment requires special skill. Whether or not the initial assessment elicits sharing of sexual problems is not always an indicator of the true situation. Perhaps no sexual problem exists, or perhaps it will take time for the patient to develop sufficient comfort and trust to share a problem. The patient may confide in a nurse when a problem does arise. Assessment should include a description of the older person's past patterns of sexual expression, recent changes in the pattern of sexual activity, knowledge of age-related changes in sexual functions, knowledge of illness-related changes in sexual functions, and beliefs about sexual expression. An individual's concern about sexuality may or may not be associated with a change in sexual function. Guidelines that can be used to facilitate an assessment of sexual concerns include the following:

- Provide privacy while conducting the assessment; assure the patient of the assessment's confidentiality.
- Prepare the patient for the assessment with an introductory statement that briefly explains the purpose of the interview. For example: "To help plan care for your health needs, I am going to ask you for some information. You may find these questions personal, but these are issues about which older individuals often have concerns."
- Help patients identify clearly and specifically any sexual concern or concerns they are experiencing. Assessment can begin with the question "Has your illness caused a change in sexual functioning?" If the patient answers yes, the next question can be "Is that a concern for you?" Those who reply yes may be invited to describe the concern.
- Allow the patient to refuse to answer. You might say, "You seem reluctant about answering that question. Would you prefer I bring it up later?"

- Give the older person a chance to ask questions: "What questions about sexual health would you like answered?"

Some suggested questions are included in Box 6-3.

If sexual activity has not been a concern for the older adult in earlier life, and is not at present, the nurse should not impose problems or needs on the individual. As important as sexual fulfillment is for some people, it is not a major concern for all. The nurse should be alert for covert signs of unmet sexual needs such as repeated references to sex, repeated inappropriate attempts to touch staff members, or reports of sexually inappropriate behavior from friends or family members.

The single most important factor in helping people with sexual concerns and questions is the ease and comfort with which the clinician handles sensitive and value-laden sexual topics. To be effective, nurses must first achieve a healthy attitude toward their own sexuality. Sexuality is an area to which many people attach strong emotions, religious ideas, and rigid opinions. Sexual attitudes, values, and behaviors that are acceptable to one person may be uncomfortable for another. Nurses must be able to clarify and acknowledge their own feelings, attitudes, and opinions about sexual issues. This self-understanding helps nurses to develop an atmosphere of acceptance and respect for the sexual beliefs and practices of others.

NURSING DIAGNOSES

Once the data collection has been completed, an analysis of the data, problem identification, and formulation of nursing diagnoses can take place. Nursing diagnoses represent actual or potential areas of alterations in patterns of human functioning that nurses are licensed to treat.

The diagnoses of sexual dysfunction and *altered sexuality patterns* encompass all situations in which an individual expresses concern regarding sexuality because of actual or per-

ceived difficulties, limitations, or changes in sexual behavior (Korb & Kupperberg, 1993). These nursing diagnoses cover a wide range of defining characteristics and contributing risk factors. Defining characteristics are the cluster of subjective and objective signs that validate the presence of a diagnostic category. Contributing risk factors are those clinical and personal situations that can change or influence health status or problem development.

Defining characteristics are the patient's verbalization of sexual difficulties, limitations, or changes; impaired expression of one's sexuality; or expression of fear of potential limitations of sexual performance. The contributing risk factors can be grouped into two categories—those related to physical or medical conditions and those related to psychosocial factors. Any disease process or illness experience can cause or contribute to an altered sexuality pattern. Psychosocial factors include psychologic, interpersonal, environmental, situational, and cultural factors such as the following:

- Past experiences with sexuality (restrictive upbringing, traumatic sexual experiences)
- Death of or separation from partner or spouse
- Disability of patient or partner
- Poor communication with partner
- Lack of privacy
- Lack of opportunity for touching or being touched
- Stressors (financial worries, conflicting values)

Three frequent diagnoses that may coexist in older patients who are experiencing an alteration in sexuality pattern are the following:

Knowledge deficit
Self-esteem disturbance
Body image disturbance

It is highly unlikely that an older person would only have a diagnosis concerning sexual functioning; rather, multiple conditions and diagnoses are the norm. Because of this complexity many health professionals either ignore or overlook the

BOX 6-3 SUGGESTED QUESTIONS TO ASSESS SEXUAL CONCERNS

SEXUAL SATISFACTION

- Have you experienced any changes in your sexual relationships lately?
- To what do you attribute this change?
- What types of sexual activities have you usually enjoyed the most, including things such as hugging, kissing, sleeping together, intercourse, masturbation, and so on?
- Do you or your partner take any prescription medications? What are they? How often do you take them? Have you experienced any changes in your level of energy since you started them? What about overall feelings of well-being? Any changes in sexual desire or activity?

For men

- Have you noticed any changes in the intensity of your ejaculations, orgasms, or ability to attain or maintain an erection?
- Have you ever had orgasms without ejaculations?
- Has your level of enjoyment from sexual relations altered as a result of these changes?
- Have you had any problems with urethral discharge or urination?

For women

- Have you experienced any vaginal soreness or irritation after sexual intercourse? How long does it last? Any problems with urgency or with burning on urination after intercourse? Have you experienced abdominal contractions or back pain after intercourse?
- Have you had any problems with vaginal discharge or itching?
- Have any of these problems interfered with your sexual pleasure?
- Have you or your partner experienced any changes in your health status recently? How have these changes affected your sexual relationship?

ALTERATIONS IN SELF-PERCEPTION

- How has growing older changed your lifestyle or things you enjoy doing?
- How has the change in your health or your partner's health altered your lifestyle or your goals?
- How do you rate your general health?
- On a scale of 1 to 10, how would you describe your satisfaction with your life?
- On a scale of 1 to 10, how would you describe your satisfaction with your sexual relationships?

RELATIONSHIPS WITH OTHERS

- Have you ever discussed sexual topics with your spouse, friends, family, or health care professional?
- Whom do you talk to when you have problems of any kind or just want someone to talk to?

ENVIRONMENT

- With whom do you live?
- Do you have a chance for privacy? To be alone? To talk with others privately if you want to?

problems in sexuality that threaten the well-being of the older person. Many times the nurse who is knowledgeable and sensitive will be the first health professional to uncover older adults' concerns regarding their sexuality.

PLANNING AND GOAL IDENTIFICATION

The following are examples of diagnoses and goals that might be formulated for sexuality problems in older adults.

Alteration in sexual patterns related to loss of husband

A long-term goal would be expression of satisfaction in sexual fulfillment.

Short-term goals would be the following:

1. Verbalization of loss of sexual pleasure (feelings of warmth, love, and intimacy)
2. Resumption of social contacts with age peers
3. Involvement with adult children and grandchildren
4. Decision making regarding living arrangements

Knowledge deficit related to physical changes of the aging process or medical treatment

A long-term goal would be acceptance of age-related physical changes.

Short-term goals would be the following:

1. Understanding of impact of medications and surgical treatment on sexual functioning
2. Verbalization to health professionals of concerns with sexual functioning
3. Participation in decision making regarding sexual health

IMPLEMENTATION

One intervention model is the P-LI-SS-IT model developed by Annon (1976). The model includes four levels of intervention: P—permission giving; LI—limited information; SS—specific suggestions; and IT—intensive therapy. The nurse can use this approach for varying levels of patient need. The model assumes that many sexual problems can be managed by using educational methods that do not require intensive therapy. Comfort (1980) states that sexual counseling and therapy depend almost entirely on permission giving and correction of false attitudes toward sexuality and aging. Some patients may need information and permission to reverse sexual problems; others benefit from direct suggestions to alleviate problem areas; and others benefit from validation that their sexual behavior is normal. For some patients, more intensive therapy is necessary to resolve problems, and the nurse may act as a referral source for these patients. It is important for nurses to be cognizant of their own comfort and skill level in order to determine how to intervene and when to refer.

In the acute care setting

The myriad of acute and chronic illnesses that bring older people to hospitals often threaten sexual health. Both medical and surgical treatments for these illnesses can present hazards to sexual functioning. The patient and spouse need to have accurate information regarding the particular illness process, the treatment interventions, and the side effects of medications. The nurse educates the patient and spouse, corrects misconceptions about normal aspects of aging, and validates normalcy of sexual feelings and behavior.

Previously held attitudes, beliefs, and religious mores regarding sexual behavior need to be explored before specific suggestions regarding sexual activities can be addressed. Not all nurses are adequately prepared to intervene at this level, and referral may be the best course of action. Specific suggestions—if appropriate for the patient and within the nurse's knowledge base—can be offered, such as the following: gradually resuming sexual activities after illness; planning sexual activity to take advantage of drug effects; promoting relaxation and pain relief by taking a warm bath or shower before sexual activity; and considering options for sexual expression other than intercourse. The nurse should always be alert to factors that may jeopardize the sexual health of older hospitalized patients.

Specific intervention strategies include the following:

- Assess patient's level of knowledge and understanding regarding sexuality
- Include partner in discussions of sexual issues; facilitate communication between partner and patient
- Encourage discussion of factors that may interfere with partner relationship or expression of sexual feelings
- Act as referral source when necessary

In the nursing home

Respect for the dignity and sexual identity of nursing home residents is the primary task of the professional nurse who responds to the enormous need for high-level nursing care in our nation's nursing homes. It is crucial to the well-being of the nursing home resident that staff members realize that sexuality is a lifelong need and it does not cease to exist because a person becomes a resident of a nursing home. Most older people stop having sex for the same reasons they stop activities such as riding a bicycle: a decline in physical abilities, fear that people will think them foolish, and for most, the lack of a bicycle (Comfort & Dial, 1991).

The staff should be educated regarding behaviors that signal possible sexual frustration, including the following: undue need for touching; vague, generalized somatic complaints; inappropriate sexual demands; and sexual jokes. Staff need to articulate their concerns and feelings regarding certain nursing home residents' desire to masturbate both in public areas and within the private confines of the resident's room. Public masturbation creates a disturbance in nursing homes because most older residents and some staff members have been taught that masturbation is a vice, sinful, and physically harmful. Staff

BOX 6-4 MAINTAINING SEXUAL INTEGRITY IN NURSING HOME RESIDENTS

1. The need for intimacy and touching may be especially critical for nursing home residents who are experiencing diminished meaningful relationships.
2. Concern related to sexual difficulties can drain patients of energy that might be used for more constructive activities.
3. The nurse should assume that the nursing home resident has unmet sexual needs.
4. Integrated living units should be arranged so that an opportunity is provided for more normal relationships, thus encouraging socially acceptable communication, warmth, and touch.
5. Nursing home staff should have opportunities to participate in classes that discuss the sexual needs of older residents.

From Hillman, J. & Stricker, G. (1994). A linkage of knowledge and attitudes toward elderly sexuality: Not necessarily a uniform relationship. *Gerontologist, 34*(2), 256-260.

members may scold and demean a resident who engages in any form of masturbation. Nurses need to be sensitive to the complexity of this issue. There must be a regard for the older resident's sexual expression, but also respect for the other residents' values and the accepted social expression of sexuality. (See Box 6-4.)

No one should demean an older nursing home resident for any form of masturbation, but if public masturbation offends other residents, the staff can assist the resident to a private space, preferably the resident's room, where no one will pass judgment on the resident's sexual behavior. The older person may then choose to return to social activity after masturbatory activity ceases. The nurse thereby models both the acceptance of the sexual need of the individual resident and acceptance of the societal norm that calls for fulfilling the need for a private setting (Shippee-Rice, 1990).

In the private or family home

Medicare financing of home health care has increased yearly by an average of 23% from 1990 to 1993. Although projected growth is lower, the demand for home care demonstrates the high level of need for home health services (Burr & Waldo, 1995). Sexual problems will rarely be the primary reason for a home visit, but sexuality should always be part of a comprehensive assessment. A major issue to consider when assessing sexual health is the availability of privacy, as well as the availability of a partner (Mulligan & Modigh, 1991).

Many older adults reside independently in their own homes, although 13% of people over age 65 live in the homes of their children or other family members. Many people over 80 live alone, and many of these older people have an informal system of social support: family that visits on a regular basis, neighbors, community services such as Meals on Wheels, or paid helpers. The nurse should always assess the adequacy of the individualized system of care.

Older adults living with adult sons and daughters may have initiated the change in living arrangements, which may be temporary or permanent, for a myriad of reasons, such as physical changes that resulted in a permanent or temporary inability to take care of themselves. With the increasing numbers of shorter hospital stays, more and more older people will need temporary assistance to allow themselves sufficient time to return to their pre-illness level of function. Other reasons that older adults live with their adult children may include financial considerations, loss of a spouse, fear of living alone, loneliness, and loss of cognitive abilities necessary to maintain independent living. In these living arrangements, older people may experience an unanticipated loss of independence and privacy that threatens their sense of self as an adult and as a healthy, attractive, sexual person.

The nurse needs to use interpersonal skills to (1) show sensitivity to the older person's need for sexual expression, (2) find opportunities to affirm the older person's attractiveness, (3) encourage the person's expression of femininity or masculinity, and (4) promote social interactions with age peers.

A critical area for nursing intervention is within the family system that is providing care and sharing their home with the older parent. The adult child, although well meaning, may have difficulty in recognizing an older parent's sexual needs. The emphasis on normalcy of sexual health throughout the life span will assist most people in overcoming their initial reluctance to accept the legitimate sexual needs of their aging parent. The nurse is able to model behaviors that affirm the sexual health of the older person and encourage discussion of factors that may interfere with the expression of sexual feelings. Most importantly, the nurse should treat all sexual concerns of the older person with the utmost respect for the person's dignity.

EVALUATION

Evaluations of nursing interventions are related to criteria identified in the planning phase and articulated in the patient's short- and long-term goals. The nurse must continually evaluate the many relationships that are established with the patient and the patient's caregivers. These relationships are critical to the nurse's ability to be an effective clinician and to assist the older adult in enjoying sexual health.

Because there are sexually active people in every decade of life, including the eighth and ninth decades, nurses who work with older adults must assume active roles in promoting sexual integrity. Three areas of special importance are the education of patients, families, and staff regarding the impact of normal aging and chronic illness on sexual function; advocacy for sensitivity to older adults' needs for closeness, touch, warmth, and meaningful relationships; and competence and comfort in conducting a sexual health assessment. Nurses who assume active roles in this area will be rewarded with new understandings of behavior.

REFERENCES

American Psychiatric Association. (1994). *Diagnostic and statistical manual of mental disorders* (4th ed.). Washington, DC: Author.

Annon, J. (1976). The P-LI-SS-IT Model. *Journal of Sex Education and Therapy, 2,* 1-15.

Barry, M.J. (1989). Pre-operative guidance for men facing prostatectomy. *Medical Aspects of Human Sexuality, 23,* 25-30.

Bolt, J.W., Evans, C., & Marshall, V.R. (1987). Sexual dysfunction after prostatectomy. *British Journal of Urology, 59,* 319-322.

Bretschneider, J.G., & McCoy, N.L. (1988). Sexual interest and behavior in healthy 80-to-102 year olds. *Archives of Sexual Behavior, 17,* 109.

Burgener, S., & Logan, G. (1989). Sexuality concerns of the post-stroke patient. *Rehabilitation Nursing, 14,* 178-181, 195.

Burr, S., & Waldo, D. (1995). Data view: National health expenditure projections 1994-2005. *Health Care Financing Review, 16*(4), 221-242.

Butler, R.N., & Lewis, M.I. (1991). *Aging and mental health* (4th ed.). St. Louis: Mosby.

Butler, R.N., Lewis, M., Hoffman, & Whitehead. (1994). Love and sex after 60: How physical changes affect intimate expression. *Geriatrics, 49*(9), 20-27.

Comfort, A. (1980). Sexuality in later life. In J.E. Birren & R.B. Sloane (Eds.), *Handbook of mental health and aging* (pp. 885-892). Englewood Cliffs, NJ: Prentice Hall.

Comfort, A., & Dial, L. (1991). Sexuality and aging. *Clinics in Geriatric Medicine, 7*(1), 1-5.

Corby, N., & Solnick, R.L. (1980). Psychosocial and physiological influences on sexuality in older adults. In J.E. Birren & R.B. Sloane (Eds.), *Handbook of mental health and aging* (p. 893). Englewood Cliffs, NJ: Prentice Hall.

Doress, P.B., & Siegal, D.L. (1987). *Ourselves growing older: Women aging with knowledge and power.* New York: Simon and Schuster.

Ebersole, P., & Hess, P. (1994). *Toward healthy aging: Human needs and nursing response* (4th ed.). St. Louis: Mosby.

Geary, E., Dendinger, T., Freiha, F., & Stamey, T. (1995). Nerve sparing radical prostatectomy: A different view. *Journal of Urology, 154*(1), 145-149.

Gibson H.B. (1992). *The emotional and sexual lives of older people. A manual for professionals.* London: Chapman and Hall.

Hillman J. & Stricker G. (1994). A linkage of knowledge and attitudes toward elderly sexuality: Not necessarily a uniform relationship. *Gerontologist 34*(2), 256-260.

Hogan, R. (1980). *Human sexuality: A nursing perspective.* New York: Appleton-Century-Crofts.

Janus, S., & Janus, C. (1993). *The Janus report on sexual behavior.* New York: John Wiley and Sons.

Jensen, S.B. (1985). Sexual relationships in couples with a diabetic partner. *Journal of Sex and Marital Therapy, 11,* 259-270.

Kane, R.L., Ouslander, J.G., & Abrass, I.B. (1989). *Essentials of clinical geriatrics* (2nd ed.). New York: McGraw-Hill.

Katzin, L. (1990). Sexuality. *American Journal of Nursing, 90*(1), 55-59.

Korb, C., & Kupperberg, C. (1993). Sexual dysfunction: Altered sexuality patterns. In G. McFarland & E. McFarlane (Eds.), *Diagnosis and interventions: Planning for patient care* (2nd ed.). St. Louis: Mosby.

Korenman, S. (1994). Erectile dysfunction: Impotence. In W.M. Hazzard, E. Bierman, J. Blass, W. Ettinger, & J. Halter (Eds.), *Principles of geriatric medicine and gerontology.* New York: McGraw-Hill.

Leiblum, S., Bachman, G., Kemman, E., Colburn, D., & Swartzman, L. (1983). Vaginal atrophy in the postmenopausal woman: The importance of sexual activity and hormones. *Journal of the American Medical Association, 249,* 2195-2198.

Levy, J. (1994). Sexuality and aging. In W.M. Hazzard, E. Bierman, J. Blass, W. Ettinger, & J. Halter (Eds.), *Principles of geriatric medicine and gerontology.* New York: McGraw-Hill.

Masters, W.H., Johnson, V.E., & Kolodny, R.C. (1988). *Human sexuality* (3rd ed.). Glenview, IL: Scott, Foresman, and Company.

McCartney, J.R., Izeman, H., Rogers, D., & Cohen, N. (1987). Sexuality and the institutionalized elderly. *Journal of the American Geriatrics Society, 35,* 331-333.

McFarlane, E.A., & Rubenfeld, M.G. (1983). The need for sexual integrity. In H. Yura & M.B. Walsh (Eds.), *Human needs 3 and the nursing process* (pp. 185-233). Norwalk, CT: Appleton-Century-Crofts.

Melman, A., Kaplan, D., & Redfield, J. (1984). Evaluation of the first 70 patients in the Center for Male Dysfunction of Beth Israel Medical Center. *Journal of Urology, 131,* 53-55.

Moore, K., Folk-Lighty, M., & Nolen, M.J. (1984). Counseling the cardiac patient. *Nursing 84, 14,* 105.

Mulligan, T., & Modigh, A. (1991). Sexuality in dependent living situations. *Clinics in Geriatric Medicine, 7*(1), 153-160.

Odom, M.J., Carr, B.C., & MacDonald, P.C. (1990). The menopause and estrogen replacement therapy. In W. Hazzard, R. Andres, E. Bierman, & T. Blass (Eds.), *Principles of geriatric medicine and gerontology* (pp. 777-782). New York: McGraw-Hill.

Papadopoulos, C. (1987). Sexual problems of the CAD patient. *Medical Aspects of Human Sexuality, 21,* 53.

Rosal, M., Downing, J., Littman, A., & Ahern, D. (1994). Sexual functioning post-myocardial infarction: Effects of beta-blockers, psychological status and safety information. *Journal of Psychosomatic Research, 38*(7), 555-567.

Schover, L.R. (1988a). *Sexuality and cancer: For the man who has cancer and his partner.* New York: American Cancer Society.

Schover, L.R. (1988b). *Sexuality and cancer: For the woman who has cancer and her partner.* New York: American Cancer Society.

Schreiner-Engel, P., Schiavii, R.C., Vietorisz, D., & Smith, H. (1987). The differential impact of diabetes type on female sexuality. *Journal of Psychosomatic Research, 31,* 23-33.

Sheahan, S.L. (1989). Identifying female sexual dysfunctions. *Nurse Practitioner, 14,* 25-34.

Shippee-Rice, R. (1990). Sexuality and aging. In C. Fogel & D. Lauver (Eds.), *Sexual health promotion.* Philadelphia: W.B. Saunders.

Starr, B.D., & Weiner, M.B. (1981). *Sex and sexuality in the mature years.* New York: Stein and Day.

Thompson, J.M., McFarland, G.K., Hirsch, J.E., Tucker, S.M., & Bowers, A.C. (1989). *Mosby's manual of clinical nursing* (2nd ed.). St. Louis: Mosby.

Turner, B.F., & Adams, C. (1983). The sexuality of older women. In E.W. Markson (Ed.), *Older women: Issues and prospects* (pp. 55-72). Lexington, MA: Lexington Books.

U.S. Bureau of the Census. (1987). Estimates of the population of the United States by age, sex, and race: 1980-1986, *Current Population Reports* (Series P-25, No. 100). Washington DC: U.S. Government Printing Office.

U.S. Department of Health and Human Services. (1993). *Vital and health statistics* (Series 3, No. 27).

BIBLIOGRAPHY

Bishop, G. (1989). Sex and UTI in older women. *Medical Aspects of Human Sexuality, 23,* 65-69.

Catalona, W.J., & Bigg, S.W. (1990). Nerve-sparing radical prostatectomy. *Journal of Urology, 143*(3), 538-543.

Frank, D., et al. (1978). Mastectomy and sexual behavior: A pilot study. *Sexuality and Disability, 1,* 16-26.

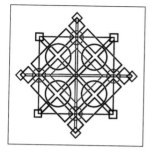

C H A P T E R 7

In fact, there's nothing that keeps its youth,
So far as I know, but a tree and truth.
There are traces of age in the one-hoss shay,
A general flavor of mild decay . . .

OLIVER WENDELL HOLMES, JR.

Sensation

■ Learning Objectives

On completion of this chapter, the reader will be able to do the following:

1. Identify age-related changes in vision, hearing, smell, and taste.
2. Assess the senses of sight, hearing, smell, taste, and touch of the older adult.
3. Recognize psychologic and sociocultural factors that interact with sensory functioning.
4. Understand the causes of sensory impairment in older people.
5. Develop a plan of nursing care for an older person with sensory impairment.
6. Provide appropriate nursing interventions for older adults with sensory impairment.

The richness of the human experience is perceived through the senses, especially through vision and hearing. Often, as people age, their ability to perceive the information received from their senses is impaired or distorted. Aging dulls the senses, and older adults must find ways to compensate for that change. A decline in sensory functioning is a silent, unnoticed process, which may occur undetected by both older adults and their families. This chapter encourages the reader to be aware of the physical, psychologic, and sociocultural indicators of sensory impairment. The senses discussed herein are sight, hearing, smell, taste, and touch.

■ Sight: Vision

Normal aging brings changes to the eye and to the sense of sight (Box 7-1). These changes affect the functional level of sight referred to as "vision." Aging brings an increase in the susceptibility to pathologic conditions that affect vision. It has been estimated that 1.3 million older adults have some loss of vision. A National Health Interview Survey of older people reported that close to 95% wore glasses, and for those over 85 years of age, only 45% reported that glasses corrected all of their vision problems (National Center for Health Statistics, 1986). For those over 85 years of age who report vision problems, 12% are legally blind.

BOX 7-1 AGE-RELATED CHANGES IN THE EYE AND IN VISION

- Cornea flattens
- Sclera becomes yellow and less elastic
- Intraocular pressure increases
- Accommodation of lens decreases
- Retina receives less light
- Capability for tearing diminishes
- Ability to gaze upward decreases
- Ability to maintain convergence diminishes
- Vitreous floaters may appear
- Arcus senilis may appear
- Visual acuity decreases
- Night vision decreases

Older adults report greater dissatisfaction with their level of visual function than do members of other age groups. The visual complaints reported by older adults are problems with seeing under low lights, difficulty processing rapidly changing displays, difficulty focusing on near-vision tasks, difficulty searching in the environment, and problems with glare and decreased night vision (Schleber, 1992).

There is a need for early intervention and rehabilitation, because many of the visually impaired older adults have conditions that are amenable to treatment. The role of the nurse is in prevention of treatable vision loss through education and screening, and rehabilitation of older adults who are subject to visual impairment.

NORMAL STRUCTURE AND FUNCTION

Vision is the result of the sense of sight being stimulated by patterns of light that are external to the person. Human sight is limited by a field of vision that excludes approximately 40% of the surrounding environment: people cannot see what is behind them at the same time that they can see what is in front of them. Light enters the eye and travels first through the cornea, the major refractive surface of the eye responsible

for most of the focusing power. The light then travels through the anterior chamber, to the pupil. The pupil regulates the amount of light entering the eye through the process of constriction and dilatation. The light rays from the visual stimulus next encounter the crystalline lens. Through the process of accommodation, the lens is able to change its shape and thereby alters its focusing power and increases the imaging power of the eye, thereby enabling individuals to view near objects. Light next passes and is imaged on the retina, where the cones and rods transduce light energy into nervous system activity (Schleber, 1992). The optic nerve then transmits impulses from the retina through the visual pathway to the occipital cortex. There, in the higher centers of the brain, the impulses from the external light rays are transformed into data that can be processed and recognized as the unique human sensation of vision for a particular moment in time and space (Figure 7-1). Vision is an amazing process that happens so quickly and so easily that it is taken for granted until it is threatened by the slow but predictable process of aging.

AGE-RELATED CHANGES

The normal eye undergoes significant age-related changes (see Box 7-1). The eye's external changes give evidence of advancing age. These changes result from multiple normal changes, such as loss of orbital fat, loss of elastic tissue, and decreases in muscle tone. The skin around the eye darkens, and wrinkles referred to as "crow's feet" appear. Some older adults lose the lateral aspect of their eyebrows; this is not a classic sign of disease, as it would be in younger adults (hypothyroidism), but rather a normal occurrence of aging. Xanthomas, cutaneous deposits of lipid material, are sometimes found at the inner portion of the lid; these may indicate elevated bloodlipid levels.

These age-related changes may give rise to two conditions: senile entropion (a condition in which the lid margin turns inward) and senile ectropion (a condition in which the eyelid mar-

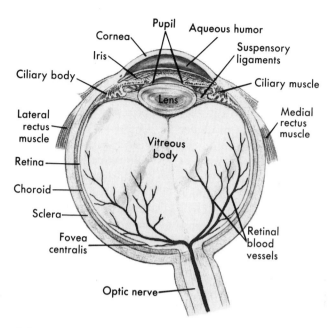

FIGURE 7-1 Cross-section of the eye. (From Thompson, J.M., et al. [1993]. *Mosby's manual of clinical nursing* [3rd ed.]. St. Louis: Mosby.)

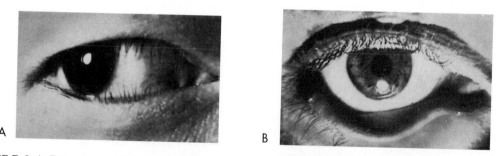

FIGURE 7-2 A, Entropion, with lashes invading the cornea; B, ectropion, in which the lower lid falls away from the globe so that the punctum can no longer function as the exit portal for tears. (From Stein, H.A., Slatt, B.J., & Stein, R.M. [1994]. *The ophthalmic assistant: Fundamentals and clinical practice* [6th ed.]. St. Louis: Mosby.)

gin turns outward) (Figure 7-2). Although not threatening to vision, these conditions may cause the older person discomfort and may become severe enough to cause psychosocial problems because of cosmetic effects. In senile entropion the turning inward of the eyelid may cause the lashes to rest against the conjunctiva, often resulting in ocular irritation. This can be corrected by a surgical procedure if the severity warrants. In contrast, senile ectropion exposes the conjunctiva and may lead to inflammation of the affected eye.

The eye itself undergoes major changes because of the aging process. The cornea, as a result of the aging process, tends to flatten, which reduces its refractory power. Also, the sensitivity of the cornea decreases, limiting its protective function. The sclera, although it remains white throughout the life span, becomes more transparent and may take on a yellow coloration because of dehydration (Michaels, 1994). The anterior chamber becomes progressively shallower. The pupil becomes smaller, and the response to different levels of illumination is lessened because of the loss of range of pupil dilation and constriction. The retina of an older individual becomes thinner because of fewer neural cells and receives only one third the amount of light that the retina of a younger person receives. This age-related change necessitates a higher level of illumination for reading. Adaptation to dark occurs more slowly and to a lesser total extent. Older people also have difficulty with color perception, especially the blue-green distinctions.

The lens of the aging eye loses its elasticity and increases in density. Surprisingly, both eyes change at the same time and the same variance (Michaels, 1994). The ability of the lens to accommodate leads to a decrease in the ability to focus near objects. By the time they are in their fifth decade, most people require glasses to be able to read fine print. This frequent condition,

resulting from the age-related changes in the human eye, is called *presbyopia.* Corrective lenses are extremely helpful in assisting the older person in maintaining visual function. Because of the change in the lens, glare becomes a more severe adaptive problem for older adults, which increases their need for sunglasses. Depth perception is also affected by the increased susceptibility to glare and the decreased contrast sensitivity (Heath, 1993). *Floaters,* opacities occurring in the vitreous humor, may appear in the older person's field of vision and may be a cause of alarm. Although floaters can be considered a normal process of the aging eye, in some instances they may be a harbinger of a serious problem, such as retinal detachment. Therefore if floaters are observed, the patient should see an ophthalmologist.

The most common, although not universal, clinical change in the cornea is *arcus senilis,* in which a grayish-yellow ring forms around the iris (Figure 7-3). This usually begins on the upper portion of the eye. It then continues to develop until the entire iris is encircled. It is caused by a

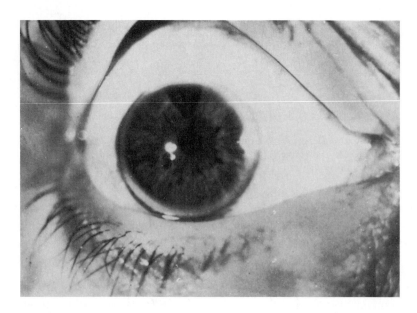

FIGURE 7-3 Arcus senilis in a patient with a peripheral iridectomy. (From Stein, H.S., Slatt, B.J., & Stein, R.M. [1994]. *The ophthalmic assistant: Fundamentals and clinical practice* [6th ed.]. St. Louis: Mosby.)

fatty invasion of the corneal margin, which blurs demarcation between the cornea and the sclera (Kasper, 1989). Arcus senilis is common in people over age 65, has no pathologic implications, does not cause any visual problems, and is not a cosmetic problem.

An accompanying age-related change that affects many minor eye problems is diminished tear secretion. Tearing, a natural protective device of the human body, slows in its ability to defend the eye against the pollution of the environment. This predisposes the eye to more infections of the conjunctiva. Many older adults use over-the-counter preparations of hydroxyethyl cellulose in solution (brand names include Hypotears, Tears Natural, and Artificial Tears) to assist in replacement of naturally occurring tears. These solutions should be used only for mild, self-limiting conditions (e.g., dry eyes) and never for infections or inflammations.

As people grow older, normal age-related changes in vision necessitate changes in behavior. These changes are minor, and most people readily adapt by taking the measures listed in Box 7-2.

COMMON HEALTH DEVIATIONS

The major pathologic causes of visual impairment in older adults are (1) cataracts, (2) glaucoma, (3) senile macular degeneration, (4) diabetic retinopathy, and (5) temporal arteritis.

Cataracts

Cataracts are the most frequent ocular disease to occur with aging, with about 50% of adults over the age of 40 years showing some signs of clouding of the lens (Heath, 1993). Any opacification of the lens is considered to be a cataract and may be the result of multiple causes (i.e., congenital, toxic, metabolic, traumatic, or senescent). This condition is a common complication of aging; although it is bilateral in nature, one eye may be involved months before the other (Michaels, 1994).

Although 95% of those over 65 years of age have some degree of cataract formation, in very

BOX 7-2 MEANS OF ADAPTING TO NORMAL AGE-RELATED VISUAL CHANGES

1. Wear eyeglasses
2. Increase the amount of light when reading
3. Allow extra time for eyes to accommodate to darkness
4. Avoid nighttime driving of vehicles
5. Wear dark glasses to reduce the impact of the sun's glare

few of that large number is the process advanced enough to cause visual disability. The process of lens opacification develops over time, with the beginning of cataract formation occurring at the periphery of the eye. This beginning phase of cataract formation usually has no significant impact on vision. However, the mature cataract is widespread, involves the pupillary area, and leads to a slow decrease in vision. The entire lens may become opaque.

The functional implications of cataracts are twofold: (1) The ability to see detail is diminished, because of the reduction in the amount of light available to the retina; this depends on the severity of the cataract. (2) The difficulty in adjusting to glare increases, so the older person with cataracts will experience significant problems with adjusting between light and dark environments. This can create major safety problems in poorly lighted environments. Interestingly, the initial development of a cataract may cause an improvement in near vision for some older adults, but this also fades as the cataract becomes more clouded (Heath, 1993).

When cataracts interfere significantly with vision, thereby diminishing the quality of life for the individual, surgery may be appropriate. Many aspects need to be considered before surgery is performed: the degree of correctable visual acuity in each eye, the physical and psychologic ability of the patient to withstand the stress of the surgery, the type of work or leisure activities in which the patient is involved, and whether the patient has a social support system available to provide immediate monitoring and care, if necessary.

After cataract removal, there are three methods of restoring vision: eyeglasses, contact lens, and intraocular implant. Special eyeglasses, rarely used after surgery, are thick and heavy, and although they allow excellent central vision, they increase object size by about 25% and seriously impair peripheral vision. Individuals must learn to turn their heads to accommodate for peripheral vision loss, and most people have difficulty adjusting to the 25% increase in image size. In fact, if one eye is normal, eyeglasses cannot be used to restore vision lost from the afflicted eye because of the resulting disparity in image size.

The second of the three methods for post-surgical restoration of vision is the use of a contact lens. The contact lens corrects the focus of the eye, permits both central and peripheral vision, and only increases object image size by 6%, which is usually a more manageable difference. Although vision is restored, the older person must be able to add the new task of handling and caring for contact lenses to the presurgical activities of daily living. Not every older person is able or willing to insert contact lenses, and only 50% to 60% of older adults are said to be capable of wearing contact lenses (Kasper, 1989).

The most frequent cataract surgery is intraocular implantation of an artificial lens. The benefits in terms of vision restoration far outweigh the minimal risk associated with having a foreign body in the eye. Careful attention to intraocular pressure and repair of adhesions with laser procedures have resulted in dramatic improvements in vision (Heath, 1993). Most of the surgeries are done in outpatient surgical units using local anesthesia, with the older patient returning home the same day. The postoperative care usually entails periodic use of eyedrops, some restrictions in activities (such as bending and lifting), and return visits to the surgeon. Most older people need another person to assist them with their postoperative care, and many may not have a readily available family member or friendly neighbor. Therefore they may not seek or may defer treatment because they lack this important human support system.

Glaucoma

Glaucoma, the leading cause of blindness throughout the world, is an eye disorder that is characterized by a significant increase in intraocular pressure, damage to the optic nerve, and a loss in the visual field. There are two major types of glaucoma: primary open-angle glaucoma and primary closed-angle glaucoma. Primary open-angle glaucoma occurs more frequently in the older population than does primary closed-angle glaucoma. Older adults with primary open-angle glaucoma may have no symptoms, and the condition is usually discovered in a routine examination checking intraocular pressures (Michaels, 1994).

Primary open-angle glaucoma develops slowly over time, so subtly that the patient is not aware of any changes. Signs and symptoms that indicate glaucoma are an increase in intraocular pressure, family history of glaucoma, blurred vision not corrected with lenses, and a halo effect around lights. The functional impairment in vision caused by glaucoma is a loss of peripheral vision. This can cause problems for the affected person, especially in driving a car.

Medical treatment consists of eyedrops that decrease the intraocular pressure or drugs such as acetazolamide (Diamox) that decrease aqueous formation. Surgical treatment is usually reserved for difficult-to-control situations.

Primary closed-angle glaucoma is characterized by an acute, rapid-onset, painful attack of increased intraocular pressure, with a marked decrease in vision. Affected patients should be referred immediately to an ophthalmologist. Medical treatment consists of first normalizing intraocular pressure by the application of eyedrops. After

BOX 7-3 STEPS FOR SELF-ADMINISTRATION OF EYEDROPS

1. Wash your hands.
2. Use adequate light.
3. Sit, stand, or lie down in front of a mirror.
4. Tilt your head back.
5. Extend your lower lid outward to make a "pocket" into which the drops can fall, and look up.
6. Insert the drops into the pocket.
7. Release your eyelid, and close your eye.

pressure is normalized, surgical treatment is required. A peripheral iridectomy is performed on the affected eye to ensure free flow of aqueous humor.

Eyedrops as a medical treatment create problems for older adults living at home, especially those who live alone. The ability to instill drops into one's own eye calls for a high level of fine-motor skill and hand-to-eye coordination, which, because of other conditions (such as arthritis or parkinsonism), may be beyond the capacity of some older adults. Nurses must skillfully assist older adults in practicing application of the drugs so as to ensure safe and appropriate care (Feinburg, 1988) (Box 7-3).

Although drugs instilled in the eye are applied topically as eyedrops, they still may be systemically absorbed and may cause side effects. It is easy to forget that these topical drugs are absorbed into the system, so the nurse must take care to note that eyedrops can be a source of adverse side effects. Table 7-1 lists major drugs used in eyedrops and their potential side effects.

Macular degeneration

Macular degeneration, an age-related disease, involves the loss of central vision and occurs over time. There is a prevalence rate of 30% in those over 75 years of age, but with only 10% experiencing any vision loss. Onset is usually earlier, at about 65 years, with the initial involvement of only one eye; within a 4-year period the second eye is involved (Heath, 1993; Michaels, 1994). The pathogenesis is little understood, and at present there is little hope for a definitive cure. However, a theory of leakage of retinal membranes has given rise to the use of laser photocoagulation with mixed results (Michaels, 1994).

The affected older adult usually will report a loss of visual acuity or distorted vision. Distortion and subsequent loss of the center of the visual field is the usual severe symptom. The patient should be referred immediately for medical care. Peripheral vision remains intact, so the patient does not lose total vision. Vision rehabilitation consists of attempts to magnify the central vision defect area. The larger the field, the less information is lost to the individual. This can be accomplished through inexpensive ocular lenses or with video enlargement (Wasson et al., 1990). It is important to refer older adults with macular degeneration to formal vision rehabilitation services (Heath, 1993).

Diabetic retinopathy

As people with diabetes mellitus live longer, the incidence of diabetic retinopathy rises, causing a significant increase in the number of people with this form of visual loss. It occurs at a rate of 7% in people who have had diabetes for less than 10 years, 26% in those who have had diabetes for 10 to 14 years, and 63% in those who have had diabetes for more than 15 years (Stefansson, 1990). Currently, in the United States, diabetic eye changes are the leading cause of blindness in the adult population (Heath, 1993). The patient with diabetic retinopathy may experience transient blurring, loss of central vision, and significant shifts in vision. On funduscopic examination, the retina of an individual with diabetic retinopathy will exhibit irregular small hemorrhages and yellow-white exudates.

At present, bilateral involvement generally occurs 10 to 15 years after the onset of diabetes.

TABLE 7-1 Ophthalmic drugs and possible side effects

Drug	Class	Side effect
Pilocarpine	Cholinergic	Bronchospasm
Timolol	Beta-blocker	Bradycardia, hypotension, confusion
Epinephrine and phenylephrine	Adrenergic	Palpitation, hypertension

Adapted from Kane, Ouslander, & Abrass. (1988). *Essentials of clinical geriatrics* (2nd ed.). New York: McGraw-Hill.

The control of the individual's diabetes does not preclude the development of diabetic retinopathy. Laser photocoagulation as a treatment has helped to alleviate some aspects of diabetic retinopathy, but definitive treatment has not yet been devised.

Temporal arteritis

Temporal arteritis, a vascular disease of older age, is an inflammatory disease of the temporal arteries and is characterized by headache, preauricular tenderness, an enlarged temporal artery, and a complaint of general malaise. The symptoms of temporal arteritis may be overlooked by the patient and family members, who may think that the symptoms are characteristics of aging rather than of disease. One half of older patients with this disease will suffer visual loss that could have been prevented. This condition is treated via steroids.

The nurse's role in the detection of temporal arteritis is to follow up on the patient's complaints, to do an accurate assessment, and to collaborate with the physician to ensure proper medical and nursing care.

■ Nursing Process

Integration of the scientific knowledge concerning age-related changes and pathologic conditions that affect the aging eye enables the nurse to use this knowledge to provide wholistic nursing care to older adults.

ASSESSMENT

Nursing assessment of vision requires an accurate history, a functional assessment of visual acuity, and a physical examination of the eye and sur-

rounding tissue. Psychosocial and environmental assessments are critical components of a wholistic approach to the nursing care of an older adult patient with a visual impairment.

History

Impairment of vision is usually a slow, insidious process that may go unnoticed by the older patient. The nurse must also consider that the older patient may think that nothing can be done to improve vision or that it is best not to complain about what the patient considers his or her minor problem. Taking an accurate history requires both interpersonal skill and scientific knowledge about normal aging and about particular conditions that affect vision.

Some older patients are excellent historians, but others require more time and more direct questioning to elicit needed information. Suggested questions include two types: open ended and direct. An open-ended question may have any number of correct answers and is open to the interpretation and concerns of the patient. An example of an open-ended approach is "Tell me what is different now about your vision." This is an appropriate way to begin the history taking. When completing the vision history, it is wise to conclude with an open-ended question such as "Is there anything else you can tell me about your vision?" If the patient is residing in the community, it is important to ascertain whether other health providers have been consulted and, if so, the approximate dates of the patient's most recent visits.

Direct questions, on the other hand, ask the patient to provide specific answers. Examples of

health care record, an in-depth nursing assessment, and conferences with family members and other health care providers. A nursing diagnosis is always made by the clustering of data that define and support the diagnosis.

Nursing diagnoses to be considered when caring for a patient with a visual impairment include the following North American Nursing Diagnosis Association (NANDA) diagnoses:

1. Alteration in sensory/visual perception
2. Impaired social interaction and/or social isolation
3. Risk for injury

The diagnosis of alteration in visual perception may be related to pathologic or other conditions, as evidenced by the following:

1. Low scores on visual screening test
2. Self-reports of limited vision
3. Inability to see near or far objects
4. Inability to recognize familiar people at a distance
5. Loss of a particular part of the visual field
6. Medical diagnosis

The diagnosis of impaired social interaction and/or social isolation may be related to visual impairment, as evidenced by the following:

1. Failure to attend usual social meetings, such as meetings of Gray Panthers, church groups, and bridge clubs
2. Failure to attend usual forms of entertainment, such as movies or concerts
3. Failure to attend usual family gatherings, such as grandchildren's birthday parties
4. Failure to visit friends

The diagnosis of risk for injury may be related to impaired vision, as evidenced by the following:

1. Hazardous living arrangement
2. Lack of cautious behavior
3. Denial of visual loss
4. Refusal to adhere to medical regimen
5. Lack of use of aids for limited vision
6. Additional functional deficits, such as limited mobility

PLANNING AND GOAL IDENTIFICATION

The planning phase of the nursing process consists of establishing realistic short- and long-term goals, based on data obtained in the assessment phase. Whenever possible, goals should be developed with the patient included as an equal member of the health care team.

Alteration in visual perception

A long-term goal is that the patient will adapt to visual loss. Short-term goals include the following:

1. Patient will be able to compensate for loss of peripheral vision by recognizing appropriate times to turn head to increase range of visual field.
2. Patient or caregiver will demonstrate ability to insert eyedrops.
3. Patient will wear clean and properly placed eyeglasses during periods of ambulation.

Impaired social interaction due to visual impairment

A long-term goal is that the patient will resume a normal range of activities. Short-term goals include the following:

1. Patient will attend Gray Panther meeting, being driven to meeting by Mr. Jones, a friend.
2. Patient will attend church services with daughter.
3. Patient will attend bridge social on Thursday evening.

These two examples illustrate the planning associated with specific diagnoses, to facilitate the reader's understanding of the specific and individualized patient-centered nature of planning.

IMPLEMENTATION

Nursing interventions that assist the older patient with visual impairment need to be specific to the defined goals, etiologies, and the defining characteristics that have been identified in the assessment phase. They also address the defining characteristics and causes that are amenable to change through interventions.

Three settings are considered to be the typical environments in which older adults receive nursing care. Two settings are institutions: (1) an acute care setting, usually a large teaching hospital or a community hospital, and (2) a nursing home. The third setting and the least restricted environment is the older person's private home. Most older people experience nursing care in at least two of these settings, and some of those who experience nursing care over a long period do so in all three settings.

In the acute care setting

Nursing care of the older adult patient with visual impairment is guided first by the condition of the patient and then by the setting in which the care is given. If the nursing care is rendered in an acute care setting, such as a hospital, the patient is probably in the setting primarily for surgical treatment, such as cataract surgery. Because most cataract surgery is performed on an outpatient basis, the nurse's role in the preoperative care and the postoperative care and teaching is important to the well-being of the patient. Both the patient and the caregiver need instruction. A caregiver will usually accompany the older patient to the surgical center and will be available after the surgery for the first 24 hours of home care. The postoperative care usually entails periodic application of eyedrops and some minor limitations on the patient's activity. The nurse needs to allow sufficient time for teaching and for answering any questions of the caregiver, who may also be an older adult.

Often when an older patient is admitted for an emergency situation that is unrelated to vision, the patient's visual deficit will go unnoticed. Glasses may have been left at home or by the bedside in the nursing home. Nurses in the hospital should be alert when they see an older patient without glasses because of the high incidence of visual impairment in the older population. The loss of corrected vision may add to the stress of a hospital stay and may deprive the older hospitalized person of the ability to see

clearly and to make sense of a strange and somewhat hostile environment.

The nurse is familiar with the sights in the hospital—the food on the dinner tray, the screen on the monitor, the person delivering pills or fixing an intravenous (IV) bag that hangs near the bed, and the faces and white coats of the medical team making rounds. For the older visually impaired patient, each new person who comes into the hospital room may pose a threat. The alert nurse can make a significant difference in the older patient's ability to maintain a sense of control and a sense of reality by making sure that eyeglasses are readily available, clean, and used by the patient.

In the nursing home

In the nursing home the nurse must be vigilant to changes that occur in the older resident's vision, must be aware of the resident's need for annual visits to an ophthalmologist, and must have an understanding of the significance of medications and their potential side effects. The care of the resident's eyeglasses should be supervised by the nurse, to ensure that they are cleaned and properly worn. It may be wise to label the glasses with the resident's name, to ensure that if they are lost, they will be returned. Residents who are confused may become more confused if their eyeglasses are lost and not replaced. The importance of maximizing the resident's visual ability should be emphasized to the staff, to the physicians, and to the resident's family.

In the private or family home

Generally, the nurse will assist the patient who lives in a private or family home in creating a barrier-free environment that allows the patient to continue to function independently. Safety is a high priority in the nurse's interventions with such patients. Besides assisting with the environment, the nurse must create a caring milieu that will facilitate the patient's acceptance of the visual impairment and will strengthen coping abilities that allow adaptation to the demands of the visual deficit.

In the private or family home, as in the nursing home, the nurse is the primary provider and must take responsibility for ensuring that all the strengths of the older person are maximized. Vision, even though it may not be the reason for the formal nursing visit, should always be assessed. The opportunity to teach older adults or couples how to improve their living environment should not be overlooked. Nurses have a responsibility to their patients to provide services that not only treat their physical conditions but also provide them with information and a caring milieu that allows continued growth, an encouraged spirit of hope, and a safe environment.

EVALUATION

In the evaluation phase the nurse examines the nursing interventions in terms of patient outcomes. Have the specific patient-centered, short-term goals been accompiished? Were these accomplished through the intervention of the nurse, or was some other unforeseen event responsible for the meeting of the goals? To what does the patient attribute the change? What about the long-term goal—has enough time passed that progress should have been made toward meeting that goal? What does the patient think? Do any of the etiologies or defining characteristics of the diagnosis still exist, and if so, how are they affecting the patient? Does the plan of care need to be revised, or has the problem been resolved?

Has the plan of care made a difference? Does the nursing documentation clearly delineate the assessment, the diagnosis, the plan of intervention, and the method of evaluation of the nursing care received by this older person? The evaluation phase of the nursing process should never be left unfinished or undocumented. Documentation is a critical factor in development of a scientific foundation for nursing practice, particularly in the compiling of data on sensory deficits such as vision or hearing impairments.

■ Hearing

The prevalence of hearing loss in the older population in the United States is significant. In the longitudinal Framingham Heart Study of adults age 63 to 95, the prevalence of hearing loss for the most important frequencies was 42% (Gates et al., 1990). Hearing loss is the third most frequently reported chronic problem in the over-65 population, and for people age 65 to 74, 24% have hearing loss, whereas in those over the age of 75, 38% experience hearing loss. In all older age groups, men have more hearing impairment than women (Jerger et al., 1995). The number of hearing-impaired adults is estimated at about 7 million people, and the number is expected to increase to at least 11 million by the year 2000 (Rees et al., 1994). In nursing home residents the prevalence of significant impairment in hearing is as high as 70% (Jerger et al., 1995). It is safe to say that hearing loss is a major factor that influences the quality of life for significant numbers of older nursing home residents.

NORMAL STRUCTURE AND FUNCTION

Hearing is a process of the transmission of sounds from the external environment through the mechanism of the ear and the auditory neural pathways to the brain's cortex (Figure 7-4). The human ear consists of three interrelated parts. The outer ear is made up of the pinna, the tragus, and the external ear canal; the middle ear contains the tympanic membrane and the three ossicles (malleus, incus, and stapes); and the inner ear is made up of the cochlea, the vestibule, and the semicircular canals. Hair cells, the auditory receptors, are located within the cochlea.

The normal auditory process includes sound entering through the external ear, proceeding through the canal, and striking the tympanic membrane. The sound then vibrates and is transmitted as neural impulses through the inner ear by the three ossicles. The purpose of the middle ear is to transform energy from the sound waves in the ear into the mechanical force needed to activate the fluid in the cochlea. The cochlea, the sensory organ of hearing, is snail shaped, filled with fluid, and located in the temporal bone. The sensory hair cells in the cochlea play a significant role in the transmission of the neural impulses to the brain along the auditory (eighth cranial nerve) neural pathway. The cochlear por-

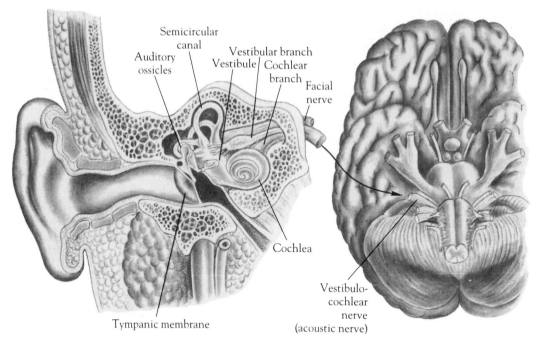

FIGURE 7-4 Components of the ear. (From Thompson, J.M., et al. [1993]. *Mosby's manual of clinical nursing* [3rd ed.]. St. Louis: Mosby.)

tion of the auditory nerve consists of about 30,000 nerve fibers, which carry information to the brain. The central auditory system is where the processing of speech occurs in the auditory cortex in the temporal lobe (Jerger et al., 1995).

The auditory process allows specific external sounds to be interpreted as meaningful communication. Hearing is fundamental to human interaction. Without the ability to hear, the older person is deprived of the total experience of life. There may be a loss of intimacy, friendship, and significant roles, such as musician or teacher. Hearing also allows the individual to discern the sounds of the external environment and to judge whether the sounds convey any danger, such as the ringing of a smoke alarm.

AGE-RELATED CHANGES

Although hearing loss is not a universal age-related occurrence, many older people experience hearing loss. Age-related changes and mani-

festations of diseases that lead to hearing loss are not well understood at this time. In spite of our lack of complete scientific understanding of this common condition, the nurse needs to know the different types of hearing loss and the terms that define hearing loss.

Common complaints of older adults concerning itching in the external ear and increase in cerumen impaction are related to changes in the number of sweat glands. Cerumen glands are modified sweat glands. Their reduction, along with a decrease in other types of sweat glands, results in dry skin and dry and hard earwax. The itching can be controlled by regular and small amounts of baby oil if there is no infection. Cerumen ear impaction can be averted by careful monitoring to avoid buildup.

Although there is a degenerative process involving the ossicular chain, middle ear changes are minimal and not clinically significant (Rees et al., 1994). Inner ear changes affecting the auditory processing system seem to increase with age and lead to an auditory processing disorder and a peripheral hearing sensitivity loss. An age-related loss of cochlear hair cells is thought by many to be a significant source of hearing loss (Rees et al., 1994). Cells of the auditory pathway have a highly specialized function and have limited regenerative ability. The length of their cell life is determined by a myriad of variables: heredity, environmental insults (noise), nutrition, cholesterol, and the body's adaptation to stress (Rees et al., 1994).

COMMON TERMS

Presbycusis is a global term used to describe hearing loss associated with normal aging. Hearing loss includes decreased hearing sensitivity caused by peripheral cochlear defects. A secondary feature of hearing loss is a defect in central auditory processing. This loss leads to (1) impairment of hearing for high-frequency tones, (2) impairment of frequency discrimination, (3) impairment of sound localization, and (4) impairment of speech discrimination (Jerger et al., 1995).

Presbycusis has been further delineated and classified based on the clinical manifestations and the current but limited understanding of the degenerative process of hearing loss.

Sensory presbycusis usually begins in middle age and is slowly progressive, and it is characterized by a loss of ability to hear high-frequency sounds (Mulrow & Lichtenstein, 1991).

Neural presbycusis is hearing loss characterized by loss of speech discrimination in excess of what would be expected in terms of loss of frequencies; it is a disorder of central processing of auditory information.

This comprehensive problem with central processing of auditory information is characterized by difficulty in understanding speech in spite of the ability to hear sounds. This type of hearing loss is related to aging changes in the auditory centers of the brain. Although not universal, it is a problem for a significant number of older adults (Jerger et al., 1995).

To be *deaf* means either to have been born without the ability to hear or to have suffered hearing loss before the advent of speech.

Tinnitus is a continuous or intermittent sound that is perceived but that is not caused by external sources; the sound is perceived in various ways, such as whistling or blowing. Frequently, people who experience hearing loss complain of tinnitus.

Approximately 20% of the population experiences tinnitus at some time in their life. The etiology of tinnitus is not clear, but factors that have been known to cause or worsen tinnitus are noise exposure, wax buildup, medications (aspirin), ear or sinus infections, allergies, and head or neck trauma. Treatments that may provide some relief are use of a hearing aid, masking of noise, biofeedback, and cognitive-behavioral therapy. Overexposure to noise, alcohol, nicotine, caffeine, and stress are all factors that have the potential to worsen tinnitus (American Tinnitus Association [ATA], 1993). The American Tinnitus Association, Post Office Box 5, Portland, OR 97207-0005.

HEARING LOSS

Hearing loss can occur at any age, as a result of many causes (e.g., otitis media, intense noise exposure, head trauma, and some drugs, such as streptomycin and gentamicin, which may have ototoxic effects) (see Box 7-6 for a list of ototoxic drugs). However, age itself also seems to be a cause of hearing loss. A loss of hearing acuity begins for most people in about the third decade of life (Heath, 1993). The functional ability of hearing is one of the fundamental skills that enables people to communicate with one another and therefore to live within a community. Without the ability to hear and to differentiate the meaning of sounds, hearing-impaired older adults are at risk for a loss of communicative skills and for resulting social isolation. Often hearing loss is undetected because the early, insidious signs and symptoms go unrecognized and untreated. For many older people with hearing loss, consonants such as *sh, f, v, t, p,* and *b* are

BOX 7-6 OTOTOXIC DRUGS (THAT CAN PRODUCE HEARING LOSS)

1. Aspirin
2. Chloroquine
3. Cisplatin
4. Erythromycin
5. Furosemide (Lasix)
6. Gentamicin
7. Indomethacin
8. Kanamycin
9. Neomycin
10. Quinidine
11. Quinine
12. Streptomycin
13. Tobramycin
14. Vancomycin

Adapted from Weinstein, B. (1989). *Geriatrics, 44*(4), 42-49.

frequently misheard, leading many times to misunderstanding (Jerger et al., 1995).

Behaviors such as withdrawal from usual social activities, increased fatigue at social gatherings, suspiciousness, and loneliness are many times considered to be normal age-related changes rather than symptoms of hearing loss that may be amenable to treatment (Bess, 1989). These significant behavioral clues to the insidious onset of hearing loss may go unnoticed by older patients and their families. This is because of the gradual, noncrisis characteristic of these behaviors and the prevailing belief that aging brings negative changes in lifestyle.

Older adults who are hard of hearing lose the ability to understand information from media sources (e.g., radio and television). They miss the intimacy of a quick and friendly comment. Establishing new friendships is increasingly difficult when communication is hindered by hearing loss, and affected people worry that they will embar-

rass themselves by responding inappropriately. It is not surprising that studies show that hard-of-hearing people are more dissatisfied with life and more depressed than are people with no hearing problems. A study conducted with a sample of older people living in their own homes found a significant relationship between hearing loss and depression (Mulrow & Lichtenstein, 1991).

The symptoms of hearing loss include gradual loss of auditory sensitivity, with perception of high-frequency sounds diminishing first. Also, there is difficulty in localizing signals and a problem in understanding speech in unfavorable situations. This loss leads to a distortion of words, and sounds become jumbled. The resultant effect is poor speech discrimination. This is characterized by the often heard remark of the hearing-impaired person, "I can hear you but I can't understand what you are saying."

Hearing loss is not uniform; some sounds are heard, whereas others are not. For example, hearing loss is worse for high frequencies than for low frequencies and is greater for consonants than for vowels. This pattern of loss makes word discrimination extremely difficult. The sentence "The thinner cat is red" may be heard as "The dinner hat is red," leading to an inappropriate response, ensuing embarrassment, and perhaps social withdrawal for the hard-of-hearing older person.

Hearing loss can have a profound effect on intimate relationships. Chmiel and Jerger (1993) found that older people with hearing loss judge their auditory handicap less severely than do their spouses. This finding supports the notion that hearing-impaired older people may not recognize the problems their hearing loss causes for those with whom they share their lives.

One form of hearing loss is referred to as "loudness recruitment." In this hearing impairment, the sounds of normal speech cannot be understood and must be made more intense to be heard; however, if the sounds exceed the individual's hearing threshold, they are heard with disturbing loudness. Thus there occurs the classic situation in which the older patient asks

Aging Alert

1. Adaptation to changes in hearing is difficult.
2. Hearing loss may be unrecognized.
3. Corrective devices (e.g., hearing aids) are not always effective.
4. Many older people consider hearing aids to be a negative sign of aging and disability.

the nurse to speak up but then bitterly complains after the request is granted, saying that it is not necessary to yell to be heard. The solution is to find the individual patient's threshold and to try to speak at that level. Another nursing intervention is to teach patients about their hearing impairment and to assist them in taking an active part in structuring communications with others.

AURAL REHABILITATION

Older people who enter an aural rehabilitation process have typically experienced hearing loss for an average of at least 10 years (Weinstein, 1989). Everyone with a hearing disorder should have an ear, nose, and throat medical evaluation to rule out a treatable condition. One common, recurring, often overlooked, compounding factor that increases hearing loss for older patients is impacted cerumen. After this and all other treatable conditions have been ruled out as causing or contributing to the hearing loss, an evaluation by an audiologist is essential for assessment of the appropriate steps for aural rehabilitation (Jerger et al., 1995). Assisted listening devices (hearing aids), instruction in speech reading (lipreading), and motivational counseling are important components of a rehabilitation program.

Only 20% of hearing-impaired people own hearing aids; older users are much less satisfied

than younger people, and use of hearing aids decreases with age (Schum, 1992). The presence of auditory processing disorder causes increased dissatisfaction with hearing aid use (Stach & Jerger, 1991). Other factors implicated in the rejection of hearing aids by older adults are denial of the condition, high cost of hearing aids (not covered by Medicare or most insurance policies), difficulty in managing the controls, and the perception that hearing aids are a stigma (Weinstein, 1989).

Despite limitations, hearing aids do improve the quality of life for many hard-of-hearing older adults. Advances in technology include mechanisms to reduce background noise and digital switching devices to accommodate different listening situations (Chmiel & Jerger, 1995). Often, older people do not know when a hearing aid will help or how to begin the process of obtaining a hearing aid. Recent literature is available from the American Association of Retired Persons (AARP) in the form of two booklets: *Have You Heard? Hearing Loss and Aging* and *Product Report: Hearing Aids*. A 1992 article entitled "How to Buy a Hearing Aid" appeared in *Consumer Reports*. Many older adults will find this article helpful, and this periodical can be obtained in most public libraries.

■ Nursing Process

ASSESSMENT

Physical examination

Examination of the external ear canal is performed by use of the otoscope. It is important to use the largest-sized speculum that the ear will accommodate to facilitate optimal visualization of the canal. The external ear canal is a narrow, winding canal, not a straight line. Before inserting the speculum, pull the auricle slightly upward and backward; this will facilitate entrance into the canal. It is best to have patients tilt their heads to the opposite shoulder; this allows a better view of the canal. The canal is sensitive, so the examiner should exercise skillful control of the otoscope and should stabilize the patient's head with the free hand to minimize unnecessary movement.

Cerumen in the canal may be seen as a brownish-yellow material, with varying degrees of consistency. The most common compounding cause of conduction hearing loss is an accumulation of cerumen. If there is no obstruction in the canal, the examiner will be able to observe the pearly gray tympanic membrane. The outline of the malleus may be seen, and a light reflex known as the "cone of light" may also be seen during the otoscopic examination of a normal ear.

Hearing assessment

Screening for hearing acuity consists of three tests: the spoken word test, the Rinne test, and the Weber test. To perform both the Weber and Rinne hearing tests, the nurse will need a 500-Hz tuning fork. The nurse should be sure that the fork is vibrating before applying it to the patient. Avoid touching the vibrating surfaces.

The spoken word test The spoken word test consists of simply standing a few feet from the patient, placing a hand in front of the mouth to conceal its movements, and whispering a short sentence. This should be done on both sides of the patient to test hearing in both ears. The patient should be asked to repeat the sentence. It is important to change the sentence when testing the second ear.

The Weber test Strike the tuning fork, check the vibration, and place the handle of the fork on the center of the patient's forehead firmly in touch with the skull bone. Ask the patient where the sound of the vibration is heard. People with sensorineural hearing loss will hear the sound in the better ear, those with conductive loss will hear the sound in the impaired ear, and those with normal hearing will hear the sound equally in both ears.

The Rinne test Strike the tuning fork, check the vibration, and place the handle of the fork firmly on the mastoid process. Ask the

Healthy People 2000 Objectives

17.17   Increase to at least 60% the proportion of providers of primary care for older adults who routinely evaluate people aged 65 and older for impairments of vision and hearing.

From U.S. Department of Health and Human Services. (1990). *Healthy People 2000: National health promotion and disease prevention objectives* (DHHS Pub. No. [PHS] 91-50212). Washington, DC: U.S. Government Printing Office.

patient to say when the sound of the vibration is no longer heard. At that point, place the still-vibrating tuning fork next to the anterior surface of the external ear. Again, ask the patient to signal when the sound is no longer heard. The principle that guides this test is that air conduction is greater than bone conduction.

Normal-hearing patients will report hearing the sound longer when the tuning fork is held in the air next to the ear. Normal-hearing patients also will report no difference in the loudness of the sound. In conductive hearing loss, the sound of the vibrating tuning fork is heard more loudly and longer at the mastoid process.

Psychosocial assessment

The psychosocial assessment for patients experiencing hearing loss is similar to that for visual loss (Box 7-7). Denial or lack of understanding may be more pronounced in a patient with hearing loss than in a patient with visual loss. The increased denial of hearing loss may be attributed to negative stereotypic images of older people not hearing well, consequently losing social status, and not being able to compensate for this loss. This image persists in spite of the many successful hard-of-hearing older adults.

BOX 7-7 PSYCHOSOCIAL ASSESSMENT OF HEARING

1. Is there any specific problem you are experiencing that is related to your hearing loss?
2. Have you changed in any way your communications with family or friends?
3. Are you having difficulties listening on the telephone or listening to the radio, television, or movies?
4. At times, does your hearing problem cause you to avoid groups of people?
5. Do you feel a loss of self-confidence because of your hearing problem?
6. At times, does your hearing problem cause you to feel depressed?
7. Is there any information you need to help you live with your hearing problem?
8. Is there anything that I have not covered that you would like to tell me about your hearing?

Nurses need to focus on the ability of hard-of-hearing older people to manage their deficit and to continue meaningful lives.

Another factor that contributes to the negative view of hearing loss is the fact that hearing aids have not been as successful in correcting hearing loss as glasses have been in correcting visual loss. Furthermore, many older patients have had experiences with relatives or friends who were unable to use a hearing aid effectively. These factors, plus the insidious nature of hearing loss, contribute to the denial of loss and increase the reticence of many older people in seeking treatment.

The nurse conducting a psychosocial assessment needs to consider the patient's attitude. Even though an attitude may be prevalent in society, one cannot assume that every individual patient subscribes to that attitude. It is also good

to recall the high level of association between depression and hearing loss and to be alert for any symptoms of depression.

With the patient's permission, include family members in the psychosocial assessment. The attitudes and behaviors of family members regarding the patient's hearing loss should always be assessed. If possible, it is also wise to ask family members the same questions asked of the patient regarding the patient's response to the hearing loss. The older patient with hearing loss has experienced a significant sensory ability loss that often goes unrecognized by both the patient and the patient's family. The nurse has an opportunity to make a contribution to the quality of life for many older adults by providing screening and early detection of hearing loss.

Environmental assessment

Because hearing loss can create communication difficulties, any environmental factor that impedes or facilitates human communication should be assessed. The major areas to assess are the placement and use of radios, televisions, and telephones. Assessment data should be obtained concerning the normal noise level and the changes in the noise level influenced by environmental factors.

The hospital and the nursing home can be difficult places for older patients who have hearing losses. Staff should be aware of the significance of hearing loss in its effects on the communication abilities of the patient. The volume of the radio or television, especially in the nursing home, needs to be adjusted to the level that is comfortable for the patient. Also, all staff should be instructed in and reminded of the procedures necessary to facilitate communication with a hearing-impaired person. Nurses must always model the correct techniques in communicating with the older patient who has a hearing loss.

Resource assessment

The use of a hearing aid is addressed in this portion of the assessment. Ask open-ended ques-

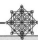

BOX 7-8 HEARING AID ASSESSMENT

1. How have you managed with your hearing aid?
2. On a normal day, how long do you wear your hearing aid?
3. Are you having any difficulties using your hearing aid?
4. Can you show me how you put in your hearing aid and how you adjust the controls?
5. Do you need assistance in using the aid? If so, is a person living with you able to help?
6. How often do you change the batteries in your hearing aid?
7. Do you have spare batteries available?
8. Where do you keep the aid when it is not in use?
9. At night, do you disengage the battery?

BOX 7-9 HINTS FOR FIRST-TIME HEARING AID USERS

1. Begin by using the aid for short periods of time, and add 30 minutes each day.
2. Start by using the aid when listening only to one person. Avoid using it when in large groups until accustomed to the aid.
3. Before placing the aid into the ear, be sure that the switch is off.
4. Practice inserting the aid and using the controls before purchasing the aid.
5. Higher volume is not always better.
6. Whistling sounds or squeals indicate too high a volume or a loose-fitting earmold.
7. Have patience, and allow for enough time to get accustomed to using the aid.

tions, such as "How have you been doing with using your hearing aid?" This type of question allows the skillful nurse to obtain pertinent data without threatening the patient (Box 7-8). Attentive listening to answers to the open-ended questions, coupled with responses to a few direct questions, will help the nurse to assess how well the older patient is adjusting to living with a hearing aid.

During this interview the nurse needs to be empathetic concerning any difficulties the patient may experience in using the hearing aid. Encouragement and positive reinforcement of behaviors that demonstrate acceptance and utilization of the hearing aid are important nursing interventions that may increase the older person's ability to overcome a hearing deficit (Box 7-9).

The economic status of the older patient will have a significant impact on the patient's ability to purchase a hearing aid, because the current Medicare provisions do not cover either eyeglasses or hearing aids. Purchase and maintenance of hearing aids can be quite expensive.

Prices and options vary, with a low of $500 to $700 for a behind-the-ear aid, and with the most sophisticated aid being digitally programmed and costing $2500 ("How to Buy," 1992). The constant replacement of batteries is both an added cost and an added chore, which may be difficult for many older adults to manage.

In addition, a hearing aid for hearing loss is not equivalent to eyeglasses for vision loss. Eyeglasses are made specifically for individual vision loss, whereas most hearing aids do not have that type of specificity. Adjustment to a hearing aid takes time and patience.

Some older adults, because of physical, cognitive, or social conditions, will be unable to use a hearing aid successfully. For example, the person may be unable to manipulate the controls of a hearing aid successfully because of arthritis, may be unable to understand instructions because of dementia, may be unable to afford the high cost of the hearing aid, or may even be unwilling to accept the necessity of wearing a hearing aid. These are reasons frequently given for not purchasing and using hearing aids. Another reason may be that the hearing aid is not effective in particular situations, such as listening to television or listening in noisy environments.

Assistive listening devices (ALDs) can be used in addition to hearing aids or even as an alternative to them. These devices enhance the older person's ability to understand speech in difficult situations. An inexpensive and easy-to-use ALD is a hard-wired system, which includes (1) a microphone that is held close to the sound source, (2) an amplifier, (3) a transducer, and (4) a headphone (Figure 7-5). The ALD (hard-wired) system can be used to facilitate interviews and history taking for hearing-impaired older adults who may have chosen not to use a conventional

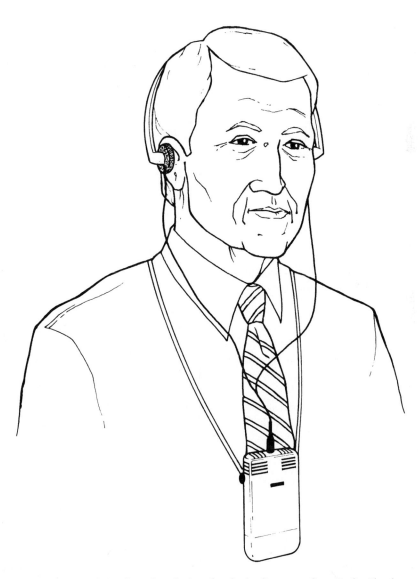

FIGURE 7-5 Assistive listening device (hard-wired) system from Radio Shack.

hearing aid. The low cost and the commercial availability of these devices make them an attractive alternative for some older people. The ALD (the hard-wired system) is available from Radio Shack and from the telephone company (Weinstein, 1989).

NURSING DIAGNOSES

NANDA diagnoses that should be considered when caring for a patient with a hearing loss include the following:

1. Alteration in auditory perception
2. Impaired verbal communication
3. Self-esteem disturbance
4. Impaired social interaction and/or social isolation

The diagnosis of alteration in auditory perception may be related to physical changes, as evidenced by the following:

1. Results of audiology testing
2. Self-reports of hearing loss
3. Reports of others concerning the patient's hearing loss

The diagnosis of impaired verbal communication may be related to hearing loss, as evidenced by the following:

1. Test results
2. Self-reports and reports by others
3. Avoidance of people individually and in groups
4. Denial of hearing difficulties
5. Reluctance to use a hearing aid
6. Blaming others for hearing difficulties
7. Increased arguments
8. Withdrawal from family

The diagnosis of self-esteem disturbance may be related to hearing loss, as evidenced by the following:

1. Expression of feelings of diminished self-worth
2. Avoidance of people
3. Suspiciousness of others

The diagnosis of impaired social interaction may be related to hearing loss, as evidenced by the following:

1. Diminished activity level
2. Avoidance of people

PLANNING AND GOAL IDENTIFICATION

The planning phase consists of compiling all the data gathered during the assessment phase and deciding on priorities of care. After the priorities have been designated, the planning team will plan appropriate nursing interventions that will ameliorate or alleviate the condition. The nursing intervention may be a referral or a consultation with a representative of another health discipline. Each planned nursing intervention is goal specific, not random.

Alteration in auditory perception

A long-term goal is that the patient will adapt to hearing loss. Short-term goals include the following:

1. Patient will accept use of hearing aid.
2. Caregiver and support system will encourage and assist patient in the beginning stages of hearing-aid use.
3. Patient will be able to care for and correctly use hearing aid.

Impaired verbal communication

A long-term goal is that the patient's verbal communication with others will be appropriate and untroubled. Short-term goals include the following:

1. Patient will not avoid communication with family and friends.
2. Arguments within the family will diminish.
3. Patient will be able to verbalize the personal reality and consequences of having a hearing loss.

Impaired social interaction

A long-term goal is that the patient will regain and maintain a pre–hearing-loss level of social interaction with family, friends, and community organizations. Short-term goals include the following:

1. Patient will attend family functions.
2. Patient will engage in personally chosen social activities.

IMPLEMENTATION
In the acute care setting

Hospitalization of older people occurs for many reasons, but usually not for treatment concerning their hearing loss; instead, the hearing loss may go undetected or disregarded. Not all older people are hard of hearing, but the functional status of hearing should be part of every nursing assessment. Also, if there is a hearing loss, the nurse must assess both how well the patient understands and accepts the loss, and how well the patient communicates, in order to be able to formulate a plan of care.

When an older patient is undergoing diagnostic testing, particularly in a hospital, the patient may be engaged in multiple interactions with a wide array of people, from the transport personnel to the technicians conducting the tests. These interactions take place in a dynamic, complex, and even frenzied environment, including crammed corridors and crowded elevators. For the older patient in a wheelchair—or worse, on a stretcher or a gurney—the environment may be frightening. In addition, for the hard-of-hearing patient, it may be difficult to understand instructions. In these situations the nurse can intervene by taking the time to explain to the patient in detail the reason for the test, the procedures involved in the test, and any other helpful information about the experience. The nurse may also intervene to alert other hospital staff to the patient's level of hearing loss; this nursing intervention often improves the diagnostic testing experience for all concerned.

When developing interventions for communicating with hard-of-hearing older patients, it is critical to allow time for the patient to process information. Without sufficient time for the inter-

---

BOX 7-10 STEPS TO EFFECTIVE COMMUNICATION WITH HEARING-IMPAIRED OLDER ADULTS

1. Be sure you have the person's attention before beginning to speak.
2. Face the person to whom you are speaking, and stand reasonably close to the listener.
3. Avoid standing in the glare of bright sunlight or other lights.
4. Lower the pitch of your voice.
5. Speak clearly and slowly.
6. Use short sentences.
7. Avoid background noise.
8. Encourage the use of nonverbal communication, such as touch.
9. Use written communication if you are unable to communicate verbally.

---

action and without knowledge and compassion on the part of the nurse, effective nursing care will not occur. Several measures can be taken to communicate effectively with hearing-impaired older adults, as seen in Box 7-10.

In the nursing home

With the large numbers of hearing-impaired people who are living in nursing homes, it is crucial that all nursing home personnel be aware of appropriate ways to communicate with hard-of-hearing residents. In addition, hearing loss may exacerbate the confusional states of many nursing home residents. Residents with dementia may also be hard of hearing. Therefore nurses must continually assess both the hearing function and the communication ability of the residents. Nurses must also use a high level of skill to communicate effectively with older residents who are afflicted with both dementia and hearing loss.

Nurses need to emphasize to the staff members the importance of (1) allowing time for the resident to respond, (2) recognizing each resident's unique abilities, and (3) acquiring and constantly using communication skills that facilitate dialogue with people who suffer from hearing loss. All levels of nursing staff should be instructed in the different ways in which hearing loss is manifested. Such awareness may help to minimize complaints that residents are just stubborn or only hear what they want to hear. The staff must understand the symptoms associated with the loss of the ability to discriminate sounds and speech, as well as those accompanying a simple loss of hearing of gross sounds. If necessary, repeatedly explain the differences to the nursing staff responsible for the daily personal care of nursing home residents. The professional nurse plans, guides, and supervises the care of the resident, and the nonprofessional staff members are educated and supervised by the professional nursing staff.

One physical aspect of hearing loss that needs constant assessment and treatment is the accumulation of cerumen (earwax). Mahoney (1993) observed impacted cerumen in 26 out of 104 nursing home residents, and 78 other residents had a large accumulation of cerumen without impaction. Although small, this study does suggest a high incidence of impacted cerumen in nursing home residents. Nurses can improve the quality of life for these older people. After checking with each patient's physician to be sure that there are no contraindications (e.g., punctured tympanic membrane), the nurse may cleanse the patient's ears. Irrigation as a method of cleansing cerumen from the external canal is usually considered a nursing function. An effective method of cerumen removal is to use either a dental waterpik or a bulb syringe for irrigation. The water should be tepid; hot or cold extremes will distress the resident. If the cerumen is difficult to dislodge, it may be necessary to use drops, such as mineral oil or a mixture of hydrogen peroxide and mineral oil, to soften the accumulation. The irrigation should be done with the resident's shoulder draped with a towel, the head tipped

toward the shoulder, and an emesis basin positioned to catch the draining water. The ear canal will need to be viewed with an otoscope both before and after the irrigation. The goal of the irrigation is a clear canal. Some improvement in hearing may result from this procedure. It is best to assess for accumulated cerumen on a monthly basis.

In the private or family home

Many of the interventions cited for the acute care and nursing home settings have relevance to the private or family home setting. The teaching of specific communication skills should focus on the family caregivers. Some caregivers may find it extremely difficult to accept any type of instruction in communication. Family members usually have a long history of communication patterns that might not be amenable to change. As is the case with hospitalized older patients, the primary reason for a home visit seldom relates to the patient's hearing loss. Nonetheless, the nurse can use expert knowledge in assessing, diagnosing, and intervening to make a significant contribution to the quality of life for the hearing-impaired older person.

Family members need an understanding of the type of hearing loss the older patient is experiencing and how it affects daily living. Also, techniques for improving communication with the older patient may be taught by the nurse both to interested family members and to the hard-of-hearing patient. Often, the authentic concern of the nurse creates a therapeutic milieu that allows and encourages older adults and their families to continue to maintain an independent living arrangement.

EVALUATION

Evaluation of nursing interventions is an essential component of the nursing process that often goes unnoticed and unrecorded. It is crucial for nurses always to include an evaluative statement in the documentation of care. For one thing, evaluation may help to determine the accuracy of assessment data, as well as to substantiate the

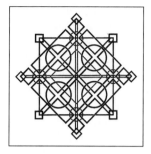

CHAPTER 8

The faces of the old are like old houses;
every line's a highway from the past.

R. McKuen, *Valentines*

Integument

■ Learning Objectives

On completion of this chapter, the reader will be able to do the following:

1. Identify age-related changes in the integument and in the oral mucous membranes.
2. Assess the older adult's integument and oral mucous membranes.
3. Recognize risk factors that lead to impaired skin integrity and alterations in oral mucous membranes.
4. Describe the causes of integumentary impairment, and oral mucous membrane impairment in older adults.
5. Develop a plan of nursing care for an older adult with integumentary impairment or with alterations in oral mucous membranes.
6. Implement appropriate nursing interventions for older adults with integumentary impairment and with alterations in oral mucous membranes.
7. Evaluate the effectiveness of nursing interventions carried out to resolve integumentary and oral mucous membrane problems.

Although the skin provides a protective barrier between the body and the environment, diseases of the skin and subcutaneous tissue do occur. Furthermore, some age-related changes in the skin and oral mucous membranes can lead to delayed healing of wounds, decreased sweating, altered temperature regulation, wrinkles, loss of dentition, and increased susceptibility to disease. These skin conditions and diseases account for high morbidity and high treatment costs. Despite advances in dental hygiene, the average person has lost ten teeth by the age of 70; more than 65% of older adults have an edentulous jaw (Kresevic & Lincoln, 1995). This chapter presents information regarding age-related skin and oral mucous membrane changes, the major causes of skin and oral mucous membrane impairment, and the nursing requirements to manage these integumentary problems when they occur among older adults.

■ Skin

NORMAL STRUCTURE AND FUNCTION

The skin is the largest organ of the body and comprises three layers: the epidermis, the dermis, and the subcutaneous. The *epidermis* is the outermost layer and consists of stratified squamous epithelium cells (keratinocytes and melanocytes). The main functions of the epidermis are to protect the body against invasion by environmental substances, to restrict water loss, and to synthesize keratin cells. Two divisions make up the epidermis: the superficial papillary dermis (connecting with the epidermal layer) and the reticular dermis (connecting with the subcutaneous fat layer). Appendages of the epidermis are the eccrine and apocrine sweat glands, sebaceous glands, hair, and nails. The *dermis* comprises the papillary layer and the reticular layer. Blood vessels and nerve elements are in the *papillary layer,* which extends into the epidermis. Elastin fibers, collagen fibers, and reticulin fibers form the *reticular layer.* The *subcutaneous layer* is composed of loose connective tissue and fat cells. Its main functions are to provide heat, insulation, and caloric reserves and to act as a shock absorber. A cross section of the skin is shown in Figure 8-1.

The major functions of the skin include protection, minimization of body fluid loss, excretion of some waste materials and toxins, temperature regulation, blood pressure regulation, tissue repair, synthesis of vitamin D, sensory perception, and expression of feelings. Increasingly, intact skin is being recognized as a key element in the prevention of disease; disruption in skin integrity provides a site for pathogens to enter (Beare & Myers, 1994). Each of these functions is described in Table 8-1.

AGE-RELATED CHANGES

As humans age, two types of predictable changes occur in the skin: (1) intrinsic aging and (2) photoaging. In intrinsic aging, there is a systemic

TABLE 8-1 Functions of the skin

Skin function	Mechanism
Protection	Intact skin covering creates a physical barrier against bacteria, minor physical trauma, and foreign substances
Synthesis of keratin	Keratinocytes are produced in the basal layer, develop, and then move to the surface of the skin
Excretion of wastes	Sweat, sodium chloride, urea, and lactic acid are excreted through the skin
Blood pressure regulation	Skin blood vessels can constrict, which promotes venous return and increases the cardiac output and blood pressure
Fluid regulation	Skin keeps fluids contained in the body
Temperature regulation	Skin blood vessels can (1) dilate to promote heat loss or to prevent tissue freezing (radiation); (2) constrict to conserve heat; or (3) regulate temperature by conduction, convection, and evaporation
Tissue repair	Skin replaces damaged skin cells and forms scar tissue
Production of vitamin D	In the presence of ultraviolet light, a precursor of vitamin D is converted to vitamin D in the skin
Sensory perception	Special sensors in the skin respond to touch, pain, heat, cold, pressure, vibration, tickling, itching, wetness, oiliness, and stickiness
Expression of emotional feelings	Surface of the skin can respond to emotions through sweating, pallor, or flushing.

often targets. About 70% of melanomas are classified as superficial spreading melanomas, 10% as lentigo melanoma (on skin areas exposed to sun), 8% as acral lentiginous melanoma, and 15% as nodular melanoma (Kurban & Kurban, 1993). Following confirmation of the melanoma by biopsy, the patient is examined for evidence of metastasis. Treatment involves deep surgical removal of the lesion, chemotherapy, and possibly radiation therapy. Follow-up examinations are essential because recurrence of malignant melanomas is common.

Radiation therapy for treatment of cancer causes damage to the normal skin and to mucous membranes. These can be classified as local or systemic effects. Locally, the effects are related to the area of skin irradiated and may include alopecia (loss of hair) and localized skin reactions. Three stages of skin reactions are (1) erythema, (2) dry desquamation with flaking, and (3) moist desquamation with shedding of surface epithelium (Beare & Myers, 1994). Treatment of radiation effects on the skin includes (1) avoiding further trauma, (2) reducing friction and exposure to the sun, (3) using nonadhesive dressings, (4) keeping the skin warm and dry, and (5) avoiding harsh chemicals and soaps. Use of over-the-counter (OTC) skin products should be discouraged, because they may contain harmful ingredients.

Pressure ulcers

A *pressure ulcer* is an area of cellular necrosis, which is an endemic problem in the debilitated patient population. In skilled care nursing home facilities, the prevalence is approximately 23% (Panel for the Prediction and Prevention of Pressure Ulcers in Adults, 1992). Pressure ulcers develop when the external pressure on the skin covering bony prominences exceeds capillary hydrostatic pressure. Generally there is agreement that local tissue perfusion and oxygenation are compromised in the pressure ulcer patient. Patients who are immobile, dependent, malnourished, and subject to friction and shearing force

are most likely to develop pressure ulcers (Kashyup, 1989). A pressure ulcer can be described in terms of stages for purposes of treatment. (See Figure 8-9 for a description of the four stages of pressure ulcers.) Sites for pressure ulcers are the sacrum, greater trochanter (hip), ischial tuberosity (buttocks), lateral malleolus (ankle), ears, and tuberosity of the calcaneus (heel) (Tierney et al., 1995). These sites account for more than 95% of all pressure ulcers; in immobile older adults the most frequent site for a pressure ulcer is the sacrum.

Assessment Numerous pressure ulcer risk assessment tools are available to identify the high-risk older adult. Two validated pressure ulcer risk assessment tools are the Braden scale (Box 8-1) and the Norton scale (Box 8-2) (Panel for the Prediction and Prevention, 1992).

Generally the assessment should focus on clustering clinical cues to provide a guide for interventions. In Sparks's study (1990), 11 assessment parameters and 20 clinical cues were identified as being characteristic of the patient who develops a pressure ulcer. See Table 8-2 for a description of the assessment parameters and clinical cues.

Pressure ulcer risk assessment using established instruments such as the Braden scale or Norton scale should be performed initially and repeated at frequent intervals to detect changes requiring implementation of pressure ulcer prevention protocols.

Family assessment Discuss the impact of skin problems with family members or significant others. Determine the adequacy of their knowledge base and the need for patient or family education to carry out prescribed skin regimens.

Environmental assessment Determine the nature of the patient's living environment and daily activity patterns. If frequent sun exposure occurs, advise the use of sunscreen and protective clothing. Find out about environmental hazards, such as wrinkled bed linen, improperly fitting shoes or clothes, uncovered heat vents, and exposure to radiation. If the patient is immobile,

BOX 8-1 BRADEN SCALE FOR PREDICTING PRESSURE ULCER RISK

Patient's Name _____ Evaluator's Name _____ Date of Assessment _____

SENSORY PERCEPTION Ability to respond meaningfully to pressure-related discomfort	**1. Completely limited:** Unresponsive (does not moan, flinch, or grasp) to painful stimuli, due to diminished level of consciousness or sedation, OR limited ability to feel pain over most of body surface.	**2. Very Limited:** Responds only to painful stimuli. Cannot communicate discomfort except by moaning or restlessness, OR has a sensory impairment which limits the ability to feel pain or discomfort over ½ of body.	**3. Slightly Limited:** Responds to verbal commands but cannot always communicate discomfort or need to be turned. OR has some sensory impairment which limits ability to feel pain or discomfort in 1 or 2 extremities.	**4. No Impairment:** Responds to verbal commands. Has no sensory deficit which would limit ability to feel pain or voice pain or discomfort.			
MOISTURE Degree to which skin is exposed to moisture	**1. Constantly Moist:** Skin is kept moist almost constantly by perspiration, urine, etc. Dampness is detected every time patient is moved or turned.	**2. Moist:** Skin is often but not always moist. Linen must be changed at least once a shift.	**3. Occasionally Moist:** Skin is occasionally moist, requiring an extra linen change approximately once a day.	**4. Rarely Moist:** Skin is usually dry; linen requires changing only at routine intervals.			
ACTIVITY Degree of physical activity	**1. Bedfast:** Confined to bed	**2. Chairfast:** Ability to walk severely limited or nonexistent. Cannot bear own weight and/or must be assisted into chair or wheelchair.	**3. Walks Occasionally:** Walks occasionally during day but for very short distances, with or without assistance. Spends majority of each shift in bed or chair.	**4. Walks Frequently:** Walks outside the room at least twice a day and inside room at least once every 2 hours during waking hours.			
MOBILITY Ability to change and control body position	**1. Completely Immobile:** Does not make even slight changes in body or extremity position without assistance.	**2. Very Limited:** Makes occasional slight changes in body or extremity position but unable to make frequent or significant changes independently.	**3. Slightly Limited:** Makes frequent though slight changes in body or extremity position independently.	**4. No Limitations:** Makes major and frequent changes in position without assistance.			
NUTRITION Usual food intake pattern	**1. Very Poor:** Never eats a complete meal. Rarely eats more than ⅓ of any food offered. Eats 2 servings or less of protein (meat or dairy products) per day. Takes fluids poorly. Does not take a liquid dietary supplement, OR is NPO and/or maintained on clear liquids or IVs for more than 5 days.	**2. Probably Inadequate:** Rarely eats a complete meal and generally eats only about ½ of any food offered. Protein intake includes only 3 servings of meat or dairy products per day. Occasionally will take a dietary supplement, OR receives less than optimum amount of liquid diet or tube feeding.	**3. Adequate:** Eats over half of most meals. Eats a total of 4 servings of protein (meat, dairy products) each day. Occasionally will refuse a meal, but will usually take a supplement if offered, OR is on a tube feeding or TPN regimen, which probably meets most of nutritional needs.	**4. Excellent:** Eats most of every meal. Never refuses a meal. Usually eats a total of 4 or more servings of meat and dairy products. Occasionally eats between meals. Does not require supplementation.			
FRICTION AND SHEAR	**1. Problem:** Requires moderate to maximum assistance in moving. Complete lifting without sliding against sheets is impossible. Frequently slides down in bed or chair, requiring frequent repositioning with maximum assistance. Spasticity, contractures, or agitation leads to almost constant friction.	**2. Potential Problem:** Moves feebly or requires minimum assistance. During a move skin probably slides to some extent against sheets, chair, restraints, or other devices. Maintains relatively good position in chair or bed most of the time but occasionally slides down.	**3. No Apparent Problem:** Moves in bed and in chair independently and has sufficient muscle strength to lift up completely during move. Maintains good position in bed or chair at all times.				
							Total Score

© Copyright Barbara Braden and Nancy Bergstrom, 1988.

BOX 8-2 NORTON SCALE

NORTON RISK ASSESSMENT SCALE

		Physical Condition	Mental Condition	Activity	Mobility	Incontinent	
		Good 4	Alert 4	Ambulant 4	Full 4	Not 4	TOTAL
		Fair 3	Apathetic 3	Walk/help 3	Sl. limited 3	Occasional 3	SCORE
		Poor 2	Confused 2	Chairbound 2	V. limited 2	Usually/Urine 2	
		Very Bad 1	Stupor 1	Bed 1	Immobile 1	Doubly 1	
Name	Date						

Reprinted with permission, Norton D., McLaren R., and Exton-Smith A.N.: *An investigation of geriatric nursing problems in hospital*, 1962, reissue 1975, Churchill Livingstone, Edinburgh.

TABLE 8-2 Pressure ulcer assessment parameters and clinical cues

Assessment parameters	Clinical cues
Activity status	Confinement to bed; confinement to chair; paralysis
Circulation	Decreased
Incontinence	Bladder; bowel
Infection	Localized infection in pressure-supporting areas
Mechanical factors	Friction; external pressure; shearing forces
Mental status	Comatose
Mobility status	Dependent
Musculoskeletal status	Skeletal prominence; loss of tissue; loss of muscle
Nutritional status	Cachexia or debilitation; dehydration; low serum albumin
Self-care ability	Dependent
Skin condition	Maceration

suggest the use of materials to prevent skin breakdown, such as cushions, mattresses, lotions, and positioning devices.

Once the nurse identifies a patient as requiring intervention for pressure ulcers (either to prevent or to treat such ulcers), the nurse must plan, implement, and monitor the appropriate interventions. The management and treatment of pressure ulcers can be divided into two categories: (1) preventive therapy and (2) treatment of existing pressure ulcers.

Preventive therapy Preventive pressure ulcer therapy requires adequate nutrition (increased protein and vitamins) and hydration, keeping the skin clean and dry, and reducing friction, shearing forces, and the amount of pressure exerted on any

Aging Alert
Warning signs of malignant melanoma in a pigmented lesion

- **Asymmetry**
- **Border irregularity**
- **Color variation or dark border color**
- **Diameter greater than 6 mm**

From Kurban, R. S., & Kurban, A. K. (1993). Common skin disorders of aging: Diagnosis and treatment. *Geriatrics, 48* (4), 30-42.

body part. Reduction of pressure may be accomplished by moving and turning the patient at least every 2 hours and by using pillows, flotation devices, special mattresses, and positioning devices.

To prevent tissue trauma from shearing force or friction, the patient must be lifted, not pulled, when repositioned in bed or in a wheelchair. Small shifts of body weight are also effective in reducing pressure. Using a "pull sheet" or reusable underpad may aid in moving the patient without causing additional tissue trauma. Shearing force can be reduced by limiting the amount of time the patient spends at an angle of 30 degrees or higher. The use of pressure-reducing devices such as foam mattresses, water mattresses, and gel-filled cushions should follow local institutional guidelines. The key to prevention is relief of pressure.

Treatment Treatment of existing pressure ulcers depends on their location and severity and the patient's condition. Pressure ulcers must be constantly monitored to detect changes in healing and the onset of infection. Pressure ulcers can be grouped into stages, according to their characteristics, and treatment may be provided according to general guidelines for each stage. It is essential to recognize that pressure relief is the key element in any treatment plan. (See Table 8-3 for an overview of treatment strategies related to the stage of pressure ulcer development.)

Two publications dealing with the prediction, prevention, and treatment of pressure ul-

TABLE 8-3 Pressure ulcer treatments

Stage	Goal	Treatment
0	Prevention of skin breakdown	Relief of pressure Eliminate shear and friction Maintain adequate nutrition/fluid Use pressure-relieving devices Turning frequently
1	Erythema resolves No epidermal breakdown	All of the above + Transparent adhesive dressings + Padding bony prominences
2	Epidermis heals No necrotic tissue	All of the above + Hydrocolloidal dressings Polyurethane foam dressings
3	Ulcer heals Free of eschar No infection	Same as for stage 0 + Treat infection Debridement—surgical or enzymatic
4	Ulcer heals No osteomyelitis	Surgical closure (skin graft or skin flap)

Aging Alert
Prevention of pressure ulcers
- Increase mobility; move or turn frequently
- Examine skin daily for areas of redness or tenderness
- Maintain nutritional status and hydration
- Reduce pressure on bony prominences
- Avoid friction and shearing forces
- Keep skin dry; pat skin, do not rub

cers are available to clinicians and patients. The first, *Pressure Ulcers in Adults: Prediction and Prevention* (Panel for the Prediction and Prevention, 1992), provides guidelines for identifying patients at risk for pressure ulcers and recommends early interventions for the prevention of pressure ulcers. *Treatment of Pressure Ulcers* (Bergstrom et al., 1992) makes recommendations in six areas: assessment, managing tissue loads, ulcer care, managing bacterial colonization and infection, operative repair, and education and quality improvement. Both publications are available as a quick reference guide for clinicians and as a patient's guide, which is available in English and Spanish. To order copies of the guidelines, call the Agency for Health Care Policy and Research (AHCPR) Publications Clearinghouse at 1-800-358-9295 or write to AHCPR Publications Clearinghouse, Post Office Box 8547, Silver Spring, MD 20907.

Venous ulcers

Venous ulcers occur when venous blood pools in the lower extremities, causing skin lesions and infections (Figure 8-10). In older adults this is most frequently caused by venous insufficiency. The incidence of venous ulcers is estimated to be 0.2% to 0.4% among the general population; the incidence is probably higher in the older adult segment of the population. These ulcers are commonly located on the medial aspect of the leg, whereas ulcers caused by arterial insufficiency are found on the lateral aspect of the leg or the malleoli (ankles). Research has shown that diffusion and exchange of nutrients are impaired following the occurrence of unrelieved venous pressure.

Preventive treatment includes education about meticulous foot care and use of aseptic technique. Strategies to improve circulation and maintain cellular nutrition, such as elevation of the feet and use of compression stockings to reduce edema, are also recommended. "Compression should achieve a pressure of 30 mm Hg below the knee and 40 mm Hg at the ankle. The stockings should not be used in patients with arterial insufficiency ... Pneumatic sequential compression devices may be of great benefit" (Tierney et al., 1995). When ulcers occur, treatment is aimed at correction of factors that impair wound healing. This includes nutritional therapy, with particular emphasis on vitamin C and zinc, if the patient is malnourished. Control of systemic diseases such as anemia, congestive heart failure, and diabetes mellitus is essential.

The ulcer is cleansed, treated with a steroid ointment, and covered with an occlusive dressing or a polyurethane foam dressing, and an Unna zinc paste boot is applied (changed weekly). The ulcer should heal in 2 to 3 months; if healing does not occur, pinch grafts may be necessary. Newer techniques, using cultured epidermal cell grafts, are being used in some cases not successfully treated with other therapy (Tierney et al., 1995).

Antibiotic therapy is usually avoided unless there are signs of cellulitis. If there *are* signs of cellulitis, hospitalization or specialized home care may be required for the administration of intravenous antibiotics. Because many patients have allergies, the nurse must exercise caution in selecting and using both topical preparations and those with systemic effect. Contact dermatitis might occur, causing pruritus and erythema, which further delay healing.

Synthetic occlusive dressings for venous ulcers are helpful in reducing pain and in stimulating granulation tissue. This type of treatment also allows the patient to be monitored in an outpatient setting. Occlusive dressings may become filled with exudate, and an unpleasant odor is often present; nonetheless, in most cases the patient is instructed *not* to remove the dressing. The dressing usually remains in place for 2 to 3 weeks, after which time it is removed and replaced with a standard dressing. If the surrounding skin is very fragile or there is extensive dermatitis, occlusive dressings cannot be used. For patients who are unable to do their own dressing changes, Unna boots may be used to dress ulcers; they are changed only once a week and are a form of occlusive therapy.

Arterial ulcers

Arterial ulcers are usually caused by atherosclerosis. They occur on the legs, ankles, and feet and are characterized by pallor, patchy bluish-purple mottling of the skin, and cold, clammy skin. Absence of arterial pulses and distortion of the toenails (onychogryposis) are also clinical signs of arterial ulcers. The ulcers are smaller than venous ulcers and are sharply defined, and muscle or tendon is often exposed. Cues for distinguishing arterial and venous ulcers are presented in Table 8-4.

Treatment is aimed at reducing peripheral vascular disease risk factors. Smoking should be strongly discouraged because the nicotinic acid in tobacco causes arteries to constrict. Hypertension, diabetes mellitus, hyperlipemia, and obesity should be controlled. Meticulous foot care is essential. The patient should be referred to a podiatrist for management of corns, calluses, and nail dystrophies. Protective foot pads may be needed to prevent injury.

Fungal infections

Fungal infections occur frequently in the compromised older adult. *Candida albicans,* a yeastlike fungus, is normally found in the body; moist skin, use of antibiotics or corticosteroids, and poor general health can lead to candidiasis (Figure 8-11). It is manifested by pruritus, burning, and red, eroded patches of skin. Treatment consists of topical and systemically acting antifungal agents such as nystatin (Mycostatin). Cool Burrow's compresses may be recommended to relieve inflam-

TABLE 8-4 Cues for distinguishing arterial and venous ulcers

Cue	Arterial ulcer	Venous ulcer
Previous history	Arteriosclerosis	Thrombophlebitis
Pain	Severe	Moderate
Characteristics		
Margins	Well defined	Ragged
Location	Tips of toes, heels, phalangeal heads, above lateral aspect of malleolus	Malleolus, pretibial area
Depth	Deep	Shallow
Tissue	Necrotic	Granulated
Skin	Shiny, dry	Edematous
Nails	Thick	Unchanged
Skin temperature	Variable	Cool or hot
Dependent position	Rubor	Unchanged
Edema	None	Common

Impaired tissue integrity: Venous ulcer

The condition may be evidenced by the following defining characteristics:

Ulceration of the lower extremity
Normal pulses
Edema

Knowledge deficit: Skin care

The condition may be evidenced by the following defining characteristics:

Verbalization of need for information about skin condition
Inaccurate follow-through on instructions for management of skin problem
Incomplete resolution of the skin problem
Readmission for the same skin problem

PLANNING AND GOAL IDENTIFICATION

The outcome identification phase of the nursing process consists of setting realistic long- and short-term goals based on nursing diagnoses. The patient is an integral member of the health care team and, if able, should be closely involved in the development of these goals.

Risk for impaired skin integrity: Pressure ulcer

A long-term goal is that the patient will have no skin breakdown. Short-term goals include the following:

1. Patient or family will verbalize an understanding of preventive skin care measures.
2. Patient or family will demonstrate preventive skin care measures.
3. Patient or family will be able to describe the relationship between risk factors and skin breakdown.

Impaired skin integrity

A long-term goal is that the patient will have healed lesions or wounds. The following may be appropriate short-term goals:

1. Patient will explain skin care regimen.
2. Patient will carry out skin care regimen correctly.

3. Patient will understand the relationship between various risk factors and skin breakdown.
4. Patient will discuss impact of skin changes on body image and self-concept.

Impaired tissue integrity

A long-term goal is that the patient will follow the skin care regimen after discharge from the hospital. Short-term goals include the following:

1. Patient will verbalize an understanding of the relationship between various risk factors and skin changes.
2. Patient will maintain peripheral circulation at baseline level (specify parameters for individual patient).
3. Patient will carry out skin care regimen, including exercise, foot care, avoidance of dependent positions, and use of antiembolism stockings.

Knowledge deficit: Skin care

A long-term goal is that the patient will verbalize an understanding of skin condition and its relationship to risk factors. Short-term goals include the following:

1. Patient will follow instructions for skin care correctly.
2. Patient will demonstrate correct skin care regimen.
3. Patient will state intention to use skin care consultants.

IMPLEMENTATION

Nursing interventions are planned to achieve the goals established for the skin care plan. They should focus on the etiology of the problem and should be specific. Interventions are carried out wherever the patient may be found—in the acute care setting, the nursing home, or the patient's private home environment. Because of the frequency of skin problems in older adults, it is likely that most or all of the measures discussed will be needed in at least one setting.

Health Promotion
Skin protection

- Examine skin daily for any changes, and report any changes in moles or lesions. Report any lesion that fails to heal.
- Avoid scratching of dry skin.
- Avoid daily hot baths or showers. Bathing 2 to 3 times per week is sufficient. Daily sponge bathing is permissible.
- Use superfatted, nondeodorant soaps.
- Use bath or mineral oils with extreme caution. These can cause slipping in the shower or tub.
- Apply emollients or lotions after bathing.
- Drink several glasses of water every day.
- Do not use rubbing alcohol on skin. This causes drying.
- Consider the use of a humidifier in winter, if dry skin is a problem.

Health Promotion
Sun exposure

- Protect skin from overexposure to the sun. Avoid being in the sun between the hours of 10 a.m. and 3 p.m.
- Wear protective clothing, such as light-colored, long-sleeved shirts, long pants, and wide-brimmed hats, when out in the sun.
- Apply sunscreen with an SPF of at least 15 before exposure to the sun. Wear sunscreen even on cloudy days (clouds do not block ultraviolet rays).
- Avoid sunburn. There is no such thing as a healthy tan!

The focus of each intervention is on achieving a specific goal. For purposes of discussion, each section describes physical care measures, psychosocial care measures, and educational measures carried out by the nurse, patient, and/or family to resolve skin problems.

In the acute care setting

The primary way to prevent skin breakdown is to decrease pressure. This can be accomplished through frequent changes in position, the use of pressure-relieving devices, and regular inspection of the skin for signs of early damage. Position changes should be made at least every 2 hours, and small shifts of body weight should be encouraged. *Bony prominences should not be massaged.* Avoid drying agents such as alcohol or alcohol-based rubs. Use moisturizing agents to prevent skin dryness. To avoid shearing force when moving patients, lift—do not pull. A complete bath can be given every 3 to 4 days, and a sponge bath can be given daily, to prevent drying of the skin. The skin should be patted dry, not rubbed, to avoid tissue trauma. Good nutrition and adequate hydration are integral components of a skin care program to maintain skin integrity. All skin surfaces should be inspected daily so that corrective action, if needed, can be initiated immediately.

Compresses or wet dressings using Burrow's solution (Domeboro powder) are sometimes used to treat skin problems. The packet is mixed with 1 qt of water, and the solution is applied using sterile gauze dressings for 30 minutes 3 times a day. The wet dressing should be wrapped with a nonporous covering to protect the rest of the patient's skin.

Pressure-relieving devices usually consist of mattresses, cushions, and body part supports (see further discussion of pressure-relieving devices in Table 8-5). For the patient at minimal

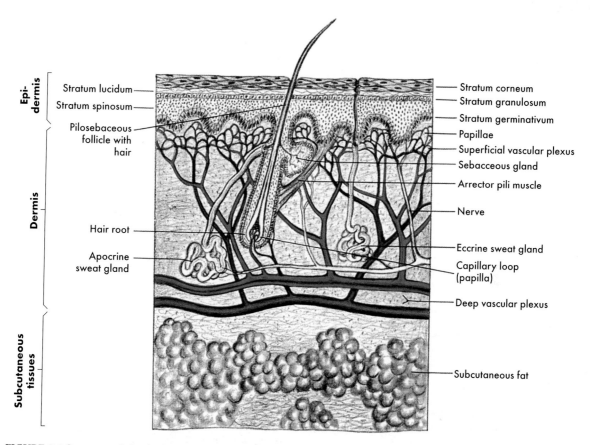

Epidermis
- Stratum lucidum
- Stratum spinosum

Dermis
- Pilosebaceous follicle with hair
- Hair root
- Apocrine sweat gland

Subcutaneous tissues

- Stratum corneum
- Stratum granulosum
- Stratum germinativum
- Papillae
- Superficial vascular plexus
- Sebacceous gland
- Arrector pili muscle
- Nerve
- Eccrine sweat gland
- Capillary loop (papilla)
- Deep vascular plexus
- Subcutaneous fat

FIGURE 8-1 Structures of the skin. (From Thompson, J.M., et al, [1993]. *Mosby's manual of clinical nursing,* St. Louis: Mosby.)

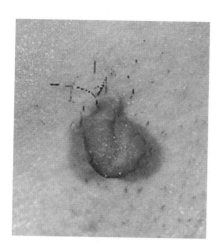

FIGURE 8-2 Acrochordon (skin tag). (From Habif, T.P. [1996]. *Clinical dermatology,* [3rd ed.]. St. Louis: Mosby.)

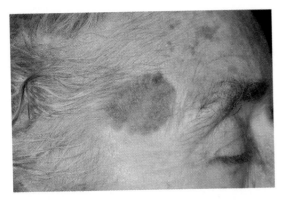

FIGURE 8-3 Seborrheic keratosis. (From Habif, T.P. [1996]. *Clinical dermatology,* [3rded.]. St. Louis: Mosby.)

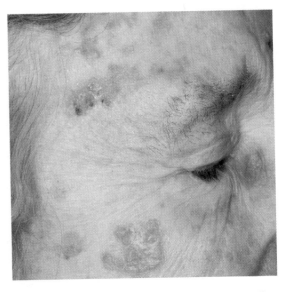

FIGURE 8-4 Actinic keratosis. (From Habif, T.P. [1996]. *Clinical dermatology,* [3rded.]. St. Louis: Mosby.)

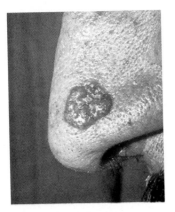

FIGURE 8-5 Basal cell carcinoma. (From Habif, T.P. [1996]. *Clinical dermatology,* [3rded.]. St. Louis: Mosby.)

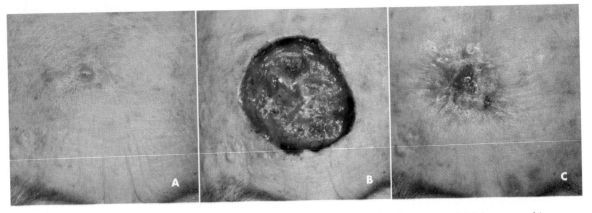

FIGURE 8-6 Basal cell carcinoma before, immediately after surgery, and 6 weeks after surgery using Mohs' micrographic surgical technique. (From Habif, T.P. [1996]. *Clinical dermatology,* [3rded.]. St. Louis: Mosby.)

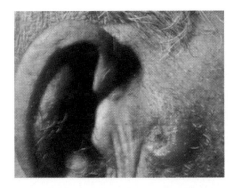

FIGURE 8-7 Squamous cell carcinoma. (From Habif, T.P. [1996]. *Clinical dermatology,* [3rd ed.]. St. Louis: Mosby.)

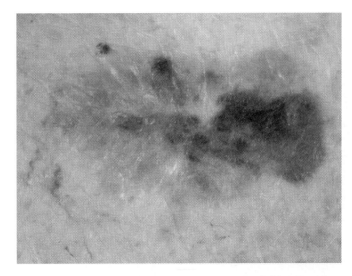

FIGURE 8-8 Lentigo malignant melanoma. (From Habif, T.P. [1996]. *Clinical dermatology,* [3rd ed.]. St. Louis: Mosby.)

Pressure Ulcer Staging

Stage 1

Nonblanchable erythema of intact skin; the heralding lesion of skin ulceration. Discoloration of skin, warmth, or hardness may also be indicators.

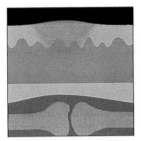

Stage 3

Full-thickness skin loss involving damage or necrosis of subcutaneous tissue that may extend down to, but not through, underlying fascia. The ulcer presents clinically as a deep crater with or without undermining of adjacent tissue.

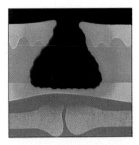

Stage 2

Partial-thickness skin loss involving epidermis and/or dermis. The ulcer is superficial and presents clinically as an abrasion, blister, or shallow crater.

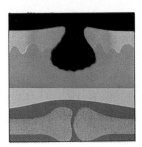

Stage 4

Full-thickness skin loss with extensive destruction, tissue necrosis, or damage to muscle, bone, or supporting structures (eg, tendon, joint capsule).

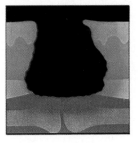

FIGURE 8-9 Stages of a pressure ulcer. (From the National Pressure Ulcer Advisory Panel and the Agency for Health Care Policy and Research.)

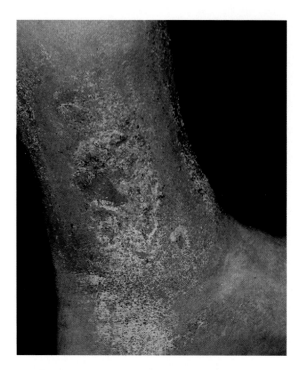

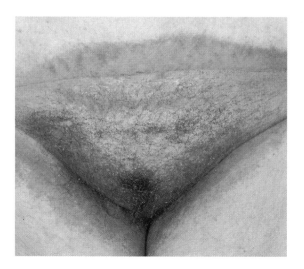

FIGURE 8-11 Candida intertrigo. (From Habif, T.P. [1996]. *Clinical dermatology,* [3rd ed.]. St. Louis: Mosby.)

FIGURE 8-10 Venous stasis ulcer. (From Habif, T.P. [1996]. *Clinical dermatology,* [3rd ed.]. St. Louis: Mosby.)

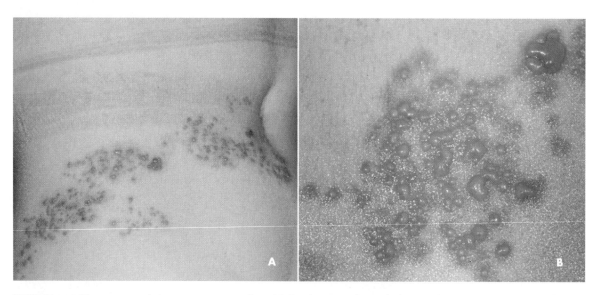

FIGURE 8-12 Herpes zoster. *A,* A common presentation with involvement of a single thoracic dermatome. *B,* A group of vesicles that vary in size. Vesicles of herpes simplex are a uniform size. (From Habif, T.P. [1996]. *Clinical dermatology,* [3rd ed.]. St. Louis: Mosby.)

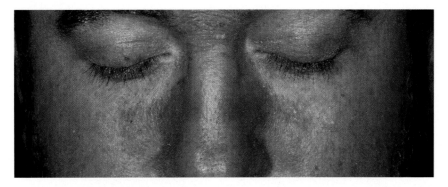

FIGURE 8-13 Seborrheic dermatitis. (From Habif, T.P. [1996]. *Clinical dermatology,* [3ʳᵈed.]. St. Louis: Mosby.)

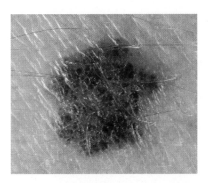

FIGURE 8-14 Dermal nevus. Surface speckling. Examination of the surface of this pigmented lesion with a hand lens reveals uniform speckling over the surface, a characteristic of a benign pigmented nevus. (From Habif, T.P. [1996]. *Clinical dermatology,* [3ʳᵈed.]. St. Louis: Mosby.)

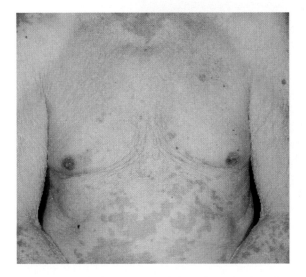

FIGURE 8-15 Vitiligo. (From Habif, T.P. [1996]. *Clinical dermatology,* [3ʳᵈed.]. St. Louis: Mosby.)

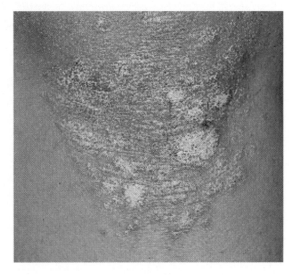

FIGURE 8-16 Psoriasis. (From Habif, T.P. [1996]. *Clinical dermatology,* [3ʳᵈed.]. St. Louis: Mosby.)

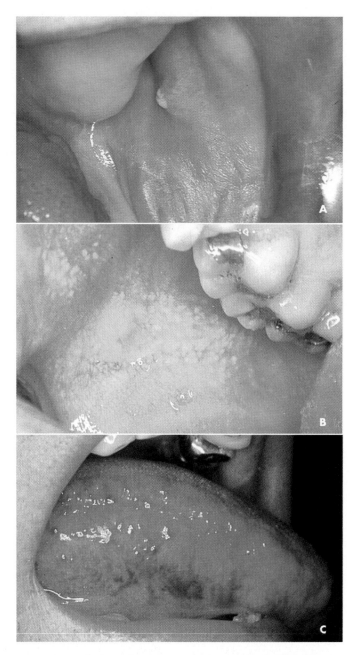

FIGURE 8-17 *A,* External pressure on the parotid gland of this client with acute bacterial sialadenitis produces pus at the parotid duct orifice. *B,* Fordyce spots–normal sebaceous glands just under the buccal mucosa. *C,* Sublingual varicosities. (From Cawson, R.A., Binnie, W.H. & Eveson, J.W. [1994] *Color atlas of oral disease: Clinical and pathologic correlations,* [2nd ed.]. London: Wolfe Publishing.)

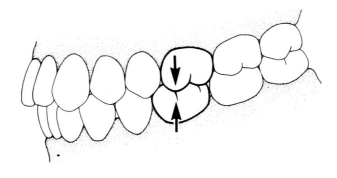

A

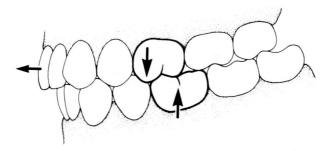

B

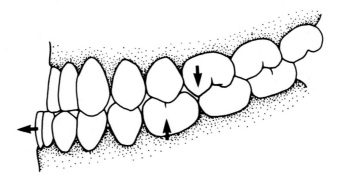

C

FIGURE 8-18 Occlusion. *A*, Class I–neutroclusion. *B*, Class II–distoclusion. *C*, Class III–mesioclusion. (From Brand, R. & Isselhard, D. [1990]. *Anatomy of orofacial structures,* [4th ed.]. St. Louis: Mosby.)

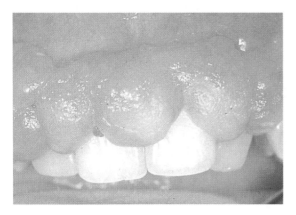

FIGURE 8-19 Phenytoin-induced gingival hyperplasia. (From Cawson, R.A., Binnie, W.H., & Eveson, J.W. [1994]. *Color atlas of oral disease: Clinical and pathologic correlations,* [2nd ed.]. London: Wolfe Publishing.)

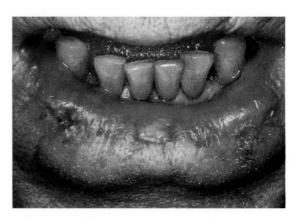

FIGURE 8-20 Squamous cell carcinoma. Several ulcerated lesions are present on the lower lip of this patient who has spent years working outdoors. (From Habif, T.P. [1996]. *Clinical dermatology,* [3rd ed.]. St. Louis: Mosby.)

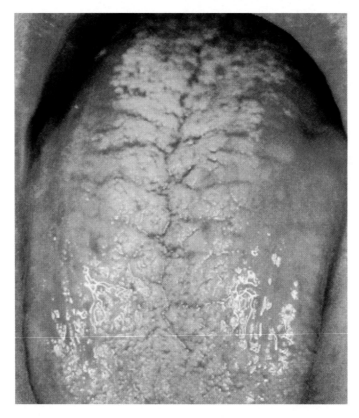

FIGURE 8-21 Oral candidiasis. (From Habif, T.P. [1996]. *Clinical dermatology,* [3rd ed.]. St. Louis: Mosby.)

Aging Alert

Three critical components of care for the older diabetic patient are exercise, diet, and medication.

patient collaboratively plan a program of care, which strongly emphasizes the self-care responsibilities of the patient, though the nurse accepts responsibility for teaching and supporting the patient in the management of diabetes. The goals of care include the following:

- Adherence to diet, exercise, and medication regimens
- Continued acquisition of knowledge about diabetes
- Maintenance of blood glucose levels within a normal range
- Prevention of DM complications

Exercise

Exercise enhances the ability of the body to use glucose, although scientists have not been able to define the mechanism by which this happens. Regular exercise improves the level of blood glucose, and it improves circulation, helps digestion, and encourages a feeling of well-being. Because of the positive effect of exercise, this aspect of treatment is strongly recommended. However, each exercise program must be individualized according to the abilities and limitations of the person. As people age, the presence of comorbidity influences treatment and care for all illnesses. From a positive standpoint, the exercise that is recommended for diabetes may also benefit the person who suffers from arthritis or from osteoporosis. In any case, however, the selection of exercises is critical. Low-impact exercises, such as walking and swimming, are usually recommended for older people and are quite

effective for them. As the older people gradually become more impaired, a home program of stretching and range-of-motion activities can be designed and taught to the patient. As with all forms of treatment, before any particular exercise program is started, the patients should be examined for any potential hazards relating to the fitness activity; they should also be advised to start slowly and to increase their level of activity very gradually.

Diet

Diet is another important factor in the care of older diabetic patients. Usually the older person has established lifelong routines and preferences for eating particular foods, in particular amounts, and at particular time intervals. Often the dietary requirements for diabetic management and control differ from those long-established eating and dietary patterns of the older diabetic patient. This aspect of diabetic care presents an immediate and major challenge to the nurse. The patient has to be convinced that adjustments in foods and dietary habits are necessary. Teaching the patient about foods and dietary habits is one challenge; an even greater challenge is to get the patient to accept and to comply with the prescribed diet and food preparation requirements. The nurse encourages the patient to believe the following: a reasonable goal is to achieve a well-balanced, consistent diet.

The food plan recommended by the American Dietetic Association (ADA) for the diabetic diet consists of wholesome food and a well-balanced selection of foods from the six food groups.

In all likelihood, patients with diabetes can eat the same food as that prepared for others in the family. However, the diabetic patient must eat the proper foods at the proper time and in the amounts recommended. The American Dietetic Association and the American Diabetes Association have prepared extensive literature about food exchanges for diabetic patients. The *food exchange* is a selection system in which the patient can choose the foods to eat at each meal from a variety of foods in each of six food groups. The following lists the food groups and the number of servings from each group to be selected for a 1500-calorie daily diet:

Food group 1: Starch and bread list   8 servings/day
Food group 2: Meat list   5 servings/day
Food group 3: Vegetable list   4 servings/day
Food group 4: Fruit list   3 servings/day
Food group 5: Milk list   2 servings/day
Food group 6: Fat list   3 servings/day

Consultation with a qualified dietitian to review food selection and to discuss food preparation can be invaluable to the diabetic patient. In fact, a positive experience related to the dietary aspect of diabetic care can sometimes make the difference in ensuring compliance that is consistent with the patient's needs and preferences, as well as specific food likes and dislikes. The variety of food choices (exchanges) available in the food exchange system can provide an arrangement of meals and snacks that will be satisfying for the patient, as well as compatible with the diabetes. See Box 9-3 for examples of food selections on each list.

If there are obstacles to the purchase or the preparation of a nutritious diet, the diabetic patient may seek the services provided by Meals on Wheels or congregate feeding programs. These programs are available to those in need of warm, nutritious meals and will assist the diabetic patient in achieving a prescribed diet regimen.

In addition to the selection and preparation of prescribed foods, the regularity of eating scheduled meals and snacks is very important for the diabetic patient. This is one means of maintaining a balanced blood glucose level.

Medication

The third essential component of self-care for the diabetic patient is medication, though diet is the cornerstone of therapy, and control of the blood glucose level by adjustment of diet is often the treatment of choice. In some instances diabetic patients can comply with a prescribed diet and can keep blood glucose levels within normal limits through food adjustment alone.

Type I (IDDM) diabetic patients Though diet, exercise, and medication are crucial to both types of diabetic patients, some differences between the two should be addressed. Type I (IDDM) diabetic patients require careful instruction and regular support to learn about insulin administration. Monitoring and support must be provided for the IDDM patient for as long as necessary if the patient is to become able to function independently in giving the subcutaneous injections of insulin on a daily basis. Clear instructions and patient demonstrations of the technique of insulin administration will enable the patient to achieve self-care and will reassure the patient and the caregiver that self-care is a reasonable, positive goal in health care.

When the type and dosage of insulin have been prescribed, the nurse assumes responsibility for teaching the patient the technique of administering the medication and making the needed regular observations. The diabetic patient must know how to detect or monitor two conditions, and how to respond if they are detected: hyperglycemia and hypoglycemia.

Hyperglycemia is a state of high blood sugar that occurs when the patient has too much food or too little insulin. Symptoms include extreme thirst, increased urination, itching, drowsiness, headache, and sometimes nausea. The onset of this complication is rather gradual. Blood glucose tests reveal a high blood glucose level. The physician should be called in the case of this reaction.

Hypoglycemia is a state of low blood sugar that occurs when the patient has too little food, too much insulin (or oral hypoglycemic medication), or too much exercise. Symptoms include shaking, tachycardia (fast heartbeat), sweating, dizziness, and hunger. The onset of this complication is sudden, and tests will reveal a very low blood glucose level. As soon as symptoms of hypoglycemia appear, the patient should drink a

BOX 9-3 SELECTED FOODS ON THE EXCHANGE LIST

Starch and bread list (One-half cup of cereal, grain, or pasta is one exchange; a 1-oz bread product is one exchange.)

Cereals, grains, and pasta
    Bran flakes .... ½ cup
    Cooked cereals .... ½ cup
    Grits (cooked) .... ½ cup
    Pasta (cooked) .... ½ cup
    Rice (cooked) .... ⅓ cup
Dried beans, peas, and lentils
    Beans and peas (cooked) .... ⅓ cup
    Lentils (cooked) .... ⅓ cup
    Baked beans .... ¼ cup
    Chick peas .... ⅓ cup
Starchy vegetables
    Corn .... ½ cup
    Corn on cob—6 inches long 1
    Lima beans .... ½ cup
    Potato—baked .... 1 small (3 oz)
    Potato—mashed .... ½ cup
    Squash—winter .... 1 cup
Bread
    Bagel .... ½ (1 oz)
    English muffin .... ½
    Pita—6 inches across .... ½
    Pumpernickel, rye .... 1 slice (1 oz)
    White .... 1 slice (1 oz)

Meat list (The list is divided into three parts, depending on the amount of fat and calories: lean, medium fat, and high fat. The following exchanges are taken from the lean meat list.)

Beef .... 1 oz
    Ground round, flank steak, tenderloin, chipped beef
Pork .... 1 oz
    Fresh ham, lean pork
Veal .... 1 oz
    Cutlets, chops, roasts
Poultry .... 1 oz
    Chicken, turkey
Fish
    All fresh or frozen fish .... 1 oz
    Oysters .... 6 medium
    Tuna—canned in water .... ¼ cup
Cheese .... ¼ cup
    Any cottage cheese
Other .... 1½ oz
    95% fat-free luncheon meat

Continued

BOX 9-3 SELECTED FOODS ON THE EXCHANGE LIST—cont'd

Vegetable list (Serving size for one vegetable exchange is ½ cup of cooked vegetables, 1 cup of raw vegetables.)

Asparagus	Beets
Beans—green, wax	Cabbage
Carrots	Sauerkraut
Eggplant	Spinach (cooked)
Leeks	Tomato—1 large
Onion	Turnips
Peppers—green	Zucchini (cooked)

Fruit list

Apple—raw, 2 inches across	1
Applesauce—unsweetened	½ cup
Banana—9 inches long	½
Cantaloupe—5 inches across	⅓
Grapefruit	½ medium
Grapes	15 small
Orange—2½ inches across	1
Pear	1 small
Strawberries—raw, whole	1¼ cup

Juice

Cranberry juice cocktail	⅓ cup
Orange juice	½ cup
Pineapple juice	½ cup
Prune juice	⅓ cup

Milk list

Skim milk	1 cup
½% milk	1 cup
1% milk	1 cup
Lowfat buttermilk	1 cup
Plain nonfat yogurt	8 oz
Whole milk	1 cup

Fat list

Unsaturated fats

Margarine	1 tsp
Mayonnaise	1 tsp

Nuts and seeds

Almonds	6 whole
Pecans	2 whole
Peanuts	20 small
Walnuts	2 whole
Olives	10 small

Saturated fats

Butter	1 tsp
Bacon	1 slice
Coconut—shredded	2 tbsp
Cream—light, coffee	2 tbsp
Cream—sour	2 tbsp

Adapted from American Diabetic Association and American Dietetic Association. (1989). *Exchange lists—For meal planning.* Virginia and Illinois: Author.

glass of orange juice (8 oz) or should eat several (about five or six) Lifesavers, one or two pieces of medium-sized hard candy, or 2 tsp of sugar or honey. With this prescribed treatment, the blood sugar levels usually return to normal within 20 to 30 minutes. When the symptoms have disappeared, the patient may appreciate having a glass of milk and a peanut butter sandwich if mealtime is not near.

IDDM patients are urged to wear an identification bracelet or to carry an identification card to notify appropriate people of the diabetic condition and insulin dependency. It is also important for IDDM patients to carry extra carbohydrate supplies with them at all times so that they can respond if symptoms of hypoglycemia appear.

Type II (NIDDM) diabetic patients   Type II (NIDDM) diabetic patients are also challenged to maintain blood glucose levels within a normal range, and they, too, need to comply with adjustments in food intake. Often, NIDDM patients are coping with an obesity problem, too, so guidance in weight reduction, as well as blood glucose control, is provided. Usually, NIDDM patients are treated with one of the sulfonylureas; these are chemical compounds that have been available to diabetic patients as oral medications since 1956. Their purpose is to stimulate insulin secretion, and if the response to these drugs is positive, patients can maintain adequate control of their diabetes with just the oral medication. The majority of diabetes patients enjoy a good response to these drugs, and this method of maintaining a normal blood glucose level has been welcomed by many diabetic patients. Regular monitoring of blood glucose levels, regular examinations to detect potential complications of diabetes, and strict adherence to prescribed diets are essential to successful control of this complex illness.

Family support

Older patients face a unique challenge in exercising control over this health problem. Some people experience diminished vision as they age, so the selection of food in the grocery store and the preparation of food at home present potential problems. Diabetic patients must carefully read food labels to determine the ingredients so that they do not buy foods that have unwanted sugar. Most diabetic patients who have recently received their diagnosis find it difficult to change from their accustomed food patterns, having to adjust or even delete some favorite recipes from their diets. Caregivers of older adults can support the older diabetic patient during the days when these adaptations are being made. Patients, families, and caregivers should be encouraged to give the assistance needed during the early days of adjusting to the illness, which will aid the compliant, interested, and motivated patient in assuming self-care.

EVALUATION

The liaison between the diabetic patient and the nurse is never ending. Positive management and control of DM depends on conscientious attention to diet, exercise, and medications. The nurse remains available to the patient, as needed, and also schedules regular meetings with the patient, to reassess patient needs and to reinforce information about diabetes and about specific self-care activities. The nurse thoroughly evaluates the extent to which specific patient problems have been and are being resolved according to the nursing diagnoses that were established at the outset of care.

The nurse assumes a heavy responsibility for teaching the DM patient how to provide the self-care that is required for DM management and why it is essential. The nurse must diligently assess the patient's need for information, as well as the patient's ability and intention to adhere to the prescriptive plan that is offered. "Nursing is a primary force for helping older [diabetic] persons comply with programs designed to enhance their health status" (Dellasega, 1990).

With adequate instruction, reasonable support, and sincere help, the older diabetic patient can usually manage the exercise, diet, and medication self-care of the diabetic regimen. The nurse provides information about these aspects of diabetes treatment so that the patient will know about the health problem and will know what to do, how to do it, and when to do it. Determining the secret to compliance for each individual patient will be a continuing challenge for those who are caregivers for older adults with diabetes.

DM poses one of the most challenging health care problems with which many older patients are coping. Whether the condition is that of IDDM or NIDDM, it usually requires major adjustments in the patient's lifestyle. The patient who has recently received the diagnosis of DM must learn to maintain an ideal body weight, must learn to regulate blood glucose levels through dietary adjustment and/or medication administration, must learn the technical skill of self-administration of insulin, and must learn to engage in activities and exercises on a regularly scheduled basis, all of which require deliberate attention and planning. Many activities of daily living (ADLs) that were performed automatically and without deliberate planning in the past now require careful consideration to ensure that all aspects of diabetic self-care are included in the activities of each day. In their effort to prevent the complications that are known to accompany increased blood glucose levels, diabetic patients are usually motivated to learn all that they need to know about diabetes and about self-care requirements. With assistance and support from nurses who know about diabetic care, most patients can successfully cope with the diagnosis of DM. Those patients who have difficulty adhering to the prescribed care regimen present a major but not impossible challenge to the nurse.

■ Temperature

COMMON HEALTH DEVIATION: DIFFICULTY IN TEMPERATURE REGULATION

Temperature is controlled through the processes of sweating, shivering, vasoconstriction, vasodilation, and hypothalamic and nervous system functions. Difficulties in temperature regulation in older adults are probably related to an increasing inability to respond adequately to change in temperature and a narrowing of homeostatic mechanisms (Abrass, 1994). Shivering decreases in older adults (Collins et al., 1981), as does the function of their sweat glands (Balin, 1990). Decreased sensitivity, sedentary lifestyle, and disorders of the cardiovascular, endocrine, and nervous systems all contribute to the vulnerability of the older person to experiencing *hypothermia* (low body temperature) or *hyperthermia* (high body temperature) (Natsume et al., cited in Abrass, 1994).

Hypothermia

Many older adults may unknowingly be quite susceptible to developing a mild hypothermia, which, unrecognized, may progress to a more severe condition. During the winter season, hypothermia, which is underreported and underdiagnosed, contributes to morbidity and, to a lesser extent, to mortality in the older adult population (MacLean & Emslie-Smith, 1977; Rango, 1984). There is evidence that in the older adult population, hypothermia (core body temperature less than 34° C) occurs during the winter season in northern climates such as in Great Britain, Canada, and the northern United States. Two large-scale surveys were conducted in Great Britain among older adults who lived in private or family homes (outside of acute care or nursing home settings), and the results demonstrated that 10% of the subjects had experienced some degree of hypothermia (Fox et al., 1973).

Because body fat contributes to the body's ability to insulate itself against the cold, thin older men are at high risk for developing hypothermia (Thorne & Wahren, 1990). Furthermore, malnutrition caused by mental confusion, homelessness, or chronic alcohol abuse increases the risk of hypothermia. These alterations, along with drugs that interfere with normal thermoregulation, account for older adults' poor adjustment to extremes in environmental temperature.

A particularly hazardous behavior in cold weather is the ingestion of alcohol. The use of alcohol blocks the vasoconstrictive response to cold and actually makes a person physically colder, contrary to the perceived sense of warmth. Factors that predispose an older adult to hypothermia are extremes of temperature (although hypothermia can occur in moderate temperatures), poor or no housing, malnutrition, increased age, multiple diseases, alcohol use, and impaired mental functioning (Robbins, 1989).

■ Nursing Process

ASSESSMENT

During a period of cold weather, when an older patient with a history of exposure to the cold or with a history of poor socioeconomic living conditions seeks treatment, the nurse caring for the patient considers the possibility of hypothermia. The older person in the early stages of hypothermia may appear fatigued, complain of weakness, have cool skin, and exhibit signs of confusion.

Early symptoms of severe hypothermia may be increased confusion and increased sensation of being cold. Consciousness is usually lost when the body temperature descends to between 30° and 28° C. The most important clinical sign is the recording of low body temperature.

NURSING DIAGNOSIS

Hypothermia related to exposure to a cold environment is evidenced by body temperature of less than 34° C and altered mental state.

PLANNING AND GOAL IDENTIFICATION

A long-term goal is that the patient will be knowledgeable concerning risk factors of hypothermia and will engage in health-promoting activities. A short-term goal is that the patient will be monitored closely until body temperature returns to the normal range.

IMPLEMENTATION

The first aspect of treatment is to remove the patient from the cold environment. If clothing is wet, it should be removed immediately and the patient should be covered top and bottom with

Aging Alert

- Older adults need protection from extremes of temperature.
- Exposure to a cold environment is especially hazardous for older people if they are malnourished, dehydrated, or wearing inadequate clothing.
- Exposure to a very warm environment can result in heat stroke for the older person.
- Ingestion of alcohol and/or medications can contribute to hypothermia or hyperthermia in the older person.

blankets. Care needs to be taken when moving these patients, because rough handling may cause arrhythmias. In mild hypothermia (32° to 34° C), treatment consists of passive warming and monitoring. More severe hypothermia is a medical emergency and requires hospitalization of the patient. Mortality for severe hypothermia is 50% or higher in older adult populations. Underlying infections are a frequent condition in older patients admitted to the hospital with hypothermia (Darowski et al., 1991).

Prevention of hypothermia is the best treatment. In the winter, any older adult who is at risk for hypothermia requires indoor temperatures that are higher than 70° F. Good nutrition, increased fluid intake, decreased alcohol intake, and adequate clothing will help protect the older person from hypothermia (McGough, 1983). Many older adults in the homeless population of large cities in the United States are at risk for hypothermia during severe winter weather.

EVALUATION

The determination of successful treatment of hypothermia is based on the clinical sign of body temperature readings that range above 34° C, and on the older patient's exhibiting diminished symptoms of confusion and sensations of cold. The need to decrease the threat of recurring hypothermia may call for a change in the living arrangements of the older person, and social services may be the appropriate referral. The care of the older person is a team effort, and all members of the health care team are utilized to bring about optimal care and to ensure the return to health of the older person.

Hyperthermia

Over 3000 deaths occur on a yearly basis in people over 60 years of age as a direct result of heat stroke. The degrees of heat illness can range from a mild state (heat exhaustion), in which symptoms include muscle cramps and volume depletion, to the more severe state of heat stroke (Robbins, 1989). Heat exhaustion often occurs when a person has engaged in exercise during days of extreme temperature and high humidity.

Hyperthermia or "heat stroke," is defined as an acute condition in which body temperature rises above 40.6° C (105° F) (Abrass, 1994). Heat stroke in the older adult is usually nonexertional and occurs in a warm climate. Death from heat stroke is not an element of the past. Studies done in the 1980s reported that in the 1984 New York City heat wave, deaths increased by almost 50% in people 75 years old and over. Women were more prone to succumbing to heat stroke than men by a three-to-two margin in heat waves in New York, St. Louis, and Georgia (Centers for Disease Control, 1984; Hope et al., 1984). A more recent experience was the heat wave of 1995 in Chicago, in which large numbers of deaths of older adults stunned the city and the nation.

The major causes of heat stroke are (1) impairment of heat loss caused by diminished sweating or the absence of sweating and (2) environmental factors. Physiologic age-related changes, disease processes, and extremes in climate all contribute to the increased risk of heat stroke in the older person. Often, cardiovascular disease in the older person is aggravated during a time of intense humidity and heat. The older person may not be physically able to respond to the stress caused by the heat wave, and death may result.

Risk factors for heat stroke are being older, being female, living alone, being mentally confused, having poor sensitivity to temperature changes, being alcoholic, having heart disease or diabetes, having reduced fluid intake, and taking tranquilizers and anticholinergic drugs (Abrass, 1994).

■ Nursing Process

ASSESSMENT

The older patient who has an elevated temperature may not be recognized as suffering from heat illness. The elevated temperature may be attributed to another factor, such as an infection. Factors that contribute to occurrence of heat illness are a prolonged heat wave, a history of exposure (such as a broken air conditioner during a heat wave), and a sensation of being warm. The patient may complain of general nonspecific types of symptoms, which can include headache, dizziness, and weakness.

Heat stroke is a serious, life-threatening condition and is manifested by classic signs and symptoms; loss of consciousness, headache, weakness, nausea, and hot skin with an elevated body temperature are the signs that will lead the clinician to consider heat stroke. The complications of heat stroke are severe and often lead to death if not corrected quickly.

NURSING DIAGNOSIS

Hyperthermia related to exposure to extreme temperature and depletion of fluid volume is evidenced by a temperature of 40.6° C.

PLANNING AND GOAL IDENTIFICATION

Long-term goals include the following: (1) the patient will be knowledgeable concerning the importance of hydration and the risks of exposure to extremes of temperature, and (2) the patient will also engage in health-promoting behaviors that reduce the risk of hyperthermia. A short-term goal is that the patient will be monitored and treated appropriately until temperature returns to the normal range.

IMPLEMENTATION

Hyperthermia is considered a medical emergency and requires immediate hospitalization and treatment that will lower body temperature. Treatment consists of lowering the body temperature—through cold water sponging of the body surface or through baths. The core body temperature should be brought to 39° C (102° F) within the first treatment hour (Abrass, 1994). There is a significant risk of shock, and many older adults do not survive an episode of severe hyperthermia. Constant monitoring is an essential nursing action during this emergency situation.

EVALUATION

Evaluation is a continuous, patient-centered, goal-oriented process. Determination of the successful achievement of the short-range goal of restoring the older person to a normal temperature range is the first step in the evaluative process. The long-term goal of educating the patient, the family, and the community is a joint goal of all health professionals.

Evaluation of achievement of the long-term goal will focus on the nurse's particular patient population: the individual patient, if the nurse has been the provider for a particular patient with hyperthermia; the nursing home residents, if the nurse is the director of nursing in a nursing home; the community, if the nurse is a public health nurse in a particular community; and the nation, if the nurse is a consultant to the federal government. Evaluation of nursing care provides a systematic, empirically based method for appraisal of interventions and for the development of standards of care that are recognized by the profession and by society as effective and appropriate for special populations.

HEALTH PROMOTION

The best treatment for both hypothermia and hyperthermia is prevention. The nurse must increase the awareness of older adults regarding their physical vulnerability to extremes of environmental temperature. The nurse's educational focus for the prevention of heat illnesses is on teaching older adults and their caregivers to engage in appropriate behaviors during warm weather, such as decreasing exercise, increasing intake of fluids, avoiding alcohol, and wearing loose-fitting clothing.

■ Infections

The risk of acquiring a serious infection increases as people age. Older adults have poorer outcomes from the treatment of infections and subsequently have higher rates of morbidity and mortality than do younger people. This section of the chapter discusses age-related changes in the body's defense system; other physical, social, and environmental factors that contribute to the increased risk of infection; and the nursing care of the older person who is at risk for infection.

THE BODY'S DEFENSE SYSTEM
First lines of defense

The mechanical barriers of the skin and the mucous membranes are the first lines of human defense against noxious agents. Once these barriers are broken and penetrated, the human body can activate two other intrinsic mechanisms to protect the person: the inflammatory process and the immune response. These are part of the body's reaction whenever cells or tissues are injured or a foreign material is introduced into body tissue.

Inflammatory process

The inflammatory process is an acute, immediate, generalized response to cell injury, which results in vasodilation and delivery of fluid and cellular material to the damaged area. The cardinal manifestations of inflammation, although muted in older adults, are redness, heat, pain, swelling, and altered function. The role of the inflammatory process is to localize, destroy, and remove injurious agents to allow for the healing process to occur.

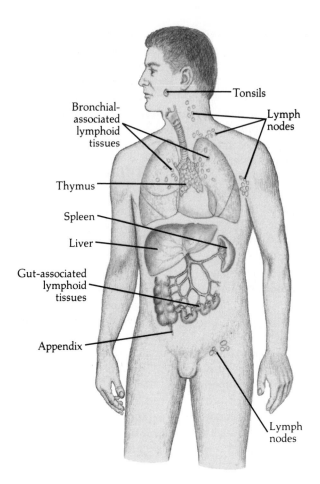

FIGURE 9-1 Organization of the immune system. (From Thompson, J.M. et al. [1993]. *Mosby's clinical nursing* [3rd ed.]. St. Louis: Mosby.)

Immune response

The immune system is a complex organization of groups of cells and tissues that function to protect the body against invasion by microorganisms, to maintain internal homeostasis, and to guard against the development of tumor cells (Thompson et al., 1993) (Figure 9-1). The immune response can be one of two types: humoral immune response or cell-mediated immune reaction. Both types of immune response are activated by the introduction of antigens into the body. *Antigens* are usually protein structures that exist as part of the complex organization of bacteria, viruses, or foreign living tissues. Immunoglobulin antibodies are formed as part of the humoral immune response to attack those antigens. Cellular immunity, a function of the cell-mediated response, occurs through the development of specifically sensitized lymphocytes. T cells (T lymphocytes) are crucial for cellular immunity, and B lymphocytes are active participants in humoral immunity. The combined immune response functions to eliminate the offending antigen. A more extensive explanation of the body's defense system is beyond the scope of this text, but the reader is advised to consult an appropriate text, if necessary, to understand the complex workings of this intricate system.

AGE-RELATED CHANGES IN THE BODY'S DEFENSE SYSTEM

There is debate in the field concerning age-related changes that are universally experienced by the human immune system. Although the older adult population shows an increase in both the number of infections and the incidence of certain diseases such as cancer, there is still not complete understanding of how age affects the immune system. There is agreement among scientists that with age there is a loss of functional cells, a decrease in the proliferation ability of T cells, a change in the ability to respond to an event, and basic changes in the pattern of response to an activation event (Adler & Nagel, 1994). There is, however, a high degree of variability of immune function among the older adult population, with some older adults having an immune function comparable to that of a younger person.

On the other hand, there is a remarkable stability in the total white count and in the number of lymphocytes of most older individuals (Adler & Nagel, 1994). One important clinical result of age-related changes in the body's defense system is a slowed response to antibiotic therapy (Yoshikawa et al., 1989). Furthermore, the element of time, the slowed response of the older immune system to events, may be the most significant factor in the increased rate of mortality and morbidity in older people. The fact remains that an older adult is more vulnerable to infection and its complications than is a younger person.

CONTRIBUTING FACTORS TO INFECTION
Physical changes

Age-related physical changes in the older person that increase susceptibility to infection are atrophic skin, decreased gastric acid, decreased pulmonary function and cough reflex, decreased mucociliary activity, and decreased elasticity of the bronchiolar musculature.

Nutrition

The nutritional status of older patients is particularly pertinent to their ability to withstand and recover from an infectious process. Depletion of protein reserves interferes with the function of the immune system. There is a consensus that serum albumin shows a steady decline throughout adult life. The normal range of serum albumin for adults is 3.8-5.0 g/dl, and the range for older adults is hypothesized to be 3.3-4.9 g/dl (Hodkinson, 1990). This age-related change might not be significant, but it is well understood that the diet of the older person is a critical factor in the prevention of and recovery from infectious illness.

Chronic disease and medications

The coexistence of chronic diseases with the need for medications that may suppress the immune response is another significant factor that affects the vulnerability of the older person to infection. Certain corticosteroid, antibiotic, nonsteroidal anti-inflammatory, and cytotoxic drugs have the potential to cause immunosuppression. Also, radiation therapy, a frequent treatment modality for cancer, destroys lymphocytes. These drugs and treatments, combined with age-related changes, decrease the ability of the older person to respond effectively to an infectious illness.

Psychosocial factors

Other factors that influence the older person's susceptibility to infection are a long history of smoking, living in an air-polluted community, having been engaged in a hazardous occupation, alcoholism, poor access to health care, and poor social support systems. In addition, mental confusion is a significant risk factor because the confused older person may not recognize signs and symptoms of a progressing infection, which may delay early detection and treatment.

The same problem of delay in seeking treatment occurs with an older adult who has an inadequate support system. Delay increases the potential for a serious infection and may be the direct result of a lack of available transportation. Gaining access to health care is difficult if there is no transportation. Usually the older person is expected to go to the health care provider, as opposed to a more reasonable treatment arrangement, which would bring the provider to the patient.

Fever

An age-related change that affects the clinical manifestation of an infection in an older adult is the increased significance of a fever. Often the older person will not have a high fever, but will have a low-grade fever that may be overlooked by the inexperienced nurse or physician. Any level of fever in an older patient is to be considered a sign of a bacterial infection until proven otherwise.

Often the older person with a serious infection may have no sign of a fever, but will show atypical signs of weakness, anorexia, and, most significantly, a change in functional status. Knowing the importance of taking an in-depth history and knowing about age-related changes that affect the well-being of the older patient are two major components of the knowledge base that guides the practice of the gerontologic nurse.

TYPES OF INFECTIONS

Infections are a leading cause of morbidity and death in those 65 years of age and older, with pneumonia and influenza being the fifth leading cause of death in this age group (U.S. Bureau of the Census, 1992). In the United States fewer than 1000 people a year die of vaccine-preventable diseases of childhood. In contrast, between 50,000 and 70,000 adults die of influenza virus infections and pneumococcal bacterial infections (National Vaccine Program, 1994). The most commonly acquired bacterial pneumonias among community-dwelling older adults are caused by *Streptococcus pneumoniae, Hemophilus influenza,* and *Mycoplasma pneumoniae.* Nosocomial pneumonias contracted in institu-tional settings are commonly caused by *Staphylococcus aureus* and by gram-negative coli such as *Escherichia coli, Klebsiella pneumoniae,* and *Pseudomonas aeruginosa.* Older adults are also particularly susceptible to pneumonia from *Legionella* and *B. catarrhalis.* Older adults also represent a disproportionally large share of reported active tuberculosis cases, primarily cases of reactivation of previous infections (Fraser, 1993).

More than 70% of the tetanus cases reported annually are in people 50 years of age or older, and nearly all of the 1 to 5 cases of diphtheria reported annually occur in unimmunized adults (*National Vaccine Program,* 1994).

Older adults are also more susceptible to urinary tract, intraabdominal, and skin and soft-tissue infections. Asymptomatic bacteriuria occurs in 20% of women over the age of 65 and in about 10% of the men (Baldasarre & Kaye, 1991). Acute diverticulitis, gastroenteritis, and appendicitis are frequent sources of intra-abdominal infections in the older adult. Alterations in skin integrity can be caused by age-related thinning of the dermis and increased susceptibility of the dermis to shear forces. Skin integrity can also be disrupted by pressure injuries, ischemia, and maceration. Immobility and fecal and urinary incontinence are major factors leading to disruption of skin integrity.

Age-related alterations in skin and mucosal barriers, decreased ciliary activity and diminished cough reflex, and decreased bone marrow reserve and diminished cellular and humoral immunity contribute to older adults' increased susceptibility to infection and increase infection-related morbidity. Diminished homeostatic reserve mechanisms, such as age-related decreased catecholamine response and decreased concentrating ability of the kidneys, also contribute to the infection-related morbidity (Fraser, 1993). The risks are even greater when malnutrition, smoking, alcohol or drug abuse, immobility, chronic disease, altered skin integrity, poor hygiene of the older adult or caregivers, and impaired cognitive function are present.

health care institutions, but such risk is still substantial. Many home care visits by the nurse are for dressing changes, and these dressings are often for a surgical wound.

The long-term goal might be that the wound will heal within 6 weeks, and the short-term goal might be to have Meals on Wheels deliver meals for 1 month. Adequate nutrition is critical for wound healing, and many older adults living alone and recuperating from hospitalizations are unable to prepare adequate meals. The need for community services is apparent, and the nurse works with the social worker to provide needed services to the older patient.

Other outcomes that may pertain to both the older adults and their caregivers include the following:

- Will be able to describe the risk of infection and potential outcomes
- Will use appropriate hand washing techniques and personal hygiene measures
- Will use only the antibiotics prescribed and in the manner prescribed
- Will have age-appropriate vaccinations
- Will wash fruits and vegetables thoroughly and use proper refrigerated storage
- Will demonstrate proper food handling and preparation techniques
- Will specify ways to minimize contact with infected individuals
- Will promptly report potential signs and symptoms of infection to the health care provider
- Will practice appropriate cleaning and maintenance procedures for humidifiers, catheters, respiratory equipment, or other devices used in daily personal care or treatment
- Will have a plan for alternative care if the caregiver develops an infection

Intervention in the private or family home

The role of the nurse as a teacher and promoter of health and well-being is a major consideration in home care nursing. The nurse assesses how the patient manages personal hygiene, and teaches the patient the importance of hand washing. Personal hygiene is an important aspect of the prevention of infection in the older person. Daily cleansing of skin, thorough drying with a clean towel, and daily use of clean, cotton undergarments decrease the likelihood of infections. The visiting home care nurse provides reassurance and support, along with the technical expertise necessary to monitor the progress of wound healing, and the ability to access community-based services.

EVALUATION

Evaluation of all nursing care is ongoing and relates to specific goals in terms of patient outcomes. For example: Was an infection prevented? Did the wound heal in the appropriate time frame? Were new methods of teaching the nursing home resident to control voiding successful? Did the patient cough and deep breathe effectively during the first 24 hours postoperatively? The answers to these kinds of questions must be legally documented in medical records. Systematic, observable evaluation must be recorded and documented appropriately.

REFERENCES

Abbey. (1990). *Diabetes care guide.* Unpublished project, Catholic University of America, School of Nursing, Adult Nurse Practitioner Program, Washington, DC.

Abrass, I.B. (1994). Disorders of temperature regulation. In W. Hazzard, et al., (Eds.), *Principles of geriatric medicine and gerontology* (2nd ed., pp. 383-412). New York: McGraw-Hill.

Adler, W., & Nagel, J. (1994). Clinical immunology. In W. Hazzard, et al., (Eds.), *Principles of geriatric medicine and gerontology* (2nd ed., pp. 60-71). New York: McGraw-Hill.

Baldasarre, J.S., & Kaye, D. (1991). Special problems of urinary tract infections in the elderly. *Medical Clinics of North America, 75*(2), 375-389.

Balin, A. (1990). Aging of the human skin. In W. Hazzard, et al., (Eds.), *Principles of geriatric medicine and gerontology* (pp. 383-412). New York: McGraw-Hill.

Blainey, C. (1986). Diabetes mellitus. In D.L. Carnevali & M. Patrick (Eds.), *Nursing management for the elderly* (2nd ed., pp. 403-422). Philadelphia: J.B. Lippincott.

Centers for Disease Control. (1984). Heat associated mortality—New York City. *Morbidity and Mortality Weekly Report, 33,* 430.

Collins, K.J., et al. (1981). Shivering thermogenesis and vasomotor responses with convective cooling in the elderly. *Journal of Physiology, 320,* 76.

Darowski, A., et al. (1991). Hypothermia and infection in elderly patients admitted to hospital. *Age Ageing, 20,* 100.

Dellasega, C. (1990, January). Self-care for the elderly diabetic. *Journal of Gerontological Nursing, 16*(1), 16-19.

Ferri, R.S. (1994). Health perception-health management pattern. In R.S. Ferri (Ed.), *Care planning for the older adult: Nursing diagnosis in long term care.* Philadelphia: W.B. Saunders.

Fisch, M.D., Jr. (1990, June). Complications of diabetes, other than those of vision, in older patients. *Aging and Vision News, 3*(1).

Fox, R.H., et al. (1973). Body temperatures in the elderly: A national study of physiological, social, and environmental conditions. *British Medical Journal, 27,* 200-206.

Fraser, D. (1993). Patient assessment: Infection in the elderly. *Journal of Gerontological Nursing, 19*(7), 5-11.

Goldberg, A.P., Andres, R., & Bierman, E.L. (1990). Diabetes mellitus in the elderly. In W. Hazzard, et al., (Eds.), *Principles of geriatric medicine and gerontology* (pp. 60-71). New York: McGraw-Hill.

Gregerman, R., & Katz, M. (1994). Thyroid diseases. In W. Hazzard, et al. (Eds.), *Principles of geriatric medicine and gerontology* (2nd ed., pp. 719-737). New York: McGraw-Hill.

Hodkinson, H.M. (1990). Alterations of laboratory findings. In W. Hazzard, et al. (Eds.), *Principles of geriatric medicine and gerontology* (pp. 241-244). New York: McGraw-Hill.

Hope, W., et al. (1984). Illness and death due to environmental heat: Georgia and St. Louis. 1983. Leads from the MMWR. *Journal of the American Medical Association, 252,* 209.

MacLean, D., & Emslie-Smith, D. (1977). *Accidental hypothermia.* London: Blackwell Scientific.

McKee, P.A., et al. (1971). The natural history of congestive heart failure: The Framingham Study. *New England Journal of Medicine, 285,* 1441.

Mersey, J. (1989). Diabetes mellitus in the elderly patient. In W. Reichel (Ed.), *Clinical aspects of aging.* Baltimore: Williams & Wilkins.

National Vaccine Program. (1994). *Adult immunization: A report by the National Advisory Committee.* Atlanta: U.S. Department of Health and Human Services, Public Health Service, Centers for Disease Control and Prevention.

Palmer, M.A. (1990). Care of the older surgical patient. In C. Eliopoulos (Ed.), *Caring for the elderly in diverse care settings.* Philadelphia: J.B. Lippincott.

Radak, J.T., Jewler, D., & Steinburg, C. (1990, September). Finding more clues. *Diabetes Forecast, 43*(9), 31-38.

Rango, N. (1984). Exposure-related hypothermia mortality in the United States 1970-79. *American Journal of Public Health, 74,* 1159.

Robbins, A. (1989). Hypothermia and heat stroke: Protecting the elderly patient. *Geriatrics, 44*(1), 73-80.

Saviteer, S., Samsa, G., & Rutale, W. (1988). Nosocomial infections in the elderly: Increased risk per hospital day. *American Journal of Medicine, 84,* 661.

Shapiro, et al. (1991). The protective efficacy of polyvalent pneumococcal polysaccharide vaccine. *New England Journal of Medicine, 325,* 1506.

Solomon, B.I. (1980, September). Symposium on endocrine disorders: Foreword. *Nursing Clinics of North America, 15*(3), 433-434.

Stolley, J.M., & Buckwalter, K.C. (1991). Iatrogenesis in the elderly: Nosocomial infections. *Journal of Gerontological Nursing, 17*(9), 30-34.

Terpenning, M.S., & Bradley, S.F. (1991). Why aging leads to increased susceptibility to infection. *Geriatrics, 46*(2), 77-80.

Terry, L., & Halter, J. (1994). Aging of the endocrine system. In W. Hazzard, et al. (Eds.), *Principles of geriatric medicine and gerontology.* New York: McGraw-Hill.

Thompson, J.M., et al. (1993). *Mosby's clinical nursing.* St. Louis: Mosby.

Thorne, A., & Wahren, J. (1990). Diminished meal-induced thermogenesis in elderly men. *Clinical Physiology, 10,* 427.

U.S. Bureau of the Census. (1992). *Sixty-five plus in America.* (Current Population Reports, Special Studies P-23-178RV.) Washington, DC: U.S. Government Printing Office.

U.S. Department of Health and Human Services, Public Health Service. (1991). *Healthy People 2000: National health promotion and disease prevention objectives: Full report, with commentary.* Washington, DC: U.S. Government Printing Office.

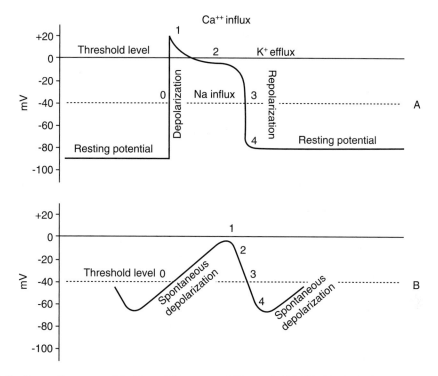

FIGURE 10-3 Cardiac action potential. (From Thompson, J.M., et al. [1993]. *Mosby's clinical nursing* [3rd ed.]. St Louis: Mosby.)

length of the cardiac muscle fiber. Preload, which is the length of the stretch of the cardiac muscle fiber, and stroke volume create the Frank-Starling curve. Blood volume, HR, SV, and peripheral resistance all contribute to the shape of the Frank-Starling curve. As one ages, the cardiac muscle begins to lose its ability to stretch and rebound as it becomes more like a worn-out elastic band, predisposing a person to congestive heart failure (CHF).

The peripheral vascular system is composed of arteries, capillaries, and veins. The oxygenated blood flows from the left ventricle of the heart into highly elastic arteries of the body, which are able to distend because of increased pressure. Constriction and dilatation of the arteries control blood flow as the body's needs change. The

arterial system holds 20% of the blood volume. Capillaries are the smallest vessels, in which the exchange of the oxygen, nutrients, and waste products occurs. The venous system collects the blood from the capillaries to return it to the heart. The venous system holds approximately 60% of the blood volume and has the ability to distend and compress as the body's needs change. One-way valves assist the veins in moving blood from the arms and legs back to the heart. Like the cardiac system described earlier, the peripheral vascular system responds to changes brought about by the autonomic nervous system and chemical agents such as drugs.

The function of the cardiovascular system is influenced by many factors. As one ages, the response to these factors is altered. The condition of an aged heart, as well as other factors such as blood volume, determines the level at which the heart will function. The following section describes the age-related changes that occur.

■ Age-Related Changes

In general, the most common change in the cardiovascular and peripheral vascular system associated with increased age is a stiffening of structures. These structural changes affect the function of both the heart and the peripheral vascular system. Lipofuscin, a yellow-brown granular material, accumulates in the myocardial cell, and amyloid deposits are seen extracellularly. As in other areas of the body, collagen and lipid deposits increase intercellularly in the heart muscle, resulting in different degrees of ventricular hypertrophy (Kenney, 1989). This decreases left ventricular (LV) stretch (compliance). The valves of the heart also become thicker and more rigid as a result of calcification. The mitral and aortic valves are most affected because of their exposure to high pressures in the vascular system. In addition, in the conduction system, the SA node is infiltrated by fat and connective tissue, resulting in a decrease in the heart's ability to regulate the rate of the sinus node, also causing a slowing of electrical impulses through the AV tissue. There is a 10% decrease in the number of pacemaker cells in the SA node by age 75 (Gawlinski & Jensen, 1991). Many of the arrhythmias seen in the older person are a result of either the decrease in pacemaker cells or the infiltration of fat in the SA node.

These physiologic and biochemical changes affect the heart's performance. Even though the resting heart rate only modestly decreases with age, there is a significant decrease in the maximum heart rate that can be achieved with exercise. Also, there is a slight increase in preload, a decline in SV, a prolonged relaxation contraction phase, and a 50% reduction in LV filling caused by stiffness (Wenger, 1992).

Data from the Baltimore longitudinal study suggests that the cardiac output during exercise remains unchanged with age. Because of the delay in diastolic filling time, there is more time for the ventricles to fill. This helps to offset, to some extent, the stroke volume decrease that occurs because of stiffening of the left ventricle. These changes associated with increased age are particularly notable when the cardiovascular system is challenged. First, the aging cardiovascular system becomes less responsive to increases in work load and has a diminished reserve capacity for managing high levels of stress. Second, resting myocardium oxygen consumption is reduced by approximately 1% per year as one ages, resulting in a decrease in exercise tolerance. The measurement of myocardium oxygen consumption is commonly used to determine functional status. Lastly, it has been shown that older people's response to beta stimulation induced by drugs or the autonomic nervous system is also decreased. A regular exercise program has been shown to improve exercise tolerance in older adults (Shephard, 1993).

The effect of normal aging on the peripheral vascular system is arterial stiffening. Vascular changes occur because of cross-linking of collagen, causing a thicker and less elastic vessel. This is related to changes in the subendothelial vascular layer, which becomes thickened with connective tissue. Fragmentation of elastin and calcification occur within the media of the vessels and contribute to increased rigidity. These changes are independent of atherosclerosis and hypertension. Generally, there is an increase in resistance in the vascular system, and the baroreceptor in the arterial tree becomes less sensitive to pressure changes (Wenger, 1992).

Overall, the age-related changes in the cardiovascular system increase the probability of disease. The rate of change with age will affect the progression of cardiovascular disease in varied and unique ways. The individual's adaptive capacity will also influence the manifestation of disease. For instance, one person with arterial

Aging Alert

1. The line between normal aging processes and disease is difficult to delineate.
2. The normal aging heart has a diminished capacity to manage high levels of stress.
3. Lifestyle influences cardiovascular function.

insufficiency may develop significant collateral circulation in the lower extremities and experience little discomfort, whereas another with the same degree of blockage in major peripheral arteries will not develop collateral circulation sufficient to prevent claudication.

The major age-related cardiovascular and peripheral vascular changes are a result of the interaction of several factors. As the vessels become thick, they are less able to respond to stressors such as illness, medications, and exercise. The following sections will review unique characteristics of common health deviations, focus on the older adult's cardiovascular and peripheral vascular concerns, and outline health promotion criteria for this population.

■ Common Health Deviations

ATHEROSCLEROSIS AND CORONARY ARTERY DISEASE

Atherosclerosis is the most commonly used term for thickening and hardening of the arteries. This condition is the leading cause of coronary obstruction, otherwise known as coronary artery disease (CAD). It is also the leading cause of death in the United States for the age group over 65 years; over 80% of all CAD is found in people over 65. Atherosclerosis is the process that leads to ischemic events. It appears to begin early in

life and progresses over the years. After menopause, women have the same rate of disease as men. Clinical manifestations of atherosclerosis of the coronary arteries include warning signs and symptoms of angina pectoris or myocardial infarction (MI), resulting in damaged heart muscle. Atherosclerosis is the common pathologic cause that leads not only to CAD but also to hypertension, stroke, renal failure, and peripheral vascular disease. These organ dysfunctions are the result of limited blood supply caused by narrowing of the arteries by atheromatous plaque. Generally, symptoms of CAD are not experienced until the vessel lumen is reduced by 50% or more. CAD is suspected in individuals who have positive cardiac risk factors such as male gender, being a postmenopausal woman, history of cigarette smoking, hypertension, hyperlipidemia, obesity, diabetes mellitus, or a family history of heart disease. Recently, physical inactivity, increased emotional stress, and type A personality have been identified as positive risk factors for CAD. Individuals who manifest signs of atherosclerotic disease elsewhere, such as those with a history of stroke or peripheral vascular disease, are likely to have CAD as well.

Many older adults, even though they may have CAD, are not symptomatic, possibly because they are sedentary or bedridden. The activity that would ordinarily produce anginal symptoms is simply not undertaken. However, symptoms may still appear if they are active or if there is a challenge, such as an infection. Angina pectoris, which is the symptomatic pain associated with the constriction of coronary arteries, is the same in the older adult population as in the younger population. However, the major complaint that drives a person to seek medical attention may be shortness of breath, syncope, sweating, or heart palpitation during exertion, rather than the traditional substernal chest tightness relieved with rest. As with angina pectoris, the older adult does not usually complain of classic symptoms for an acute myocardial infarction. The symptoms frequently reported are confusion, syncope, vertigo, weakness, progressive shortness of breath, abdominal pain, and cough. Other explanations for the lack of stated symptoms of pain are that there may be an altered pain sensation, or that the older adult may dismiss the pain as something that is normal and expected with age.

To prevent the progression of CAD, risk factor modification is the treatment of choice. Factors such as age, gender, and genetics cannot be altered, but the reversible risk factors can be reduced. There is evidence to suggest that there can be some regression of atherosclerosis with treatment (Gamble, 1994). However, the best situation is for steps to be taken early in life to prevent atherosclerosis.

Primary prevention includes a lifestyle of regular exercise, maintenance of ideal body weight, no tobacco use, limited alcohol use, a low-fat, low-cholesterol, and low-salt diet and stress reduction techniques. Secondary prevention includes screening methods, such as blood pressure (BP) measurements and cholesterol testing, to determine those at risk for CAD. Once CAD risk factors, such as elevated blood pressure, are identified, a person can control the risk factor to prevent disease progression. Other risk factor modification programs include decreasing cholesterol levels, participating in a smoking cessation program, adhering to a low-fat, low-cholesterol, and low-salt diet, and participating in a formalized exercise program (Box 10-1).

There is strong evidence that controlling one's serum cholesterol, decreasing low-density lipoprotein (LDL), and increasing high-density lipoprotein (HDL) reduce the risk of CAD. The damage from hypercholesteremia begins in middle age and continues to progress as one ages, resulting in CAD. Based on current studies, it is believed that hypercholesteremia levels of over 240 in older adults constitute a risk factor for CAD. It is recommended that all adults strive to meet the guidelines set by the National Heart, Lung, and Blood Institute's National Cholesterol Education Program (Table 10-1).

BOX 10-1 CARDIOVASCULAR RISK FACTOR PROFILE

Family history of heart disease
Sex
    Male (35 to 55 years)
    Female (over 50 years or after menopause)
Hypertension
Smoking
Excessive weight or obesity
Elevated serum level of lipids and fats
Diabetes mellitus
Physical inactivity; sedentary lifestyle
Stress
For women over 50 years: use of estrogen
    (i.e., birth control pills) and smoking

Obesity has been directly related to CAD, as well as to hypertension, hypercholesterolemia, and hyperglycemia. Weight reduction or maintenance of ideal body weight reduces the risk of CAD, as well as that of these other medical conditions. The American College of Sports Medicine recommends a brisk walk 4 times a week to improve cardiovascular function (U.S. Department of Health and Human Services [USDHHS], 1994). In one study, high-level physical activity (in excess of 2000 kcal per week) in people age 65 to 79 was associated with improved survival, as compared with that in peers with lower physical activity levels. In addition to preserving myocardial oxygen consumption, exercise is also beneficial in reducing LDL levels, increasing HDL levels, improving mental processing, improving glucose tolerance and insulin sensitivity, improving functional status in people with arthritis, and reducing the risk of fractures from osteoporosis (Shephard, 1993).

Diabetes mellitus is another risk factor associated with CAD. Although the genetic compo-

BOX 10-2 WARNING SIGNS OF POOR NUTRITION

The Warning Signs of poor nutritional health are often overlooked. Use this checklist to find out if you or someone you know is at nutritional risk.

Read the statements below. Circle the number in the yes column for those that apply to you or someone you know. For each yes answer, score the number in the box. Total your nutritional score.

DETERMINE YOUR NUTRITIONAL HEALTH

	YES
I have an illness or condition that made me change the kind and/or amount of food I eat.	2
I eat fewer than 2 meals per day.	3
I eat few fruits or vegetables or milk products.	2
I have 3 or more drinks of beer, liquor, or wine almost every day.	2
I have tooth or mouth problems that make it hard for me to eat.	2
I don't always have enough money to buy the food I need.	4
I eat alone most of the time.	1
I take 3 or more different prescribed or over-the-counter drugs a day.	1
Without wanting to, I have lost or gained 10 pounds in the last 6 months.	2
I am not always physically able to shop, cook, and/or feed myself.	2
TOTAL	

Total Your Nutritional Score. If it's —

0-2   **Good!** Recheck your nutritional score in 6 months.

3-5   **You are at moderate nutritional risk.** See what can be done to improve your eating habits and lifestyle. Your office on aging, senior nutrition program, senior citizens center, or health department can help. Recheck your nutritional score in 3 months.

6 or more   **You are at high nutritional risk.** Bring this checklist the next time you see your doctor, dietitian, or other qualified health or social service professional. Talk with them about any problems you may have. Ask for help to improve your nutritional health.

These materials developed and distributed by the Nutrition Screening Initiative, a project of:

 AMERICAN ACADEMY OF FAMILY PHYSICIANS

 THE AMERICAN DIETETIC ASSOCIATION

 NATIONAL COUNCIL ON THE AGING, INC.

Remember that warning signs suggest risk, but do not represent diagnosis of any condition. Turn the page to learn more about the Warning Signs of poor nutritional health.

Reprinted with permission by the Nutrition Screening Initiative, a project of the American Academy of Family Physicians, the American Dietetic Association, and the National Council on the Aging, Inc., and funded in part by a grant from Ross Products Division, Abbott Laboratories.

BOX 10-3 DIETARY GUIDELINES
FOR AMERICANS*

1. Eat a variety of foods.
2. Maintain a healthy weight.
3. Choose a diet low in total fat (less than 30% of calories), saturated fat (less than 10% of calories), and cholesterol.
4. Choose a diet with plenty of vegetables, fruits, and grain products (five or more servings daily).
5. Use sugars only in moderation.
6. Use salt and sodium only in moderation.
7. If you drink alcoholic beverages, do so only in moderation (no more than one drink daily for women or 2 drinks daily for men). Women who are pregnant or planning to become pregnant should not drink at all.

From U.S. Department of Agriculture and U.S. Department of Health and Human Services.
*Use these dietary guidelines with the Food Guide Pyramid.

substitute seasonings can be very helpful in ensuring that food still tastes good. If the patient uses prepared foods, encourage the use of frozen foods low in salt instead of canned or packaged foods.

The zeal to control cardiovascular risk should not lead to a decrease in the overall quality of nutritional intake or to a compromise in nutritional status. The overall goal of maintaining an ideal body weight can usually be achieved if the diet and exercise guidelines described previously are observed. If an older person's weight is not within the recommended range for his or her age and height, it may be necessary to provide additional support group activities and dietary information to assist him or her in achieving this goal.

Another important part of educating older adults is providing clear and complete information regarding medications. Older people may be taking several prescribed drugs as well as several over-the-counter (OTC) medications because of multiple medical problems. Education should cover the name of the medication, dosage, interval for taking the medication, and why the medication was prescribed. Special precautions should be discussed (Box 10-4). Medications that are of timed-release form should never be broken or crushed. Ask the patient to restate medication information before leaving an office visit or hospital. This intervention provides an opportunity for questions and clarification of the specific medication regimen. Older adults may benefit from an audiotape schedule of the medication regimen, or a written schedule that can be placed on the refrigerator or medicine cabinet as a reminder. Containers should have an easy-open lid and typing on the label that is large enough to read. In addition, the older patient should have a pocket-sized list of medications to be carried daily in case of an emergency and that can be reviewed at office and home care visits.

Nurses can be very instrumental in educating patients, evaluating their progress, and offering support. Many times a creative individual program jointly designed by the nurse and the patient is necessary to ensure compliance. Building a relationship to assist older patients in incorporating new behaviors into their day-to-day activities may be a challenge, but the overall benefits are worth the effort. The use of every interaction to teach or clarify a health promotion activity will convey the nurse's interest in patients' well-being and provide an opportunity for positive feedback and encouragement on a job well done.

■ Nursing Process

Obtaining an accurate and complete picture of a problem from an older adult is challenging at times. Changes that occur in older adults are often insidious and heightened by the combina-

Healthy People 2000 Objectives

To reduce heart disease and stroke, by the year 2000 . . .

15.1 Reduce coronary heart disease deaths to no more than 100 per 100,000 people (a 26% decrease). (Age-adjusted baseline: 135 per 100,000 in 1987.)

15.2 Reduce stroke deaths to no more than 20 per 100,000 people (a 34% decrease). (Age-adjusted baseline: 30.3 per 100,000 in 1987.)

15.4 Increase control of high blood pressure to at least 50% of people with high blood pressure (a 108% increase). (Baseline: 11% controlled among people aged 18 through 74 in 1976-80; an estimated 24% for people aged 18 and older in 1982-84.)

15.6 Reduce blood cholesterol to an average of no more than 200 mg/dL (a 6% decrease). (Baseline: 213 mg/dL among people aged 20 through 74 in 1976-80, 211 mg/dL for men and 215 mg/dL for women.)

To increase physical activity and fitness, by the year 2000 . . .

1.3 Increase moderate daily physical activity to at least 30% of people (a 36% increase). (Baseline: 22% of people aged 18 and older were active for at least 30 minutes 5 or more times per week and 12% were active 7 or more times per week in 1985.)

1.5 Reduce sedentary lifestyles to no more than 15% of people (a 38% decrease). (Baseline: 24% for people aged 18 and older in 1985.)

To improve nutrition, by the year 2000 . . .

2.3 Reduce overweight to a prevalence of no more than 20% of people (a 23% decrease). (Baseline: 26% for people aged 20 through 74 in 1976-80, 24% for men and 27% for women; 15% for adolescents aged 12 through 19 in 1976-80.)

2.5 Reduce dietary fat intake to an average of 30% of the calories (a 17% decrease). (Baseline: 36% of calories from total fat and 13% from saturated fat for people aged 20 through 74 in 1976-80; 36% and 13% for women aged 19 through 50.)

From U.S. Department of Health and Human Services. (1990). *Healthy People 2000: National health promotion and disease prevention objectives.* (DHHS Pub. No. [PHS] 91-50212). Washington, DC: U.S. Government Printing Office.

tion of normal changes of aging, pathologic processes, and pharmacologic therapies. The most important concept on which to base nursing care is to remember the effect of these combined changes on the functional capacity of the older adult. As a person ages, the functional impact from cardiovascular disease can be profound.

ASSESSMENT

An appropriate assessment of cardiovascular function will include both a history and a physical examination, although the most useful data collected from the assessment will be from the history. The patient's energy available for providing historical information may be extremely limited. People with severe cardiovascular problems may suffer from both physical and mental decrements. When the patient is a poor historian, the family, friends, or other responsible parties may be of significant help. Information may also be obtained from the health record, if it is available. Some older patients may not report clear symptoms

BOX 10-4 COMMONLY USED DRUGS FOR CARDIOVASCULAR PROBLEMS

Digoxin
  Indications
    Heart failure
    Atrial fibrillation
  Actions
    Positive inotropic action
    Negative chronotropic action
    Decreases conduction through AV node
  Selected side effects
    Anorexia
    Nausea and vomiting
    Arrhythmias, both fast and slow
    Yellow or green vision disturbances
    Muscle weakness
    Central nervous system alterations; confusion and depression
  Precautions and special considerations
    Narrow therapeutic window
    Eliminated more slowly in older adults
    Hypokalemia may enhance digoxin toxicity
    Loading and maintenance dose to be started at half the recommended adult dose
    Monitor pulse rate, rhythm, edema, and changes in weight
Beta-adrenergic blockers (atenolol, metoprolol, propranolol, sotalol, timolol)
  Indications
    Hypertension
    Angina pectoris, due to coronary atherosclerosis
    Cardiac arrhythmias
    Myocardial infarction
  Actions
    Reduce myocardial work load and oxygen consumption
    Decrease heart rate, myocardial contractility, and BP
  Selected side effects
    Exacerbation of CHF, AV block
    Hypotension
    Lightheadedness
    Bronchospasm
    Masking of symptoms of hypoglycemia
  Precautions and special considerations
    Should not be used in patients with CHF, chronic obstructive pulmonary disease, asthma, heart
      block, or SSS
    Use with caution in insulin-treated diabetic patients and patients with PVD
    Should be withdrawn slowly in patients with angina
    Instruct patients to rise slowly from lying down and avoid prolonged standing

eral vascular examination of the lower extremities should also include assessment of the skin for color changes, decreased temperature of one limb versus the other, skin atrophy (shiny, thin skin), and a decreased distribution of hair on the lower legs and toes. The feet should also be carefully assessed for any evidence of erythema, blisters, calluses, sores, infections, or ulcerations, and the toenails should be examined for thickening or pitting. Capillary refill time elicited by pressing on the nail bed of a toe should normally be less than 15 seconds. When refill takes more than 40 seconds, severe vascular disease may be present. Pedal or lower leg edema may be present in patients with venous insufficiency or right-sided heart failure. Edema should be graded as to severity on a scale of 1 to 4, with 4 being the most severe. The level of edema should also be determined.

7. Peripheral neuropathy should be evaluated by testing deep tendon reflexes, sensory function (light touch), and motor function (pinprick, proprioception, and vibratory sense). Arterial occlusion of the lower legs should also be evaluated by assessing response to light touch on the toes, and the ability to move and dorsiflex the toes, especially the large toes.

8. A mental status examination (MSE) should be routinely performed on older patients because some changes in mental status may be important signs of disease and/or may indicate the presence of a reversible delirium.

It is important to keep in mind that in older patients, signs of cardiovascular disease may be minimal or undetectable through physical examination. This may be particularly true in the case of unsymptomatic CAD, hypertension controlled with medication, and CHF.

Psychosocial assessment

A critical component of any assessment is to ask individuals, if competent, whom they would like to have make decisions for them if they should become unable to make decisions about their care themselves. This is particularly important for individuals with cardiovascular problems because of the significant risk of their experiencing a life-threatening event, with subsequent initiation of life support treatment that may range from artificial feeding and hydration through a gastric tube to artificial ventilation. Many individuals have strong feelings about what they would and would not want to have happen to them should a massive stroke or myocardial infarction occur, and it is clearly in the patient's best interest that these wishes be explored and put in writing. Individuals in nursing homes or in private or family homes may not want to be hospitalized even if they are experiencing an acute life-threatening event. Because of the risk of cardiac arrest, an assessment of whether the patient would want to be resuscitated is very important. If possible, older adults should be encouraged to give their durable power of attorney for health to someone of their choice. If this is not possible, they should at least identify someone whom they can trust to speak for them. Careful documentation of the person's desires is extremely important.

The patient's fears concerning the possible occurrence of a stroke or heart attack, or the possibility of an amputation of a leg because of PVD, should be assessed. Many older adults fear debilitation and dependency more than death. Another common fear is that something will happen to them while they are alone and that they will remain alone and injured or ill for a long time before someone finds them.

A very broad concept of family is frequently useful when considering the family assessment of an older adult. (See Box 10-5 for considerations in assessing the patient's family.) It is not unusual for older adults to have survived their spouses, their siblings, and even their children. The closest family member may be a grandchild, a niece, or a nephew. For those living in their own

BOX 10-5 FAMILY ASSESSMENT

1. Are the family members whom the patient has designated to be involved in health care decisions aware of this expectation?
2. Who are the family members who provide care, and what is their role in caring for the patient's cardiovascular needs?
3. What kinds of stress does caring for the patient impose on the individual family members?
4. What is the level of knowledge among family members about the patient's condition, and who is their primary source of information?
5. How do family members feel about the patient's decisions regarding resuscitation orders and life support interventions?
6. What barriers block the participation of family members in the care of the patient?

homes, the home health aide may be the only "family" the older adult has. Similarly, the nursing staff of a nursing home may serve as surrogate family members for older adults needing nursing home care. Finally, a court-designated responsible party may have the decision-making prerogative that is traditionally reserved for relatives.

An individual with cardiovascular problems may need assistance in obtaining medications and in taking them correctly. If dietary modifications are part of the care plan, those who shop for and prepare food need to be included in the patient-family education and planning.

It is important to assess how cardiovascular problems have affected the patient's self-concept and ability to function. The following topics would be appropriate to discuss:

1. The patient's perceptions of the cardiovascular problem (or problems)

2. The patient's perceptions of the effects of cardiovascular problems on normal activities of daily living and on instrumental activities of daily living
3. The patient's fears about the effects of the cardiovascular problem
4. What the patient sees as his or her future
5. The cultural or spiritual meaning to the patient of the experience with the cardiovascular problem
6. The effect of the cardiovascular problem on the psychologic functioning of the patient—is there a feeling of hopelessness, anxiety, or depression?
7. What the patient does that is pleasurable each day and what the patient would like to do that he or she is not currently doing
8. The patient's knowledge of and ability to manage the medical and nursing treatments
9. How the patient's body image or feeling of attractiveness has been affected by the cardiovascular problem

Environmental assessment: Living arrangement

The environment in which the older adult with cardiovascular problems lives can either support the maximal functioning of the individual, or present barriers that may cause unnecessary dependency, especially in the patient's home. The environmental assessment for a private or family home specific to cardiovascular problems is presented in Box 10-6. Environmental assessment should also be performed for individuals in nursing homes or hospitals. The assessment in these settings specific to cardiovascular problems should include the following questions:

1. Do noise levels exist that might cause extreme stress and sleep deprivation, such as from noisy roommates or noise from patient care equipment?
2. Is the temperature level comfortable? Too warm an environment may exacerbate CHF, whereas too cold an environment may cause further circulatory compromise in someone with PVD.

BOX 10-6 ENVIRONMENTAL ASSESSMENT

1. What is the length of the hallway from the patient's apartment to the elevator or building entrance?
2. Are there stairways, and how many times a day does the patient have to climb the stairs?
3. If oxygen is needed, is there space for the equipment in the patient's bedroom? Can the oxygen be moved easily to a different room, if necessary, and can it be taken out of the home if the patient leaves?
4. Is there a suitable stool, chair, or sofa on which the patient can prop up his or her legs if pedal edema is a problem?
5. Are there sharp edges on the furniture or loose scatter rugs that could cause injury to the patient with arterial insufficiency, syncopal episodes, or orthostatic hypotension?
6. Is a telephone or other lifeline means of communication within easy reach should an emergency occur, such as severe chest pain?
7. Are the kitchen facilities designed for safety?
8. Does the bathroom have an elevated toilet seat, bars to assist in getting off the toilet, and bars in the shower or bath to assist in getting in and out of the shower, and is the bathroom free of hazards that would result in a fall?
9. Are laundry facilities accessible?
10. Is there a community environment for walking and interacting with other people?

Resource assessment

Older adults with cardiovascular problems may need the use of community resources either to stay in their homes or to return to their homes after a hospitalization. The types of community resources frequently needed are equipment, such as oxygen or a hospital bed in which the head can be easily elevated, or adaptive devices, such as a bedside commode to allow the patient to avoid strain. There may be a need for a home health aide who can do grocery shopping and meal preparation, as well as assisting with activities of daily living. There may be a need for a prosthetic device following a limb amputation due to PVD. The patient who has had an amputation also may need a physical therapist to come into the home, for further rehabilitation related to the use of a prosthesis.

The resources used will depend in large part not only on the availability of a service but also on the ability to pay for the service. Some services provided through community resources are covered through private insurance plans, Medicare, or Medicaid. To be eligible for Medicaid, an individual must meet the income requirements of the state in which the individual lives. Medicare, the federally sponsored program, pays for a number of services provided in the home. The support system of friends, family, volunteers, home health aides, and nurses and other professionals is critical for older adults, regardless of where they live, but particularly when they are living alone in their own homes or apartments.

NURSING DIAGNOSES

After completing the history and physical examination of the patient, with assistance from a family member or significant other, the clinician can formulate a diagnosis and develop a plan of care with individualized interventions to best address the needs of the older patient. The following three nursing diagnoses are frequently used to reflect cardiovascular problems in older adults:

1. Alteration in tissue perfusion due to interruptions in arterial and venous flow
2. Alteration in health maintenance due to lack of adequate resources and perceived threat to health
3. Alteration in comfort due to pain from cardiac ischemia and impaired circulation to the extremities

Alteration in tissue perfusion

The alteration may be evidenced by cardiopulmonary, cerebral, or peripheral signs and symptoms:

> Cardiopulmonary—shortness of breath, tachycardia, rales, S_3, S_4, dry cough, peripheral or sacral edema, arrhythmia, chest pain, hypotension, cold or clammy skin
> Cerebral—altered mental status, restlessness, symptoms of TIAs, syncope
> Peripheral—changes in skin color and texture, temperature, hair distribution, sensation, edema, leg pain or tenderness, intermittent claudication, diminished healing capability

Alteration in health maintenance

The condition may be evidenced by unhealthy and incompetent behavior. Defining characteristics include but are not limited to the following (McFarland & McFarlane, 1993):

- Poor diet
- Need for alcohol, drugs, or tobacco
- Lack of adequate immunizations
- Inability to take responsibility for basic health practices
- Lack of knowledge of basic health practices
- Failure to manage stress

Alteration in comfort

The alteration may be evidenced by chest pain, intermittent claudication or arterial occlusion, venous insufficiency or edema, thrombophlebitis, and/or symptomatic arrhythmias.

PLANNING AND GOAL IDENTIFICATION

The planning phase determines a plan of action to assist the patient toward the goal of optimal wellness, based on the highest level of fulfillment. Both short- and long-term goals are developed for the older patient. Expected outcomes are designed with input from the patient, the patient's family or other responsible party, and the clinician.

Alteration in tissue perfusion

The long-term goal is that the patient will alter activities of daily living to minimize the effects of alterations in cerebral, peripheral, and cardiopulmonary tissue perfusion. The outcomes can be grouped into three areas (McFarland & McFarlane, 1993):

1. There will be adequate blood flow in the affected vessels.
2. Tissue needs will be reduced.
3. Patient and family will understand the cause of the problem.

The long-term goal may be achieved by reaching the following short-term goals:

1. Patient will have adequate tissue perfusion and cellular oxygenation of the cardiovascular, cerebral, and peripheral system.
2. Patient will be able to modify lifestyle activities to prevent cardiopulmonary, cerebral, and peripheral signs and symptoms.
3. Patient or caregiver will appropriately control metabolic needs by administration of medications, understanding their actions, dosage, and common side effects, and by avoiding stress-related activities.

Alteration in health maintenance

The primary goal is for the affected patient to understand that lifestyle modification is necessary to assist in the control of the aging process response of the cardiovascular, peripheral vascular, and cerebral systems. Patients should actively participate in the planning. A long-term goal would be the following: Patient will be able to modify cardiac risk factors, incorporating new behaviors into his or her lifestyle.

Short-term goals are the following:

1. Patient will be able to verbalize fears and perception of the cardiovascular, peripheral vascular, and cerebral disease.
2. Patient will engage in health behaviors such as adherence to a low-fat and low-salt diet, compliance with the medication regimen, and follow an appropriate exercise program to improve quality of life.
3. Patient will be able to identify probable future health maintenance needs.

Alteration in comfort

The long-term goal is to control the factors that intensify the symptoms: Patient will be able to describe measures to control chest pain, claudication, and dizziness.

Short-term goals are the following:

1. Patient will take appropriate medications to control pain.
2. Patient will schedule frequent rest periods.
3. Patient will monitor activity.

IMPLEMENTATION
In the acute care setting

On admission to an acute care setting, a patient with a cardiovascular problem serious enough to warrant admission may experience anxiety. The older patient in the hospital setting is frequently not included in treatment decisions. Patients who lose control of the situation often become resentful. Other issues that can add to the anxiety are fear of death or pain, and financial complications. Calmly sitting with the patient to gain an understanding of the nature of the anxiety will assist the nurse in planning interventions to alleviate the anxiety. Individuals who have been accustomed to doing things in their lives in a particular way or to eating particular foods may resist changes. It is important to discuss with the patient any changes that are likely to affect the usual way of doing things, or any special likes and dislikes. Allowing the patient to decide what to eat and when to shower or take a walk may seem like a small thing, yet to a patient it is very important. You can also arrange for a social service representative to come by and speak to the patient regarding financial concerns.

Another commonly seen condition in a seriously ill patient admitted to an acute care setting is confusion. It is easy for the nursing staff of a hospital to assume that this person has chronic dementia and will always be confused. The multiple effects of the cardiovascular problems, medical treatment, and changes in environment frequently cause delirium. Interventions aimed at orienting patients after they have been stabilized are often successful in producing remarkable mental status improvements. Explaining the time of day at each meal and having a clock and calendar in the room can help the patient achieve orientation.

Older individuals with cardiovascular problems are more likely to die or develop adverse outcomes related to hospitalization than are members of any other age group. This is because older adults have significantly compromised reserve capacity for adapting physically or emotionally to acute illness and to the trauma of hospitalization. In the hospital setting it is important to have advance directives on record, if at all possible, particularly because cardiac arrest is a significant risk in older adults with cardiovascular disease. Family and significant others should be included in decision making about diagnostic testing and treatment.

In the nursing home

The primary interventions specific to nursing home care of the resident with cardiovascular problems are the following: (1) maintaining or improving a resident's functional abilities, (2) enhancing the resident's sense of autonomy while fostering a safe environment, (3) monitoring the conditions related to the cardiovascular problems of the resident, and (4) providing specific therapies that will improve the resident's cardiovascular functioning. The reason that the older adult is in a nursing home may not necessarily be related to a cardiovascular problem. The reason usually relates to the effect of the multiplicity of disease processes linked with the normal effects of aging to diminish the person's functional capacity to such an extent that the person can no longer live in a private or family home without assistance. Many older individuals may not have family members living or may not have family members available who can provide the often extensive care needed to maintain someone in the private or family home.

Assisting residents with cardiovascular problems in maintaining autonomy should include supporting those activities that they can do themselves. It may include ensuring that a portable oxygen tank is available so that the resident can attend activities that are enjoyable. A sense of autonomy is usually clearly linked to making decisions about oneself. This includes being involved in the resident care conference, being informed about the status of the cardiovascular problem, and participating in care-planning decisions.

Monitoring the resident is critical in early detection of acute problems related to the cardiovascular system. Periodic monitoring of the vital signs is one of the best ways of identifying impending problems. Changes in heart rate and rhythm, in respiration, and in BP can provide clues to the need for further assessment. The nurse should validate vital signs and reinforce with the assistant nursing staff the importance of accurately assessing vital signs and weights. Staff should be properly educated in the importance of promptly reporting a change in vital signs or weight so that an additional assessment can be started. Mental status should also be monitored. A resident who is having an acute cardiovascular episode such as a myocardial infarction without complaints of chest pain may show signs of confusion or increased lethargy.

Effectiveness of drug therapy, as well as side effects of drugs, should be monitored. This is particularly important because the frail older person with cardiovascular problems will probably be taking at least one, if not more, medications.

In addition to the preceding therapies, encouraging the resident to elevate the legs if fluid accumulates and elevating the resident's head while the resident is in bed if breathing is a problem can ease the symptoms of cardiovascular and peripheral vascular disease. Teach the resident proper use of the emergency call system in the room, bathroom, and common area. The resident may also have periods of anxiety or depression about the effects of the diseases. Talking with the resident and understanding the basis of these feelings are important. When doing so, sit at eye level with the resident. Avoid the use of placating phrases such as "everything will be fine" or "you have nothing to worry about." Older adults have significant concerns that should never be discounted.

In the private or family home

A major consideration in the care of older adults at home is establishing a monitoring system to assess significant and possibly life-threatening changes. Many older adults live alone and have little in the way of home health services available. Because problems affecting the cardiovascular system may impair patients' ability to monitor and interpret changes in their own condition, it is helpful to identify a person who is willing to visit the patient on a regular basis or to call to see that the patient can at least answer the telephone. The person who will be monitoring the patient will need to know the signs that suggest a problem (Box 10-7).

In addition, a nurse may temporarily monitor the patient. The payment mechanism through Medicare for home health services allows only visits that can be justified on the basis of need for specific types of nursing services. Most older adults cannot afford to pay out of pocket for a nurse to provide monitoring services.

If the patient is living with a family member, that family member must also be clear about the

BOX 10-7 CARDIOVASCULAR MONITORING PARAMETERS FOR HOME CARE PROVIDERS

- Confusion
- Lack of appetite
- Pain or discomfort
- Feelings of anxiety
- Fatigue
- Disheveled appearance
- Hallucinations
- Rapid breathing
- Rapid pulse
- Diaphoresis
- Pallor
- Edema

signs that suggest a deterioration in the older adult's status. It is also helpful to have patients be clear, if possible, about any advance directives they may want in writing, such as not wanting to be admitted to a hospital. Family members should be aware of these advance directives.

Arrangements may need to be made for items such as a hospital-type bed or commode to be brought to the home. Being able to raise the head of a bed may help a person who has orthopnea to sleep more easily. There may also be a need for oxygen. The nurse may need to make arrangements with a home care supply company to bring in oxygen equipment. There is a great variation in charges for this equipment. Knowing the costs may save the patient or family from considerable financial burden, because Medicare will only pay a specific amount for the equipment.

For older adults who have a high anxiety level about needing help and not being able to obtain it, such as may happen with a heart attack or stroke, establishing a link with emergency community services may alleviate some anxiety. Some communities have a lifeline program, in which a direct line is established with an emer-

gency service. Contact can frequently be made simply by pushing a button that sets up an automatic response system at the emergency service site. For communities that do not have this sophisticated type of service, it may be desirable to establish linkages to a family member, friend, or volunteer service that can act on the patient's behalf in an emergency.

EVALUATION

Evaluation is an integral phase of the nursing process. Reassessment and replanning may be the result of an evaluation, if the patient's short-term goals are not met in a timely fashion. Interventions are evaluated in terms of their acceptance by patients and their families and in terms of their ability to assist in the accomplishment of the planned goals. Documentation and validation of goal attainment, including health promotion and education, is an essential component of the evaluation phase of the nursing process.

REFERENCES

Applegate, W.B., & Rutan, G.H. (1992). Advances in management of hypertension in older persons. *Progress in Geriatrics, 40,* 1164-1174.

Aronow, W. (1995). Treatment of ventricular arrhythmias in older adults. *Journal of the American Geriatrics Society, 43,* 688-695.

Bierman, E.G. (1994). Aging and atherosclerosis. In W.M. Hazzard, E. Bierman, J. Blass, W. Ettinger, & J. Halter (Eds.), *Principles of geriatric medicine and gerontology.* New York: McGraw-Hill.

Bruno, A. (1993a). Ischemic stroke: 1. Early, accurate diagnosis. *Geriatrics, 48*(3), 26-34.

Bruno, A. (1993b). Ischemic stroke: 2. Optimal treatment and prevention. *Geriatrics, 48*(3), 37-54.

Cohn, J. (1992). The prevention of heart failure—A new agenda. *New England Journal of Medicine, 327,* 725-727.

Dalen, J.E. (1994). Atrial fibrillation: Reducing stroke risk with low-dose anticoagulation. *Geriatrics, 49*(5), 24-32.

The fifth report of the Joint National Committee on detection, evaluation, and treatment of high blood pressure. (1993). *Archives of Internal Medicine, 153,* 154-183.

Gamble, C.L. (1994). Lipid disorders: When—and why— you should treat at-risk adults. *Geriatrics, 49*(10), 33-37.

Gawlinski, A., & Jensen, G.A. (1991, November). Cardio-vascular aging. *American Journal of Nursing,* 26-30.

Giordano, J.M. (1983). A practical approach to peripheral vascular disease. *Modern Medicine, 51,* 105-116.

Juul-Möller, S., Edvardsson, N., & Rehnquist-Ahlberg, N. (1990). Sotalol versus quinidine for the maintenance of sinus rhythm after direct current conversion of atrial fibrillation. *Circulation, 82,* 1932-1939.

Kelley, W.N. (1989). *Textbooks of international medicine.* Philadelphia: J.B. Lippincott.

Laupacis, A., et al. (1992). Antithrombotic therapy in atrial fibrillation. *Chest, 102,* 426S-433S.

Luchi, R., Taffet, G., & Teasdale, T. (1991). Congestive heart failure in the elderly. *Journal of the American Geriatrics Society, 39,* 810-825.

Massie, B.M. (1994). First-line therapy for hypertension: Different patients, different needs. *Geriatrics, 49*(4), 22-30.

McFarland, G.K., & McFarlane, E.A. (1993). *Nursing diagnosis and intervention: Planning for patient care* (2nd ed.). St. Louis: Mosby.

Pearson T., et al. (1994). Primer in preventive cardiology. Dallas: American Heart Association.

1996 physicians genRx: The complete drug reference. (1996). St. Louis: Mosby.

Pritchett, E.L.C. (1992). Management of atrial fibrillation. *New England Journal of Medicine, 326,* 1264-1271.

Shephard, R.J. (1993). Exercise and aging: Extending independence in older adults. *Geriatrics, 48*(5), 61-64.

Thiele, B.L., & Strandness, D.E., Jr. (1994). Peripheral vascular disease. In W.M. Hazzard, E. Bierman, J. Blass, W. Ettinger, & J. Halter (Eds.), *Principles of geriatric medicine and gerontology.* New York: McGraw-Hill.

U.S. Department of Health and Human Services. (1994). *Clinicians handbook of preventive services.* Washington, DC: U.S. Government Printing Office.

Wenger, N.K. (1992). Cardiovascular disease in the elderly. *Current Problems in Cardiology, 17*(10), 609-690.

BIBLIOGRAPHY

Baer, M., & Goldschlager, N. (1995). Atrial fibrillation: An update on new management strategies. *Geriatrics, 50*(4), 22-29.

Cacciabaudo, J.M., & Pecker, M.S. (1995, May-June). Hypertension: Managing the silent killer. *Contemporary Nurse Practitioner,* 24-30.

Cannon, L.A., & Marshall, J.M. (1993). Cardiac disease in the elderly population. *Clinical Geriatric Medicine, 9*(3), 499-525.

Elnicki, M., & Kotchen, T.A. (1993). Hypertension: Patient evaluation, indications for treatment. *Geriatrics, 48*(4), 47-62.

Gamble, C.L. (1994). Lipid disorders: Tailoring diet and drug therapy for individual needs. *Geriatrics, 49*(11), 52-58.

Jensen, G.A. (1991). The complications of cardiovascular aging. *American Journal of Nursing, 91*(11), 26-30.

Kenney, R.A. (1989). Physiology of aging chicago: Year Book Medical Publishers.

Krumholz, H.M., et al. (1994). Lack of association between cholesterol and coronary heart disease mortality and morbidity and all-cause mortality in persons older than 70 years. *Journal of the American Medical Association, 272,* 1335-1340.

Larson, E.B., & Bruce, R.A. (1987). Health benefits of exercise in an aging society. *Archives of Internal Medicine, 147,* 353-356.

Leaf, D.A. (1994). Lipid disorders: Applying new guidelines to your older patients. *Geriatrics, 49*(5), 35-41.

Malasanos, L., et al. (1990). *Health assessment* (4th ed.). St. Louis: Mosby.

Masiello Miller, M. (1994). Current trends in the primary care management of chronic congestive heart failure. *Elsevier Science Inc., 19*(5), 64-70.

Poole, R.M., & Chimowitz, M.I. (1994). Ischemic stroke and TIA: Clinical clues to common causes. *Geriatrics, 49*(6), 37-42.

Silva-Smith, A. (1994). Reducing the risk of stroke in patients with chronic, nonvalvular atrial fibrillation. *Elsevier Science Inc., 19*(2), 38-44.

Thompson, J., et al. (1993). *Mosby's clinical nursing* (3rd ed.). St. Louis: Mosby.

U.S. Department of Health and Human Services. (1992). *Healthy People 2000: National health promotion and disease prevention objectives.* Washington, DC: Author.

U.S. Preventive Services Task Force. (1989). *Guide to clinical preventive services.* Williams & Wilkins.

Vogt, A.R., Funk, M., & Remetz, M. (1994). Comparison of symptoms, functional ability, and health perception of elderly patients with coronary artery disease managed with three different treatment modalities. *Cardiovascular Nursing, 30*(5), 33-38.

Wei, J.Y. (1992). Age and the cardiovascular system. *New England Journal of Medicine, 327*(24), 1735-1739.

Wei, J.Y. (1994). Disorders of the heart. In W.R. Hazzard, R. Andres, E.L. Bierman, & J.P. Blass (Eds.), *Principles of geriatric medicine and gerontology* (3rd ed.). New York: McGraw-Hill.

Weinberg, M. (1993). Renal effects of angiotensin converting enzyme inhibitors heart failure: A clinician's guide to minimizing azotemia and diuretic-induced electrolyte imbalances. *Clinical Therapeutics, 15,* 3-15.

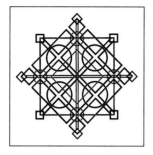

*Each step in the path oxygen takes from the air to the
metabolizing cell is vulnerable to aging.*

R.A. KENNEY, *Physiology of Aging*

Respiration

■ Learning Objectives

On completion of this chapter, the reader will be able to do the following:

1. Explain the normal structure and function of the respiratory tract.
2. Identify age-related physiologic changes of the respiratory system.
3. Identify and describe the common pathophysiologic changes that affect the respiratory system of older adults.
4. Assess the respiratory functioning of older adults.
5. Recognize the psychosocial and environmental factors that influence the nursing management of older adults with respiratory problems.
6. Develop nursing diagnoses and a plan of care for an older person with respiratory impairment.
7. Provide appropriate nursing interventions and evaluations for older adults with respiratory impairment.

The respiratory system stretches from the nasal cavity to the lungs. The system is divided into the upper and lower respiratory tracts. The normal structure and function of the respiratory system is reviewed here before addressing its age-related changes.

■ Normal Structure and Function

UPPER RESPIRATORY TRACT
The upper respiratory tract begins at the nasal cavity and extends to the vocal cords, which are located within the larynx (Figure 11-1).

Nasal cavity

When a person inhales, air passes through two openings, termed *external nares* or *nostrils.* A vertical partition, the *nasal septum,* divides the two nasal cavities, which have six main functions: conduction of air, filtration, temperature control, humidification of inhaled air, voice resonance, and olfaction.

Pharynx

Next the inhaled air passes through the pharynx. The *pharynx,* also known as the "throat," is

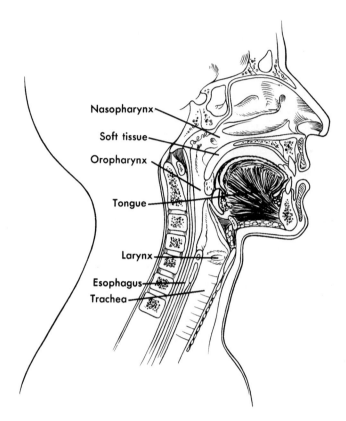

FIGURE 11-1 Upper respiratory tract. (From Phipps, W., Cassmeyer, V., Sands, J., & Lehman, M.K. [1995]. *Medical-surgical nursing: Concepts and clinical practice* [5th ed.]. St. Louis: Mosby.)

divided into the following three sections: nasopharynx (upper section), oropharynx (middle section), and laryngopharynx (lower section). The pharynx is a long, tubelike structure with two main functions: (1) serving as a passageway for air to travel to the trachea and for food to travel to the esophagus and (2) aiding in the formation of vocal sound.

Larynx

The *larynx,* which connects the pharynx with the trachea and is known as the "voice box" because of its major role in the production of sounds, is a major structure of the upper respiratory tract.

LOWER RESPIRATORY TRACT
Trachea

The *trachea,* or the "windpipe," is a tubular passageway approximately 11 to 12 cm long and 2.5 cm in diameter, located in front of the esophagus. It extends from the cricoid cartilage of the larynx to about the seventh thoracic vertebra. It is here, at the carina, that the trachea divides into the left and right main bronchi.

Bronchi, bronchioles, and alveoli

The left and right main *bronchi,* which branch from the trachea, deliver the inhaled air to the lungs. Each main bronchus divides several times,

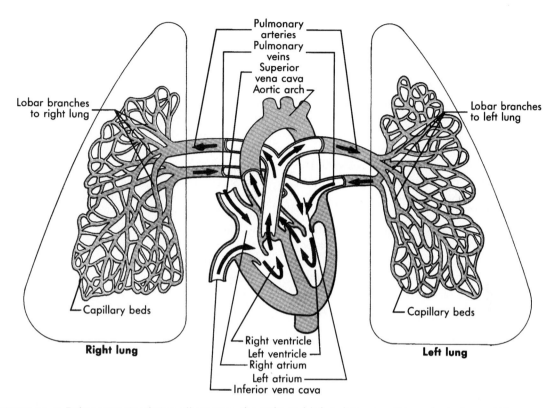

Pulmonary
arteries
Pulmonary
veins
Superior
vena cava
Aortic arch

Lobar branches
to right lung

Lobar branches
to left lung

Capillary beds

Capillary beds

Right lung

Left lung

Right ventricle
Left ventricle
Right atrium
Left atrium
Inferior vena cava

FIGURE 11-2 Pulmonary circulation, illustrating the right and left pulmonary veins and arteries and the branching capillaries. (From McCance K. & Huether, S. [1994]. *Pathophysiology: The biologic basis for disease in adults and children* [2nd ed.]. St. Louis: Mosby.)

ultimately giving rise to tiny *bronchioles.* These bronchioles subdivide many times, forming terminal and respiratory bronchioles. Each *respiratory bronchiole* subdivides into several alveolar ducts that end in clusters of small, thin-walled air sacs termed *alveoli.* Often, several alveoli open into a chamber termed an *alveolar sac.*

All structures distal to the terminal bronchiole make up the terminal respiratory unit (TRU), sometimes referred to as the *acinar unit,* or the *acinus.* This is considered the basic unit of the lung. The alveolus is the most distal structure within the TRU at which gas exchange occurs (Figure 11-2).

Lungs

The two lungs are elastic cone-shaped organs, with the apex of each lung fitting into the thoracic cavity behind the clavicle. The base of each lung rests on the surface of the diaphragm. The left lung has two lobes, as well as a concavity for the heart on its medial surface; the right lung has three lobes.

The space between the two lungs is termed the *mediastinum.* Besides separating the left and right lung, the mediastinum also accommodates several important structures: the heart, the aorta, the venae cavae, the pulmonary vessels, the esophagus, part of the trachea and bronchi, and the thymus gland.

Pleura

The *pleura* is a double-walled sac, one of which encloses each lung. It consists of two layers: the *visceral pleura* adheres firmly to the lungs, whereas the *parietal pleura* lines the walls of the thoracic cavity. The pleural cavity is the extremely narrow area between the two layers of the pleura. The pleural cavity is filled with pleural fluid, which is secreted by the pleura and acts as a lubricant, reducing friction between the two layers during respiratory movements.

Respiratory membrane

The very thin respiratory membrane separates the air in the alveoli from the circulating blood. Oxygen and carbon dioxide diffuse across this membrane during respiration, while maintaining the integrity of the vascular system.

PULMONARY CIRCULATION

For the deoxygenated blood to pass through the lungs, it must be pumped from the right ventricle, through the pulmonic valve, and into the *pulmonary artery,* also called the "pulmonary trunk." The pulmonary artery divides into two branches: (1) the right pulmonary artery, supplying the right lung, and (2) the left pulmonary artery, supplying the left lung (Figure 11-3).

Each pulmonary artery follows the bronchi to the terminal bronchioles, where the *arterioles,* small arteries, branch into capillaries in the alveolar walls. A vast and dense network of pulmonary capillaries, termed the *pulmonary capillary bed,* surrounds the alveoli and provides the contact necessary for gas exchange to occur between the alveoli and the blood.

Once gas exchange has occurred at the pulmonary membrane, oxygenated blood collects in small venules, which unite to form four large veins, termed the *pulmonary veins.* The pulmonary veins drain into the left atrium.

The most distinguishing features of the pulmonary circulation are its low pressure and its low resistance. These features result from the great distensibility of the vessels and from the low resistance to blood flow of the pulmonary vascular beds.

The pulmonary circulation connects with the bronchial circulation deep within the lung tissue; the bronchial circulation system is relatively small, receiving only 1% to 2% of the total cardiac output. Its primary function is to provide a continuous supply of nutrient blood to the conducting airways and terminal respiratory units so that the lungs can carry out their many functions.

Bronchial arteries follow the airways into the lung parenchyma, elaborately branching along the way and rejoining to form networks around the bronchi. Upon reaching the end of the conducting airways and the beginning of TRUs, these vessels anastomose with pulmonary artery capillaries from the pulmonary circulation. Blood returns to the heart via true bronchial veins, flowing into azygous veins, and eventually to the superior vena cava, and then the right atrium. Approximately 65% to 75% of the bronchial circulation flows into the pulmonary veins.

THE PROCESS OF RESPIRATION

The process of respiration can be defined in terms of three distinct events that occur with breathing: ventilation, diffusion or external respiration, and gas transport or internal respiration.

Ventilation

Ventilation is the mechanical movement of air into and out of the lungs, between the atmosphere and the lung alveoli. Ventilation involves two phases: *inspiration* (movement of air into the lungs) and *expiration* (movement of air out of the lungs). Ventilation is influenced by mechanical (muscular), neurologic, physical, and chemical events.

Muscles of respiration The act of breathing occurs through muscular actions that change intrapulmonary and intrapleural pressures and result in air volume change within the lungs. Normal, quiet inspiration is accomplished almost entirely by the diaphragm, which is the major muscle of this phase of respiration.

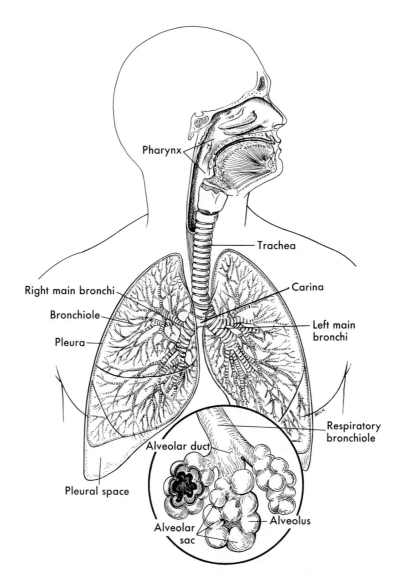

FIGURE 11-3 Structures of the pulmonary system. The circle denotes the acinus, in which oxygen and carbon dioxide are exchanged. (From Thibodeau G. [1990]. *Anthony's textbook of anatomy and physiology* [ed 13.]. St. Louis: Mosby.)

Other muscles involved in inspiration are the external intercostal muscles, which increase the anterior-posterior diameter of the thorax by elevating the ribs. The accessory muscles of inspiration include the scalene and sternocleidomastoid muscles in the neck and are responsible for raising the clavicles, upper ribs, and sternum. These muscle groups are not usually involved in normal, quiet respiration but are needed in some disease states.

Expiration is normally a passive action, resulting from the recoil tendency of the lungs through the relaxation of the inspiratory muscles. However, when increased levels of expiration are required, the abdominal and internal intercostal muscle groups are used (Levitzky, 1991).

Neurologic regulation Breathing is regulated by the central nervous system. The respiratory centers are groups of neurons that function together as a unit to regulate inspiration and expiration. The medullary respiratory center is located in the medulla oblongata, and the apneustic and pneumotaxic centers are located in the pons. These centers are involved in the regulation of the respiratory rate and depth. Impulses travel down the phrenic nerves to the diaphragm, and then via the intercostal nerves to the intercostal muscles, where changes in the rate and depth of respiration occur.

Conscious control of breathing, through nerve impulses from the motor areas of the cerebral cortex, can override the involuntary respiratory centers. This mechanism adjusts voluntary breathing to meet increased oxygen needs that result from changes in activity.

Physical forces The diaphragm and intercostal muscles contract as a result of stimulation from the central nervous system. Respiratory muscles alternately compress and distend the lungs, which causes the pressure in the alveoli to rise and fall. Gas moves from an area of greater pressure to one of lesser pressure. The pressure in the lungs and thorax must be less than atmospheric pressure for inspiration to occur. Expiration is passive, as muscles relax; intrathoracic pressures rise, and air moves out of the lungs to the atmosphere. Very little pressure change is required to move air into and out of the lungs.

Physical forces are also involved in effective gas movement. The elasticity of the lung tissue (i.e., *resistance*), the size of the large air passages, and the *compliance* of the chest wall affect respiration and can alter the work of breathing. *Surfactant,* a lipoprotein, is secreted by the epithelial cells in the alveoli. The presence of this substance contributes to lung elasticity, thereby increasing lung compliance (Levitzky,

1991). These factors are especially altered by the process of aging.

Chemical control The chemical centers that influence respiration involve central and peripheral chemoreceptors that signal the respiratory centers to change the rate and depth of respiration. Central chemoreceptors are located in the medulla and are sensitive to changes in carbon dioxide and to the acid base balance in the blood and the cerebrospinal fluid. Peripheral chemoreceptors are located in the aortic bodies near the aortic arch and in the carotid bodies near the bifurcation of the common carotid arteries. These receptors are sensitive to changes in oxygen levels in the blood and in the interstitial fluid surrounding the receptors.

Alveolar ventilation

One of the most important factors in the respiratory process is alveolar ventilation. Air can travel through the large air passages, but if the alveoli are not open, as is the case in atelectasis or pneumonia, true ventilation does not take place. Respiratory rate and volumes are important in that they affect alveolar ventilation.

Diffusion or external respiration

Ventilation refers to the mechanical movement of air into and out of the lungs. *Diffusion,* the next step in the process of respiration, is the actual transfer of oxygen into and carbon dioxide out of the blood. It is also termed *external respiration.*

During normal inspiration the alveoli fill with air. The concentration of oxygen in the alveoli is higher than the concentration of oxygen in the blood. The concentration of carbon dioxide in the alveoli is lower than that in the blood. Oxygen diffuses into the blood and carbon dioxide diffuses out of the blood across the alveolar capillary membrane until equilibrium is reached. The rate of diffusion is altered in the presence of pathophysiology. Diffusion is altered in the aging lung as a result of a decrease in functional alveoli and a reduced pulmonary capillary blood flow (Timiras, 1994).

Gas transport or internal respiration

Oxygen transport, or *internal respiration,* the third event in the process of respiration, begins after diffusion takes place. During internal respiration, oxygen moves into the cells and carbon dioxide leaves the cells to enter the blood. Arterial blood transports oxygen to the tissues, either in plasma or bound to hemoglobin. Oxygen has an affinity for the iron molecules of hemoglobin. Approximately 97% of oxygen in the blood reaches the tissues bound to hemoglobin. This concentration is determined by the oxygen level of the inspired air and the hemoglobin level in the blood. Oxygen resists being dissolved in plasma, and only 3% is carried to the tissues by this method.

Carbon dioxide transport is more complicated. Carbon dioxide is released by the tissues into the bloodstream. It travels to the lungs in three ways: (1) as a gas, dissolved in plasma (7%), (2) combined with hemoglobin (23%), and (3) combined with water in the form of carbonic acid (70%). Blood moves through the capillaries into the venous system, where carbon dioxide is reformed. This gas is diffused into the alveoli (external respiration) and is excreted in the lungs.

When oxygen-rich arterial blood reaches the body tissue cells, internal respiration, or gas exchange between systemic capillaries and interstitial fluid, takes place. This involves pressure gradients, as is the case in the diffusion process. Oxygen is transported into the interstitial fluid to nourish the cells. Age-related changes or pathophysiology of the respiratory system can affect the rate of transfer and the amount of oxygen that is given off to the tissues by making the unloading of oxygen more difficult.

■ Age-Related Changes

It is difficult to differentiate among the effects of the aging process, the lifelong environment of the individual, and disease on the respiratory system. In healthy older adults, breathing is usually sufficient to supply oxygen for normal function (Hogstel, 1994). However, this supply- and-demand balance is frequently altered when stress or pathology increase oxygen need and consumption.

An understanding of the normal changes that can be expected to occur as the adult lung ages will provide the necessary framework for the nursing process as it develops into an individualized treatment plan for the patient with respiratory disorders. These age-related changes are classified as being either "structural" or "functional."

STRUCTURAL CHANGES

Structural or anatomic changes in the aging lung are described as being either *extrapulmonary* (of skeleton and muscle) or *intrapulmonary* (of the lung parenchyma). Both result in a decrease in potential expansion, which alters the flow of air into and out of the lungs (Timiras, 1994).

Skeletal changes

Osteoporosis of the ribs and the vertebrae and calcification of the costal cartilages cause increased stiffness or rigidity, decreased rib mobility, and reduced compliance of the chest wall. Degeneration of the intervertebral disks may be seen clinically in the development of kyphosis and scoliosis. These skeletal changes of the thoracic region of the spine produce a shorter thorax with an increased anterior–posterior diameter. In severe cases, the rib cage may rest on the pelvic bones and cause marked limitation of thoracic movement.

The trachea and large bronchi are also increased in diameter because of the calcified cartilage changes. These large airway structures serve as reservoirs to conduct air from the atmosphere to the alveoli. The overall effect is both an increase in "dead space," where no diffusion takes place, and a decrease in the volume of air that actually reaches the alveoli in the aged lung.

Muscular changes

The muscles involved in respiration, like other muscles in the body, weaken with age. The result is less forceful contraction, which decreases inspiratory and expiratory effort. Atrophy of the muscles supporting the rib cage is also involved in the development of kyphosis in older adults. The combination of increased stiffness of the chest wall and decreased muscle strength results in less efficient breathing. Older people may depend more on accessory abdominal muscles to compensate for weakened thoracic muscles.

The diaphragm does not appear to lose mass with aging. This muscle continues to contribute significantly to changes in thoracic cage volume. The breathing patterns of the older adult are even more dependent on changes in intra-abdominal pressure and may be greatly affected by increased abdominal pressure or body position.

Lung parenchyma changes

The age-related changes in the lung parenchyma, where gas exchange takes place, alter respiratory efficiency and have the greatest functional effect. The lung becomes less elastic as it ages, as a result of changes in the collagen substance surrounding the alveoli and alveolar ducts. This substance has a major role in the elastic recoil properties of the lungs. During aging, the collagen stiffens and forms cross-linkages that interfere with the lung's elastic ability to expand with inspiration and contract with expiration (Timiras, 1994). This actually increases lung tissue compliance, but the effect is outweighed by that of the decreased compliance of the rib cage. With advanced age the overall compliance of the respiratory system decreases.

Changes in the lung parenchyma are also seen in the terminal bronchioles, alveolar ducts, alveoli, and capillaries. These changes begin in the third decade and continue over the remaining years. The total number of alveoli remains constant throughout the life span, but there is a decrease in the number of functioning alveoli. There is a thinning of the walls, accompanied by a progressive loss of the interalveolar septum. This results in larger alveoli and dilated bronchioles, with a decreased air exchange surface for

external respiration to take place. The aged lung looks like an emphysematous lung on chest x-ray and is referred to as "senile lung."

Changes in pulmonary vessels

The process of aging also affects the pulmonary blood vessels. In the young adult, the thin-walled pulmonary vessels have relatively low pressure because of their high distensibility and low resistance. In older adults the vessels become more fibrous and less distensible. There is also an increase in the diameter and thickness of the pulmonary artery and a consequent increase in pressure and pulmonary vascular resistance.

The mucosal bed of the alveolar capillary membrane thickens which affects the surface area available for diffusion of gases to take place. The number of capillaries declines, resulting in decreased alveolar vascularity. This combines with a diminished cardiac output to cause a decrease in pulmonary capillary blood volume.

It is unclear whether the aging process affects pulmonary surfactant. Surfactant is a lipoprotein secreted by epithelial cells in the alveoli (type II alveolar cells). This substance increases the surface tension in the alveoli and reduces the alveoli's normal tendency to collapse. Many pulmonary disease processes interfere with surfactant production. Older adults have a higher incidence of lung disease than do other adults, and they are at a greater risk for alveolar collapse secondary to decreased surfactant than are their healthy peers.

FUNCTIONAL CHANGES

The structural changes previously discussed affect respiratory function by altering the volume of air conducted to the alveolar surface, and the rate at which it is conducted, consequently affecting the volume and rate of diffusion or gas exchange in the alveoli.

Lung volumes and rate of airflow

Older adults develop altered lung volumes secondary to changes in elastic recoil and musculoskeletal changes in the chest wall. Although the change in total lung capacity is minimal in the older adult, variations are seen in the specific components of lung volume. The decreased compliance of the bony thorax accounts for major differences in residual volume and expiratory reserve volume. Residual volume increases with age by as much as 50% as a result of loss of elastic recoil. However, vital capacity decreases by 25% as the chest wall becomes less mobile and the inspiratory-expiratory capabilities are decreased (Miller, 1994). Inspiratory capacity is reduced as the ability to deep breath decreases with age. The loss of elastic recoil tends to increase total lung volumes, but this gain is offset by reduced muscle power and increased stiffness of the chest wall.

The rate of airflow from the atmosphere to the alveoli is influenced by the size of the airways, the resistance in the airways, the muscle strength, and the elastic recoil. Although airway resistance is unchanged in the healthy older person, the decrease in efficiency of elastic recoil results in early closure of the small airways and accounts for reduced rate of airflow during expiration (Timiras, 1994). In addition, the reduced muscle strength and shallow breathing patterns that usually are seen in older adults result in an increased residual volume. This problem is intensified by the supine position. For this reason, nursing plans for older adults must include both deep breathing and activity in the upright position.

Pulmonary function tests

Pulmonary function tests measure these volumes and are useful in determining the presence and degree of lung impairment, especially in the absence of overt pulmonary symptoms. For example, these tests are useful in assessing lung function in older adults who need to undergo surgical or other invasive procedures that will increase stress on respiratory patterns. They are useful in developing a specific plan of activity according to the older person's functional ability. These tests require the use of a spirometer. Because of compromising musculoskeletal changes, not all functionally impaired older adults will be able to participate in the testing methods. The older adult will also take longer to complete pulmonary function tests, even when free of lung disease.

Gas exchange

Gas exchange is the primary function of respiration, and it includes distribution of ventilation and blood flow to ventilated areas. Optimum gas exchange requires a closely matched balance of ventilation and perfusion (V-Q ratio). The shallow breathing pattern of an older person may result in hypoventilation, which decreases the V-Q ratio and is ineffective in achieving maximum gas exchange.

Measurements of partial pressure of oxygen in the arterial blood (PaO_2) and partial pressure of carbon dioxide in arterial blood ($PaCO_2$) are indicators of gas exchange adequacy in the adult. Research demonstrates a gradual decrease in arterial oxygen in the aging person, at the rate of 4 mm Hg per decade (Britt, 1993). A PaO_2 measurement of 90 would be normal in a healthy 20-year-old, whereas a value of 75 would be acceptable by age 70 (Timiras, 1994).

Several factors related to ventilation can be identified to account for the change in PaO_2: decreased areas of lung ventilation (dependent areas), early airway closure, and a decrease in functioning alveolar surface area. Other factors affect perfusion, such as decreased cardiac output and age-related hemoglobin reduction, which decreases the oxygen-carrying capacity of the blood.

Control of respiration

Central and peripheral chemoreceptors respond to hypoxemia and hypercapnia. The control of respiration by these receptors is markedly altered in older adults (Timiras, 1994). Responses to hypercapnia (increased PCO_2) and hypoxia (reduced PO_2) are reduced by 50% in the aged as compared to the young (Timiras, 1994). Normally the clinical response to hypoxemia is an increase in respiratory rate and depth. However, the older person may not exhibit the normal respiratory response to hypoxia because of age-related changes. Nursing assessment must include observation of other symptoms, such as mental confusion and restlessness. It is also important to remember that minor increases in oxygen demand will cause hypoxic symptoms more quickly in older adults and that older adults will respond more slowly to treatment for hypoxia.

Altered defense mechanisms

The older person is at increased risk for developing both upper and lower respiratory tract infections for several reasons. Both cough forcefulness and the number of cilia decrease with age. The so-called mucus escalator (which helps to move mucus and foreign materials up the respiratory tract and facilitates the coughing of mucus out through the oral cavity) is impaired. As a result, inhaled foreign material is not cleared as effectively from the large air passages. Mucus plugging of the small air ducts is also more common with aging. The alveolar macrophages, the final line of defense at the alveolar level, are less efficient (Britt, 1993). Another factor contributing to reduction of the body's defensive abilities is a decrease in IgA, the secretory immunoglobulin of nasal and respiratory mucosal surfaces, which normally neutralizes viruses (Britt, 1993).

■ Common Health Deviations

There are two types of pulmonary pathology: obstructive diseases and restrictive diseases. *Obstructive diseases* are characterized by increased resistance to airflow from one or more pathologic processes. These processes are either from inside the airway (lumenal obstruction), from outside the airway (peribronchial obstruction), or from within the wall of the airway (intrinsic airway narrowing).

Restrictive diseases are produced by a variety of disorders and diseases that affect the chest wall, pleural space, lung parenchyma, and other areas that are peripheral to the lungs. These diseases are characterized by a decrease in lung volume caused by limited lung expansion, as demonstrated by a pattern of abnormal function on the pulmonary function tests.

OBSTRUCTIVE PULMONARY DISEASES

The major obstructive pulmonary disease prominent in older adults is chronic obstructive pulmonary disease (COPD). *COPD* is an encompassing term applied to a group of pulmonary conditions that includes chronic bronchitis, pulmonary emphysema, and bronchial asthma. Usually, chronic bronchitis and pulmonary emphysema coexist in a patient, making differential diagnosis impossible. These disease entities are all of long duration and are characterized by increased resistance to or obstruction of airflow either entering or exiting the lungs as the main pathophysiologic feature.

The following facts about COPD were published by the U.S. Department of Health and Human Services (USDHHS) in a 1993 publication by the National Institutes of Health: More than 13.5 million Americans are thought to have COPD. It is the fifth leading cause of death in the United States. Between 1980 and 1990, the total death rate from COPD increased by 22%. In 1990, it was estimated that there were 84,000 deaths caused by COPD, approximately 34 per 100,000 people. Although COPD is still much more common in men than in women, the greatest increase in the COPD death rate between 1979 and 1989 occurred in women. These increases reflect the increased number of women who smoke cigarettes.

COPD attacks people at the height of their productive years, disabling them with constant shortness of breath. It destroys their ability to earn a living, causes frequent use of the health care system, and disrupts the lives of the victims' family members for as long as 20 years before death occurs. In 1990 COPD was the cause of approximately 16.2 million office visits to doctors and 1.9 million hospital days. The economic costs of this disease are enormous. In 1989 an estimated $7 billion was spent for care of people with COPD and another $8 billion was lost to the economy by lost productivity caused by morbidity and death from COPD.

Chronic bronchitis

Chronic bronchitis is defined as excessive production of mucus in the bronchi and is manifested by a chronic cough and production of mucoid or mucopurulent sputum for a minimum of 3 months per year for at least 2 consecutive years, or for 6 months during 1 year, in the absence of any other known conditions that could produce these symptoms. According to a 1993 publication by the National Institutes of Health, an estimated 12.1 million Americans have chronic bronchitis.

Middle-aged men are most often afflicted, and smoking is the most important etiologic factor. The prevalence of chronic bronchitis increases as the lifetime cigarette consumption increases beyond approximately 8 pack years of exposure, pack years being calculated by multiplying the number of packs/day times the number of years smoked (Cooper, 1993). However, environmental pollution and occupation may also play a role in the development of this disease.

The onset of bronchitis is generally insidious. It usually appears as a chronic cough that the patient, if a smoker, attributes to smoking. The course of the disease may be slow, with breathing problems not becoming apparent for many years.

Pathophysiologically, there is hypertrophy of the bronchial mucous glands and the goblet cells, and effective cilia are reduced. Death is generally due to bronchopneumonia, respiratory insufficiency, and right-sided heart failure, which occurs years after the onset of symptoms.

Pulmonary emphysema

Emphysema can only be diagnosed with certainty during a postmortem examination because it is defined morphologically as abnormal and permanent dilatation of the terminal air spaces of the lungs, combined with destruction of the alveolar wall (Cooper, 1993). The alveoli of the lungs become distended to the point of rupturing. Loss of lung elasticity accompanies this distention or rupture. The number of individuals with emphysema in the United States is estimated to be 2 million (National Institutes of Health, 1994).

On the basis of the patient's clinical picture and pulmonary function test results, a presumptive diagnosis can be made. The symptoms are slow in onset and resemble normal age-related changes in the respiratory system.

Clinically the patient develops chronic dyspnea on exertion, with or without cough. As the disease progresses, the patient demonstrates a look of anxiety, has a large hyperinflated chest, and is thin and often emaciated because of the inability to eat sufficient amounts related to the chronic dyspnea. The patient struggles to breathe, unconsciously utilizing pursed-lip breathing techniques in an effort to rid the lungs of excess trapped air. The expiratory phase of breathing is prolonged, often with wheezes (Cooper, 1993). If a cough is present, it is usually nonproductive.

Emphysema causes trapping of air in the lungs and decreases gas exchange. The trapping of air is caused by the loss of normal elastic recoil within the lungs. This loss of elasticity decreases the support and increases the collapsibility of the noncartilaginous terminal airways. This, in turn, regionally decreases lung ventilation. Decreased gas exchange leads to both pulmonary diffusion and pulmonary perfusion abnormalities.

Asthma

Asthma is a disease usually associated with childhood. However, in the older adult patient, asthma can either be of recent onset or a chronic disease from younger years. Data on the prevalence of asthma among older adults in the general population are available from several studies and are remarkably similar. Various estimates state that between 27% and 38% of adults with childhood remission of asthma have a recurrence of the disease after 45 years of age (Bardana, 1993).

There are two main types of asthma: (1) *Extrinsic,* or *IgE-triggered asthma* is primarily an allergic reaction mediated by antigen-antibody responses and is more common in the young. (2) *Intrinsic,* or *nonallergic, asthma* usually begins after the age of 35 years and may occur even later in life. This type is more commonly found in older adults. The common precipitating factor is respiratory infection. However, exposure to cigarette smoke, dust, polluted air, or just a change in temperature can precipitate an attack.

Acute exacerbation of the disease is characterized by bronchoconstriction, tracheobronchial mucosal edema, and increased secretion of thick, tenacious mucus. Local obstruction of airways can cause ventilation-perfusion mismatch. Large mucus plugs can cause complete airway obstruction.

As a result of the presence of other chronic problems, especially other cardiopulmonary disease, the older asthmatic patient has some special problems. Characteristic of moderate to severe asthma is hypoxemia. In the older adult, hypoxemia may exacerbate cardiac ischemia, as well as adversely affecting the patient's mental status.

Survival of patients with COPD is closely related to the level of their lung function at the time of diagnosis and the rate at which they lose this function. Overall, the median period of survival is about 10 years for patients with COPD who have lost approximately two thirds of the normally expected lung functioning capacity at diagnosis (National Institutes of Health, 1994). Although symptomatic relief may be obtained through pulmonary rehabilitation and education, progressive deterioration is inevitable in most patients.

RESTRICTIVE PULMONARY DISEASES

Restrictive pulmonary diseases are classified in terms of (1) whether they are acute or chronic and (2) where the pathology is located. If the primary etiologic or pathologic areas lie outside the lungs, peripheral to the visceral pleura, the disease is *extrapulmonary.*

Pulmonary restriction applies to those etiologies that lie within the lung tissue itself and that involve, to varying degrees, the alveolar and interstitial spaces, the capillary bed, or both. The major pathologic processes include loss of lung tissue, loss of functioning alveoli, and decreased lung and chest wall compliance.

Pneumonia

Pneumonia is an inflammatory process of the lung parenchyma, most commonly caused by infection. Infections of the lower respiratory tract, such as pneumonia and influenza, are a major cause of morbidity and death in older adults. The infectious agent is often present among the normal flora of the respiratory tract. Therefore the development of pneumonia can be attributed to an impaired immune system, which often occurs with aging (Timiras, 1994).

In fact, approximately 80% of deaths attributable to pneumonia and influenza occur in people older than 65 years (Fein et al., 1991). Pneumonia is the leading infectious cause of death and the fourth most common cause of death overall in older adults (Dobson & Ruben, 1993).

Sir William Osler (1892) summed things up well when he wrote that "pneumonia is the special enemy of old age. In the aged, chances are against recovery. So fatal is it in this group that it has been called the natural enemy of old man."

Today more than 800,000 hospital admissions are attributed to pneumonia each year, at a cost to the American health care system of about $1.5 billion. Approximately 37% of this figure is directed specifically at managing pneumonia in older adults (Lynch, 1992).

Pneumonia is second in frequency to urinary tract infections in older adults living in long-term care facilities. This high frequency is in part caused by the closed environment of a long-term care facility which can set the stage for periodic

All of the recommended drugs may have significant toxic effects, especially in older adults. It is very important that the nurse caring for the older patient with TB assess patient compliance with the drug regimen. Although ensuring close adherence to the drug regimen for a long time is difficult, it is essential if this disease is to be cured.

Lung cancer

Lung cancer, also referred to as bronchogenic carcinoma, is a major disease in older adults. Peak incidence for this disease occurs in the population 55 to 65 years of age. Most cases of lung cancer are seen in patients between the ages of 35 and 75 years. Each year more than 170,000 people learn that they have lung cancer (National Cancer Institute, 1993). In 1993 it was estimated that 88% of patients with a diagnosis of lung cancer would ultimately die from this disease (Perry, 1994).

The incidence of lung cancer continues to rise at remarkable rates. This form of cancer continues to be the most common fatal malignancy in men. However, increased smoking among women has resulted in a predictable increase in lung cancer in the female population. The risk of death from lung cancer is related to the degree of cigarette abuse. Fifteen or more years must elapse after a person stops smoking for the risk to approach that of nonsmokers (Perry, 1994).

Although the exact etiology of lung cancer is unknown, it is believed that the disease process begins with inhalation of carcinogenic pollutants by a susceptible host. Inhalation of such carcinogenic agents as tobacco smoke, industrial hazards, and air pollution accounts for an increase in incidence. Of these agents, tobacco smoke appears to play the major role. Lung cancer is 10 times more common in smokers than in nonsmokers.

There are four types of lung cancer: (1) squamous cell carcinoma, (2) adenocarcinoma, (3) small cell (oat cell) carcinoma, and (4) large cell carcinoma. The most common type is squamous cell. Lung cancers are classified according to the tumor node metastasis (TNM) staging system. There are five stages, 0 through 4, reflecting increasing extent or dissemination of the disease. Generally, non–small cell carcinomas respond to surgery, and small cell carcinoma responds to chemotherapy and/or radiation therapy. For all types of lung cancer, metastasis may occur in multiple sites, but bone, bone marrow, the liver, the lymph nodes, and the brain are the most common sites (Perry, 1994). Particularly low survival rates occur with small cell cancer. Life expectancy for this type of carcinoma is often given in weeks or months rather than in years, depending on staging of the disease.

The onset of lung cancer is insidious, producing either no signs and symptoms or signs and symptoms resembling those of pneumonia or other respiratory diseases that are common in the older population. Therefore, it is not uncommon for such signs to be ignored or to be attributed to other causes—smoking or bronchitis, for example. The most common early signs are cough, chest pain, and streaky hemoptysis.

The disease is more likely to be localized at diagnosis in older patients than in middle-aged patients. Localized cancers are generally more readily resectable and thus potentially curable (Perry, 1994).

The older patient facing tumor resection surgery poses a challenge to nursing. The nurse must supplement and reinforce the patient's understanding of the disease and the surgical procedure, as told by the physician. Preoperative teaching of techniques to prevent postoperative complications, as well as explanation of expected postoperative care and side effects of radiation therapy and chemotherapy, is necessary.

PULMONARY VASCULAR DISORDERS

Pulmonary vascular disorders rank among the most serious complications of respiratory or cardiovascular disease. Left untreated, these disorders cause severe lung damage that can dramatically impair or threaten a patient's lifestyle. The disorders that are commonly seen in the older patient are pulmonary edema, which usually stems from cardiac disease, and pulmonary embolism, which is caused by thrombus formation originating in the venous system.

In pulmonary vascular disorders, the pressure within the pulmonary circulation must be great enough to overcome pulmonary vascular resistance, to ensure adequate lung perfusion for gas exchange to occur. The human body reacts with two mechanisms to compensate for pulmonary vascular resistance: tachycardia and tachypnea. However, if pulmonary vascular resistance becomes chronic, these two mechanisms lead to further complications.

Pulmonary embolism and infarction

Pulmonary embolism (PE) is an obstruction of the pulmonary arterial bed by a dislodged thrombus or by foreign matter. It is known to be a complication of venous thrombosis. Pulmonary embolism is a common pulmonary complication and an important cause of morbidity and death in the older population. Of people with deep vein thrombosis, 500,000, or 10%, develop PE; 50,000 of these cases prove fatal (Mosher, 1994). PE is difficult to diagnose clinically. Pulmonary angiography is the most definitive test used for diagnosis.

Pulmonary infarction (tissue death) results when the PE is extensive enough to produce necrosis or death of lung parenchyma. This occurs in about 10% to 30% of PE patients. Pulmonary infarction is most likely to occur in patients (1) of advanced age, (2) with septic embolism and the associated inflammatory process in the lungs, (3) with already diseased pulmonary arteries from conditions such as COPD and pulmonary vasculitis, and (4) with reduced blood flow to the bronchial arteries supplying the lungs, which occurs in CHF and prolonged shock. Pulmonary infarction may evolve from PE, especially in patients with chronic cardiac or pulmonary disease.

Three basic factors relate to the development of venous thrombosis and subsequent PE: (1) venous stasis or slowing of the blood flow, (2) injury to the vein wall, and (3) hypercoagulability (Hunninghake, 1994). Risk of thrombus formation is increased by (1) obesity, (2) heart failure, (3) varicose veins, (4) abdominal infection, (5) cancer, and (6) prolonged inactivity or immobility. PE occurs predominantly in bedridden patients because of their immobility. The single condition that most predisposes a person to venous thrombosis is CHF. This is important to keep in mind when caring for older people, who frequently have some form of CHF. Prophylaxis to prevent the development of venous thrombosis is especially important in the gerontologic population (Hunninghake, 1994).

The classic presentation of PE is dyspnea, apprehension, anginal or pleuritic chest pain, hemoptysis, and a pleural friction rub in the setting of thrombophlebitis (Hunninghake, 1994). The older patient may not be able to describe the type or intensity of pain being experienced. If the patient has underlying respiratory or cardiac disease, such symptoms could be common to those diseases. The older person might ignore the symptoms or attribute them to other pathologic conditions.

Pulmonary edema

Pulmonary edema refers to accumulation of serous fluid in extravascular lung spaces. It can occur as a chronic condition, or it can develop quickly with death rapidly ensuing. It is a common complication of many cardiopulmonary diseases. Pulmonary edema usually results from left ventricular failure (LVF). Common causes of LVF include arteriosclerotic, cardiomyopathic, hypertensive, and valvular cardiac diseases which result in increased pulmonary capillary hydrostatic pressure.

Pulmonary edema can also occur in diseases that result in decreased colloid osmotic pressure in the lungs. This type is commonly referred to as noncardiogenic pulmonary edema or adult respiratory distress syndrome (ARDS). This syndrome is associated with such clinical disorders as severe malnutrition, burns, trauma, pancreatic or hepatic disease, nephritis, hematologic disorders, inhalation of noxious gases, liquid aspiration, and inflammation or infection (Matthay & Hopewell, 1994). Any lung injury that interferes with the diffusion of oxygen consequently results in tissue hypoxia, which further increases the tendency toward pulmonary edema.

In the early stages of this process, evidence of pulmonary edema reflects interstitial and alveolar fluid accumulation and diminished lung compliance. Dyspnea on exertion, paroxysmal nocturnal dyspnea, and orthopnea are the usual presenting signs and symptoms. Respirations become labored and rapid, with coughing productive of the classic "frothy pink-tinged or bloody sputum." The patient may also start to show signs of a decreased level of consciousness and of confusion as gas exchange becomes increasingly impaired.

The treatment for pulmonary edema is diuretic therapy. Such therapy will improve gas exchange and myocardial function by reducing extravascular fluid. It is also important to correct the underlying pathologic process.

■ Nursing Process

ASSESSMENT

The multidimensional status of the older patient is the focus of assessment. Essential for conducting a successful assessment of the respiratory system is the development of a complete and accurate data base.

The nurse, as the examiner, must be able to set up effective communication with the patient to obtain a complete and accurate health history. When caring for the older adult, this may be very difficult to achieve because of other medical and possibly cognitive problems.

Should the older patient be a poor historian, it is important to seek other means of obtaining information. Information can be obtained from family members, friends, previous health records,

Aging Alert

- Efficiency in collecting patient data is enhanced by developing and maintaining trust between the patient and the nurse.
- Carefully listening to the patient's responses ensures the collection of complete and pertinent patient data.
- The nurse uses inspection, palpation, percussion, and auscultation to assess the patient's respiratory status.

or other health care professionals. Having family members describe the patient's condition is helpful because they may be able to provide needed information.

Often, older patients neglect to report symptoms because they believe that their symptoms are a result of aging and are not amenable to treatment. The nurse needs to be skillful in directing questions and in carefully listening to the older patient's responses.

History

A health history is the first element of the data base. It is the single most important element in establishing the patient's problems. A comprehensive health history gives the examiner a picture of the patient's past and current problems.

To adequately assess the respiratory status of the older person, the nurse must determine three important points: (1) the presence and extent of signs and symptoms that indicate pulmonary disease or impairment, (2) the presence of environmental factors (particularly smoking) that interfere with respiratory function, and (3) the extent to which the patient's normal lifestyle and activities of daily living (ADLS) have changed or have become limited as a result of impaired respiratory function.

Important questions when assessing overall respiratory functioning include the following:

1. Do you have a history of respiratory problems, such as asthma, pneumonia, chronic lung disease, influenza, or frequent colds?
2. Do you take any prescription medication for respiratory problems?
3. Do you take any over-the-counter (OTC) preparations for coughs, colds, or allergies?
4. Do you smoke now, or have you ever smoked? Do you live with a smoker?
5. Do you now live, or have you ever lived, in a neighborhood where there was a lot of pollution from traffic or industry?
6. Have you ever been employed where you were exposed to air pollutants, dust, or fumes?
7. Do you ever have difficulty breathing or get short of breath? Does this occur when doing particular activities, such as walking or climbing stairs?
8. Do you ever feel as though you can't catch your breath or you're not getting enough air?
9. Do you have trouble breathing that is related to changes in the weather or temperature?
10. Do you ever wheeze?
11. Do you have coughing spells? If so,
    a. When do they occur?
    b. How long do they last?
    c. What brings them on?
    d. Are they dry, or do they produce sputum?
    e. What does the sputum look like?
12. Do you use more than one pillow at night? Do you change your position frequently because of difficulty in breathing?
13. Do you get tired or fatigued easily?
14. Do you have any other chronic diseases, such as hypertension, arthritis, or cardiac disease?
15. Have you recently had a chest x-ray, arterial blood gas analysis, or any pulmonary function tests?
16. Have you ever had immunizations for pneumococcal pneumonia or influenza?
17. Have you ever had TB or contact with anyone with the disease?
18. Have you ever had a positive TB skin test?

Physical examination

When examining older people, it is important to properly and thoroughly prepare the patients. Explain your actions; help them to relax; answer any questions they may have; do not rush; make sure the examination room is well lighted, warm, and quiet; and provide privacy to the patients.

Examination of the respiratory function of the patient requires use of the four key techniques: inspection, palpation, percussion, and auscultation. Equipment necessary to evaluate the respiratory system in the older adult is a stethoscope. Using a tape measure to determine the diameter of chest expansion is a waste of time because of the normal age-related changes.

Inspection or observation   To inspect the patient properly, observe everything, including the patient's behavior. The following areas should be included in the inspection phase of the physical examination.

Head and neck

1. Mental state—Delirium, confusion, or hallucinations may mean severe hypoxia or hypercarbia. With older patients, be cautious not to attribute disorientation to age. Fearfulness, restlessness, and an anxious facial expression are often seen in patients with acute respiratory distress.
2. Color—Observe for pallor, flushing, cyanosis of the buccal mucosa and lips, and extremely pink or ruddy skin.
3. Lips—Look for breathing out through pursed lips or circumoral cyanosis.
4. Nose—Look for nasal flaring.
5. Neck—Look for retraction of accessory muscles, vein engorgement, and trachea position.

Chest

1. Movement—Look for inspiratory intercostal retractions or bulges, use of accessory muscles during respiration, and abdominal breathing.
2. Sternal abnormalities—Look for pigeon, barrel, or funnel chest.
3. Spinal abnormalities—Look for kyphosis, scoliosis, or kyphoscoliosis.

Barrel chest and spinal abnormalities may be attributed to normal age-related changes. However, further investigation is warranted to make a differential diagnosis.

Extremities

1. Skin—Look for elevated temperature, diaphoresis, or clamminess.
2. Fingers and toes—Look for clubbing, asterixis, or nail bed cyanosis.
3. Legs—Look for signs of thrombophlebitis: Check the patient's calves for redness, swelling, warmth, and positive Homan's sign; check for ankle edema.

Palpation Inform the patient that you are about to put your hands on the patient's back. Be aware of the following areas: expect limited chest expansion in the older adult because of the normal age-related changes of stiffness of the rib cage and decreased muscle strength; check for increases or decreases in intensity of tactile fremitus, both anteriorly and posteriorly; palpate for abnormal masses or lumps; watch for tender areas, because rib fractures are common in older adults.

Percussion The lungs of the healthy older patient may sound resonant on percussion. Hyperresonance is usually a sign of an abnormal increase in the amount of air in the lungs, as in emphysema. Dull or flat sounds can be signs of areas of possible consolidation, tumor, or effusion.

Auscultation The older patient may not be able to take the deep and frequent breaths needed for auscultation of the lung fields. The nurse must remember that the sounds heard over normal lung tissue are no different in older versus younger adults. The breath sounds of older patients with scoliosis or kyphosis will sound distant in affected areas. All adventitious sounds—such as rales, rhonchi, wheezes, and rub—are abnormal and are heard only if disease is present.

Diagnostic studies

The complete patient data base also includes findings from diagnostic studies. Depending on the information obtained from the history and physical examination, some appropriate diagnostic studies are the following:

1. Arterial blood gas analysis
2. Pulmonary function test
3. Chest roentgenogram
4. TB skin test
5. Laboratory values
6. Sputum examination
7. Lung scan
8. Pulmonary angiography
9. Insertion of a Swan-Ganz catheter
10. Exercise tolerance test
11. Mental status examination (MSE)
12. Electrocardiogram (ECG)

Values assessment

The nurse's assessment should also help to identify the patient's values and should serve to assist the patient in providing advance health care directives on the basis of those values. If the patient is competent to make such decisions, it is important to have these stated directives put in a legal document, such as a living will or medical durable power of attorney. This is particularly important in the current age of modern technology, in which increasingly complex ethical dilemmas occur in hospitals and in long-term care facilities.

Older patients who are suffering from a chronic respiratory disease are faced with making decisions that will affect their quality and length of life, such as decisions regarding the following:

1. Resuscitation in the event of cardiopulmonary arrest
2. Performance of a tracheostomy in the event that the older patient cannot adequately clear the secretions from the lungs
3. Placement on a life-support system, such as a ventilator, because the older patient is unable to sustain adequate breathing because of a worsening disease process or patient fatigue
4. In the event of placement on such a life support system, determining whether the device should be maintained indefinitely or should be withdrawn when no clinical sings of improvement are demonstrated

Many individuals have very strong feelings about what they would and would not want to have done for them. It is clearly in the patient's best interest that these wishes be explored beforehand and that they be put in writing, as well as being discussed with family members who may be ultimately responsible for making such decisions about the patient's care.

Psychosocial assessment

Psychosocial assessment evaluates cognitive function, affective function, and the social support system. The psychosocial assessment can be focused to gather information pertinent to a specific area of nursing concern. One area to consider when caring for an older patient with a chronic respiratory condition is that person's ability to take prescribed medications correctly.

Older adults face specific risks in each area of psychosocial functioning. In the area of cognitive functioning, older adults are most likely to complain of or to experience memory impairments. It is difficult but crucial to differentiate between changes that are related to age and those that are related to respiratory disease.

Assessment of affective functioning is essential in planning appropriate interventions. If older patients are depressed, anxious, feeling hopeless, or otherwise psychosocially impaired, they will be unable to comply with the plan of care and many needed interventions.

The patient's social support system includes the social network of family and friends who are available to the patient for different types of support. Questions about economic resources and religious affiliation can be included in this section of the assessment. The purpose of a nursing assessment of the patient's social support system is to identify resources that are available to meet basic needs and to improve the quality of life for the patient.

The older individual with respiratory disease may need assistance in obtaining, as well as in correctly taking, medications. The nurse needs to consider the following:

1. Does the patient have the monetary resources or health insurance coverage to pay for the medications?
2. Does the patient have the transportation to get to a pharmacy?
3. Is the patient competent to take the medications as prescribed?
4. Is someone available to assist the patient in obtaining, taking, and monitoring the effects of medications?

Environmental assessment

The well-being of older adults is influenced by the environment, whether in the home, the hospital, or a long-term care facility. The environmental assessment specific to respiratory problems is presented in Box 11-1.

NURSING DIAGNOSES

Upon completion of a thorough history and physical examination, the nurse prepares to analyze the data and formulate appropriate nursing diagnoses. Following the nursing diagnoses, a plan of care with individualized interventions that best address the needs of the older person is developed. Input into the plan of care is elicited from the patient, family members, or significant others involved in caring for the patient.

Britt, T. L. (1993). Elderly patients. In J. M. Clochesy, C. Breu, S. Cardin, E. B. Rudy, & A. A. Whittaker (Eds.), *Critical care nursing* (pp. 1351-1372). Philadelphia: W. B. Saunders.

Centers for Disease Control and Prevention. (1994). Prevention and control of influenza: 1. Vaccines. *Morbidity and Mortality Weekly Report, 43*, RR-9.

Chapman, K., Love, L., & Brubaker, H. (1993). A comparison of breath actuated and conventional metered-dose inhaler inhalation techniques in elderly subjects *Chest, 104*, 1332-1337.

Cooper, D. (1993). Patients with chronic obstructive pulmonary disease. In J. M. Clochesy, C. Breu, S. Cardin, E. B. Rudy, & A. A. Whittaker (Eds.), *Critical care nursing* (pp. 569-588). Philadelphia: W. B. Saunders.

Couser, J. (1994). Interpreting tuberculin skin tests in the elderly. *Journal of Respiratory Diseases, 15*, 869-870.

Dettenmeier, P. A. (1992). *Pulmonary nursing care* (pp. 385-439). St. Louis: Mosby.

Dobson, M. E., & Ruben, F. L. (1993). The special challenge of pneumonia in the elderly. *Journal of Respiratory Diseases, 14*, 1145-1164.

Ely, E. W., Pegram, P. S., & Haponik, E. F. (1994a). Managing and preventing pneumonia in the elderly. *Journal of Respiratory Diseases, 15*, 295-311.

Ely, E. W., Pegram, P. S., & Haponik, E. F. (1994b). Working up the elderly patient with pneumonia. *Journal of Respiratory Diseases, 15*, 222-234.

Fein, A. M., Feinsilver, S. H., & Niederman, M. S. (1991). Atypical manifestations of pneumonia in the elderly. *Clinical Chest Medicine, 12*, 319-336.

Ferguson, G. T., & Cherniack, R. M. (1993). Management of chronic obstructive pulmonary disease. *New England Journal of Medicine, 328*, 1017-1022.

Health benefits of smoking cessation: A report of the surgeon general. (1990).

Hogstel, M. O. (1994). *Nursing care of the older adult.* New York: Delmar.

Hunninghake, G. W. (1994). Interstitial lung disease, hypersensitivity pneumonitis, and pulmonary vascular disease. In W. Hazzard, E. Bierman, J. Blass, W. Ettinger, & J. Halter (Eds.), *Principles of geriatric medicine and gerontology* (pp. 597-606). New York: McGraw-Hill.

Influenza 1994-95: Now's the time to prepare. (1994). *Journal of Respiratory Diseases, 15*, 675-687.

Levitzky, M. G. (1991). *Pulmonary physiology* (3rd ed.). New York: McGraw-Hill.

Lynch, J. P. (1992). Community-acquired pneumonia: What new trends mean in practice. *Journal of Respiratory Diseases, 13*, 1619-1643.

Maloney, S. K. (1992). *Smoking among older adults: Findings from three surveys.* American Association of Retired Persons Health Advocacy Services.

Mangura, B. T., & Reichman, L. B. (1994). Tuberculosis: Guidelines for preventive therapy. *Journal of Respiratory Diseases, 15*, 109-121.

Mathewson, M. D., & Kovac, A. L. (1994). Update on inhaled steroids. *Respiratory Care, 39*, 837-839.

Matthay, M. A., & Hopewell, P. C. (1994). Critical care for acute respiratory failure. In G. Baum & E. Wolinsky (Eds.), *Textbook of pulmonary diseases* (5th ed., Vol. 2). Boston: Little, Brown and Company.

McArthur, M. A., Simor, A. E., Campbell, B., & McGeer, A. (1995). Influenza and pneumococcal vaccinations and tuberculin skin testing programs in long-term care facilities: Where do we stand? *Infection Control and Hospital Epidemiology, 16*(1), 18-24.

Miller, C. (1994). *Nursing care of older adults: Theory and practice* (2nd ed.). Philadelphia: J. B. Lippincott.

Mosher, K. M. (1994). Pulmonary embolism. In G. Baum & E. Wolinsky (Eds.), *Textbook of pulmonary diseases* (5th ed., Vol. 2). Boston: Little, Brown and Company.

National Cancer Institute. (1993, June). *What you need to know about lung cancer* (NIH Pub. No. 93-1553). Washington, DC: U.S. Department of Health and Human Services.

National Institute on Aging. (1994). *Pneumonia prevention: It's worth a shot* (AGE PAGE). Washington, DC: U.S. Department of Health and Human Services.

National Institutes of Health, National Heart, Lung, and Blood Institute. (1994, November). NIH Pub. No. 93-2020. Washington, DC: U.S. Department of Health and Human Services.

Niederman, M. S. (1993). Pneumonia in residents of long-term care facilities: A guide to diagnosis and management. *Long-term Care Forum, 3*(2), 1:12-15.

O'Donnell, D. E., Webb, K. A., & McGuire, M. A. (1993). Older patients with COPD: Benefits of exercise training. *Geriatrics, 48*(1), 59-66.

Osler, W. (1892). *Principles and practice of medicine.* New York: D. Appleton and Company.

Perry, M. C. (1994). Lung cancer. In W. Hazzard, E. Bierman, J. Blass, W. Ettinger, & J. Halter (Eds.), *Principles of geriatric medicine and gerontology* (pp. 607-613). New York: McGraw-Hill.

Poe, R. H., & Israel, R. H. (1994). Theophylline: Still a reasonable choice? *Journal of Respiratory Diseases, 15*(1), 19-30.

Richman, L. (1992). A looming public health nightmare. In *Lungs at work.* American Lung Association.

Schapira, R. M., & Reinke, L. (1995). The outpatient diagnosis and management of chronic obstructive pulmonary disease. *Journal of Geriatric Internal Medicine, 10,* 40-55.

Stead, W., & Dutt, A. (1994). Tuberculosis: A special problem in the elderly. In W. Hazzard, E. Bierman, J. Blass, W. Ettinger, & J. Halter (Eds.), *Principles of geriatric medicine and gerontology* (pp. 575-582). New York: McGraw-Hill.

Timiras, P. S. (1994). *Physiological basis of aging and geriatrics* (2nd ed.). Boca Raton, FL: CRC Press.

Toogood, J. H. (1994). Helping your patients make better use of MDIs and spacers. *Journal of Respiratory Diseases, 15,* 151-166.

U.S. Department of Health and Human Services. (1992). *Healthy People 2000: Public health service action* (DHHS Pub. No. [PHS] 91-50212). Washington, DC: U.S. Government Printing Office.

U.S. Department of Health and Human Services. (1993, January). *Nurses: Help your patient stop smoking* (NIH Pub. No. 92-2962). Washington, DC: U.S. Government Printing Office.

Wade, W. E. (1993). Managing pneumonia in the elderly. *Clinical Consult, 12*(1), 1-7.

Yoshikawa, T. (1992). Tuberculosis in aging adults. *Journal of the American Geriatrics Society, 40,* 178.

BIBLIOGRAPHY

Allen and Hanburys. (1994). *Patient's instructions for use of inhalation aerosol* (Pamphlet No. RL-164). Author.

Alspach, J. G. (1991). *Core curriculum for critical care nursing* (4th ed.). Philadelphia: W. B. Saunders.

Kenney, R. A. (1989). *Physiology of aging.* Chicago: Yearbook Medical.

McCance, K., & Huether, S. (1994). *Pathophysiology: The biologic basis for disease in adults and children* (2nd ed.). St. Louis: Mosby.

Phipps, W., Cassmeyer, V., Sands, J., & Lehman, M. K. (1995). *Medical-surgical nursing: Concepts and clinical practice* (5th ed.). St. Louis: Mosby.

Thibodeau, G. (1990). *Anthony's textbook of anatomy and physiology* (13th ed.). St. Louis: Mosby.

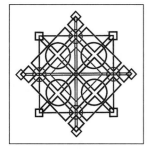

C H A P T E R 12

Give me a young man in whom there is something of the old, and an old man with something of the young: guided so, a man may grow old in body, but never in mind.

CICERO

Mobility

■ Learning Objectives

On completion of this chapter, the reader will be able to do the following:

1. Define mobility.
2. Understand the anatomy and physiology of the musculoskeletal system.
3. Know the physical and psychosocial aspects of mobility in the older adult.
4. Recognize normal age-related changes and common health deviations in the musculoskeletal system that affect mobility of the older adult.
5. Specify common psychosocial problems in relation to health deviations in mobility.
6. Assess functional mobility of the older adult.
7. Use the nursing process in determining the care of people with problems in mobility.
8. Develop methods for promoting healthy mobility throughout the adult life span.

The ability to move from one point to another without fear of pain or injury is one most adults take for granted. In the life of a small child the event of the first step is welcomed with a great deal of parental pride and trepidation. The parents' mixed feelings originate in the realization that the ability to stand and walk is the beginning of the child's ability to express free and independent action. This independent state and the freedom of choice is the hallmark of adult life. To be free to walk or run wherever you want, whenever you want, and at whatever speed you want is one of the unrecognized gifts of life. For the older adult, the ability to run is

severely limited or nonexistent; the ability or the will to walk may be limited or just more difficult to initiate and to sustain.

Mobility is defined as the independent ability to move or to be moved—a body capable of locomotion. This definition does not preclude mobility achieved through assistive devices, such as a motorized wheelchair, specially equipped automobile, or artificial limbs. In a more traditional view, assessment of mobility both clinically and for research purposes may be achieved by measurement of three physical activities: walking, climbing stairs, and transferring (Ettinger, 1994).

At first the concept of mobility seems simple and uncomplicated. On further investigation, however, the complexity of mobility in the older adult becomes apparent. Necessary ingredients for mobility are (1) cognition and motivation, (2) a skeletal system that is capable of supporting the body's weight, (3) muscles with enough strength to move the body, and (4) a neurologic system that is capable of interaction with the musculoskeletal system (Figure 12-1).

Factors that impede mobility in the older adult can be physical, psychologic, social, or environmental. Myriad physical age-related changes, such as slowed neurologic response and decreased muscle strength, can make mobility a physical challenge for the older adult. Abnormal gait and poor balance increase the challenge of safe mobility in older adults.

A psychologic condition that affects some older adults is the fear of injury. Often the older adult makes a realistic appraisal of the physical and environmental conditions and concludes that there is an increased risk of injury. How the older adult accommodates for the increased risk is the paramount issue. If the response to the risk is not to walk, not to cross the street, or not to travel, thereby significantly diminishing the risk of injury, the older adult may no longer be mobile or independent.

Related to the fear of injury is the fear of embarrassment. Actually, it is difficult to separate the two emotional responses of older adults as

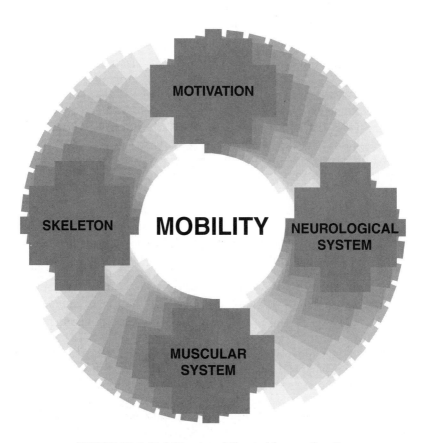

FIGURE 12-1 Mobility: A multifaceted human function.

they cope with the loss of physical vigor and agility. Planning for a day of shopping, which most people do with ease, is quite a different experience for older adults who have limited mobility. The difficulties encountered by older adults who are trying to maintain their independence and their pride in spite of impaired mobility relate to transportation, environmental obstacles, and public opinion.

Transportation is a major issue: Is there public transportation? If so, can the older adults step on and off the bus or van? Is there a relative or friend who will provide transportation and take them shopping? Can the older adults still safely drive or afford a taxi? Is there a local program that offers van transportation for people in wheelchairs?

Unexpected changes in the weather also may create a hazard for older adults, particularly those with limitations in mobility. Physically, older adults are more susceptible to the extremes of cold or heat and are at higher risk for falls during icy and rainy weather.

Other environmental factors encountered during a shopping trip are stores with difficult entrances, inclines that are slanted and poorly lighted, electric doors that are poorly marked, items that are on high shelves, fast-moving escalators, and corridors and shops that offer no place to sit and rest.

Many older adults find themselves embarrassed by either or both of the following extremes of public opinion: At one extreme is the clerk or fellow shopper who has little patience for the slow pace of the older adult shopper, or the clerk who is indifferent in providing the extra assistance needed to reach the items higher on the shelf. Either of these may cause the older adult to lose a sense of confidence. At the other extreme is the overprotective person who treats older adult shoppers as if they are 5-year-olds who have lost their mothers. As one older woman with limited mobility remarked, "Just because I've lost the ability to walk doesn't mean I've lost the ability to think." It is difficult to maintain mobility while overcoming the fear and

embarrassment that result from everyday experiences.

As with many aspects of life, mobility becomes increasingly difficult for many older adults. It is a testimony to the unrecognized strengths of older adults that the majority remain mobile, active, and occupied with all aspects of living. Nurses have the opportunity and the responsibility to recognize the strengths of older adults, provide encouraging comments about their ability to meet the challenge of maintaining mobility, and contribute to increasing their self-esteem.

The next sections of this chapter present the normal musculoskeletal system, the normal age-related changes that occur in this system, and the common health deviations that affect the mobility of many older adults.

■ Normal Structure and Function

The musculoskeletal system consists of bones, muscles, tendons, ligaments, joints, and bursae. The contribution of the skeleton to mobility is to provide structure to the human form and to facilitate movement. The skeleton is made up of bone, which is continuously involved in the processes of formation and resorption throughout the life cycle. Bone growth is partially regulated by mechanical stimuli, such as physical activity and weight bearing. Diet and genetic factors also contribute to bone growth. Skeletal mass increases during the growth years, and a peak in bone mass usually is reached between the ages of 20 and 30 years. Bone formation is the major process that contributes to the growth of bone mass.

There are two significant types of bone tissue: (1) *Trabecular bone* forms the majority of bone in the vertebral body and in the flat bones. (2) *Cortical bone* forms most of the long bones. Bones are composed of an organic matrix, 95% of which is collagen fibers and ground substance (bone salts). The bone salts principally comprise calcium and phosphate, with smaller amounts of magnesium, sodium, potassium, and carbonate ions. Calcium provides bone with its great compressional strength.

Bone gives shape to the musculoskeletal system, but other structures supply connections, strength, and flexibility. *Ligaments* are flexible bands of strong connective tissue, which connect the articular extremities of bone and which allow freedom of movement. *Tendons* are fibrous cords of connective tissue that serve as the mechanism for connecting muscle to movable structures such as bone. *Joints* provide the point of articulation between bones. *Bursae* are small, fluid-filled sacs surrounding the points of friction in joints.

There are three identifiable types of skeletal muscle fibers: type I (slow-twitch, high-oxidative fiber), type II (fast-twitch, high-oxidative fiber), and type IIB (fast-twitch, slow-oxidative fiber). The slow-twitch muscle fibers can sustain tension for long periods, are slow to fatigue, and have high aerobic capacity (high oxidation). The fast-twitch fibers, on the other hand, develop high tension rapidly but with no endurance over time and have anaerobic capacity (slow oxidation) (Schwartz & Buchner, 1994).

In conjunction with the skeletal system, muscles interact with the neurologic system to produce body movements: flexion, extension, abduction, adduction, pronation, supination, and both internal and external rotation. Disuse of muscles leads to *atrophy*, which decreases both the size and the strength of muscles.

■ Age-Related Changes

The normal musculoskeletal system undergoes various age-related changes that affect mobility (Box 12-1). Between the ages of 30 and 50 years, an equilibrium is established, in which the processes of formation and resorption stabilize the amount of bone mass. After age 50 this equilibrium shifts, and an incremental process of bone resorption without the successful formation of new bone mass leads to a gradual bone loss. That is, from age 50 on, the resorption of bone gradually extracts calcium and destroys the bone's organic matrix, thereby diminishing bone mass.

Aging-changes in cortical bone, which accounts for 75% of the skeletal weight, leads

BOX 12-1 AGE-RELATED CHANGES IN THE MUSCULOSKELETAL SYSTEM AND MOBILITY

1. Gradual loss of bone mass
2. Diminished muscle strength
3. Decrease in reaction time
4. Decrease in speed of movement

to a reduction in cortical thickness and an increase in porosity resulting in progressive cortical thinning. Trabecular bone accounts for the remaining 25% of bone weight. Aging affects trabecular bone by thinning and destruction of the bone (Baylink & Jennings, 1994).

The initial, significant loss of bone mass occurs in trabecular bone, which leads to a susceptibility to compression fractures in the vertebral column. Cortical bone loss occurs later than trabecular bone loss, and this loss leads to a susceptibility to fractures of the femur.

In normal, healthy older adults the regulation of calcium blood levels remains in a normal range. The exchange of calcium is a complex interaction among the extracellular fluid, the intestine, the skeleton, and the kidney. Calcium metabolism is influenced by parathyroid hormone (PTH), phosphate, vitamin D, and calcitonin (a thyroid hormone). In older adults the PTH levels have shown an increase, and vitamin D and calcitonin levels a decrease. Because bone and calcium metabolism are highly integrated, the age-related calcium loss from bone results from the body's need to maintain normal calcium levels (Baylink & Jennings, 1994).

In women, major bone loss determinants are estrogen deficiency, calcium malabsorption, lifestyle factors, and genetic history. The first 5 to 8 years after menopause is when major bone loss occurs. Lifestyle factors that influence bone volume are calcium intake and exercise. Estrogen replacement therapy has risks and benefits, and each woman must make a decision based on accurate, individualized, and current information.

Aging brings a decline in numbers of muscle fibers, which results in a reduced muscle mass. As people age, there is a decrease in total muscle mass, a decrease in number and size of type II (fast-twitch) muscle fibers, and a decrease in the metabolic and oxidative capacity of muscle cells (Schwartz & Buchner, 1994). For many older adults there is a sequential loss in muscle strength. The degree of loss varies greatly among muscle groups, and changes attributed to the aging process are significantly less where the muscle group has been used. In different groups of older adults, studies have shown that regular exercise, especially resistance training (weight lifting), demonstrates a reduced rate of muscle strength decline (Buchner et al., 1992; Fiatrone et al., 1990). The decline in muscle function depends on other systems, such as the neurologic and the musculoskeletal systems. As a result of age-related changes in the neurologic system, there is a progressive decrease in reaction time and speed of movement, and this adversely affects muscle function.

The loss of muscle strength creates a cycle of debilitating events as people begin to think that, because they are older, they have lost strength and cannot exercise, when actually the loss of strength is compounded by a lack of exercise. The body's adaptability to exercise remains unimpaired with aging. Recent investigations support the proposition that much of what has been attributed to aging is a result of inactivity. Recovery from exercise may take longer for older adults, but under proper guidance, an effective exercise program can lead to increased muscle strength. The axiom "Use it or lose it" directly relates to aging muscle.

Many health professionals unquestioningly accept stereotypic descriptions of older adults, such as "kyphotic," and "having muscular rigidity," because of their experience with institutionalized, inactive older adults. They come to accept the debilitative condition of institutionalized older adults as a result of the aging process and

Aging Alert
1. Disuse of muscles leads to loss of muscle strength.
2. Physical inactivity is a major threat to health.
3. Exercise is a vital component of a healthy lifestyle.

chronic disease. This is a mistake. It would be more accurate to ascribe this condition at least partly to inactivity and inappropriate care. A treatment plan that does not provide for exercise or for activities for all older adults is neglectful. Lack of appropriate care contributes to the loss of strength and the loss of spirit that lead to a loss of mobility, a triple jeopardy for institutionalized older adults.

Inactivity, bed rest, and subsequent immobility lead to a rapid loss of muscle size and strength. To prevent this type of loss, the nurse, along with other members of the health care team, needs to be aware of the potential problems that can arise because of prolonged muscle disuse.

■ Common Health Deviations

OSTEOPOROSIS

Osteoporosis is a disease of multiple etiologies. A common element in all cases of the disease is reduction of bone mass to a level leading to fracture, especially of the vertebrae, distal radius, and femur. Skeletal osteopenia refers to bone mass reduction. Inasmuch as bone loss is universal, osteoporosis as a clinical entity occurs only if there is an associated fracture.

Osteoporosis is a common occurrence in the older population, leading to an estimated 1.5 million fractures per year. The cost and burden of suffering associated with this condition have

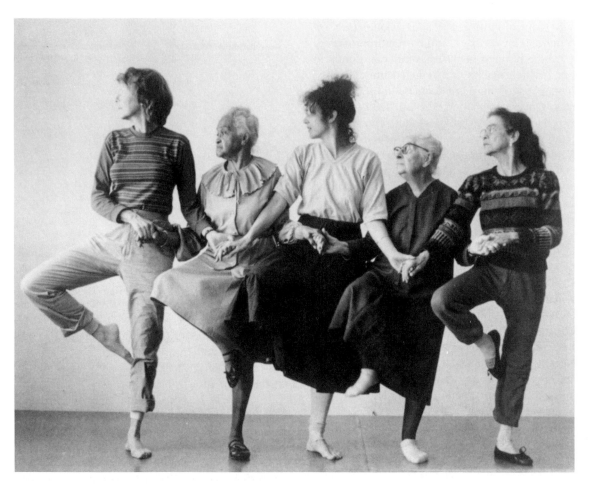

Dancers of the Third Age (DTA), a multigenerational modern dance company, is one of many programs sponsored by The Dance Exchange. The Dance Exchange, founded by dancer-choreographer Liz Lerman, is a nonprofit arts organization whose work is based on the inseparable concerns of artistic excellence and community involvement. By bringing dance to senior adults, people in hospitals, children, people without homes, and women in shelters, as well as concert stage audiences, The Dance Exchange demonstrates its philosophy that dance is for everyone. (Printed with permission of The Dance Exchange, Inc., 1746-B Kalorama Road, NW, Washington, DC 20009.) *Photo by Dennis Deloria.*

become a public health concern. Of women who are now 35 years of age, 8% will experience a hip fracture in their lifetime. The mortality rate for hip fractures is as high as 20%. Thirty percent of women and 15% of men over the age of 60 years have clinical osteoporosis. Risk factors that influ-ence the development of osteoporosis are the level of bone mass at maturity, gender, age, diet, disease, alcoholism, smoking, medications, and mobility (Chestnut, 1994) (Figure 12-2).

Skeletal mass at maturity is less for women than for men; 18-year-old women have 20% less

RISK FACTORS FOR OSTEOPOROSIS

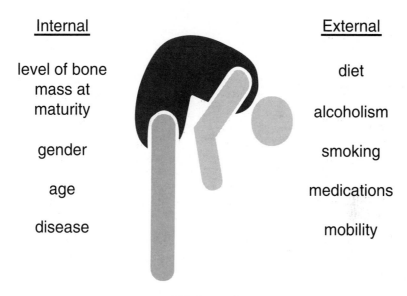

Internal

level of bone
mass at
maturity

gender

age

disease

External

diet

alcoholism

smoking

medications

mobility

FIGURE 12-2 Risk factors for osteoporosis.

bone mass than 18-year-old men. Women lose bone mass more rapidly than men. Following the cessation of menses, the rate of bone loss is accelerated for approximately 5 to 8 years. The type of bone lost in this initial high-loss period is trabecular bone, the loss of which is associated with compression fractures of the spine. Cortical bone is lost at a slower rate, and its loss is more directly associated with fractures of the femur. With bone loss there is a decrease in bone strength, and there is a thinning of the vertebral body in the spine. For many older adults, this thinning process leads to decreased height and to increased vulnerability to compression fractures of the spine, caused by only minor degrees of trauma.

Estrogen deficiency in postmenopausal women is thought to be one cause of accelerated bone loss. Estrogen replacement therapy may be medically recommended in women who are not at risk for the detrimental side effects of such therapy, who have no contraindications, and who will adhere to a careful follow-up program that includes annual mammography (Culliton, 1987). The estrogen compounds prevent the loss of bone mass but do not restore previously lost bone mass. Their value seems to be prophylactic. Side effects of estrogen therapy include endometrial cancer and thromboembolic disease, and there is a possible association with gallbladder disease and breast cancer (Chestnut, 1994). The combined use of estrogen and a progestational agent decreases the risk of endometrial cancer but causes repeated episodes of uterine bleeding. The combination therapy of estrogen and progesterone also decreases the efficiency of estrogen in providing protection for the cardiovascular system.

Vitamin D levels have also been found to be lower in osteoporotic women than in nonosteoporotic women. A multivitamin with 400 to 800 IU of vitamin D is therapeutic for postmenopausal women (Chestnut, 1992). The pallor of many older adults is the result of a lack of exposure to sunshine. Vitamin D deficiency can be alleviated by encouraging and helping older adults to spend some time outdoors. When the individual is adequately dressed, exposure to fresh air and sunshine offers physical and psychologic benefits.

The demonstrated need for an increase in calcium in the diet of older adults, especially women, has created an increased awareness of this nutrient as a requirement. Calcium intake is deficient in teenage, perimenopausal, and postmenopausal American women. Although data are conflictual on the efficacy of increased calcium intake as a preventive measure against hip fractures, it is generally thought that perimenopausal and postmenopausal women need a minimum of 1000 to 1500 mg of calcium a day. Milk, dairy products, and calcium carbonate supplements are adequate, available, and reasonably priced sources of calcium.

Calcitonin is an anti–bone resorption agent that has been shown to slow bone loss and increase bone mass. Negative aspects of the drug are the expense, the route of administration (injection), and the short duration of efficacy (2 to 3 years). For some women calcitonin will be a safe prophylactic and a reasonable alternative to estrogen therapy until a more viable method of administration is developed. Recent development and use of a calcitonin nasal spray has shown encouraging results (Overgaard et al., 1992).

It is known that immobility leads to osteoporosis even in healthy young men. Inactivity is associated with a dramatic loss of strength. Studies in older adults have shown a consistent but variable gain in muscle strength through resistance exercise programs. Endurance training such as riding a stationary bike has resulted in a 10% to 25% functional improvement in arthritic patients (Minon et al., 1989). The need to avoid a sedentary lifestyle is an especially important factor to consider in the care of older adults. Prevention of osteoporosis should begin at an early age, with emphasis on lifestyle variables that may alleviate the progression of bone loss.

ARTHRITIS

Table 12-1 describes some of the data relevant to two common forms of arthritis—osteoarthritis (OA) and rheumatoid arthritis (RA).

TABLE 12-1 Osteoarthritis and rheumatoid arthritis differences

	Osteoarthritis	Rheumatoid arthritis
Morning stiffness	Lasts for a few minutes	Lasts for an hour or more
Pain	Usually follows activity	Occurs even at rest
Joint involvement	May be asymmetric; interphalangeal and metacarpophalangeal joints always involved	Symmetric; knees, hips
Synovial fluid	Viscosity decreased	Viscosity normal
Weakness	Usually follows activity	Often severe
Fatigue	Not usual	Usually pronounced
Emotional depression	Not usual	Common

Adapted from Calkins, E., Reinhard, J., & Vladutiu. (1994). Rheumatoid arthritis and the autoimmune rheumatic disease in the older patient. In W.M. Hazzard, E. Bierman, J. Blass, W. Ettinger, & J. Halter (Eds.), *Principles of geriatric medicine and gerontology.* New York: McGraw-Hill.

Osteoarthritis

The incidence of osteoarthritis (OA) increases with age; this condition affects up to 40 million Americans and is the second leading cause of disability (Fife, 1994). Osteoarthritis is a noninflammatory disease of movable joints, characterized by deterioration of articular cartilage and commonly known as "degenerative joint disease (DJD)." Although the definitive cause of OA is not known, there are a number of risk factors: obesity, repetitive mechanical overuse of a joint, and a familial tendency. Certainly nothing can be done concerning a person's genetic makeup, but health teaching concerning obesity and the need to protect joints used in work or sports is an area in need of nursing's input.

The clinical manifestations of OA are joint pain, swelling, decreased range of motion of the joint, and crepitus. Typically the large weight-bearing joints (hips and knees) are affected, as well as joints of the hand. Heberden's nodes, lateral enlargements at the distal interphalangeal joints, are diagnostic of osteoarthritis. The frequency and severity of the disease increase markedly with age, particularly in women. Osteoarthritis of the knee is 3 times more prevalent in older women than in older men, and hip involvement is twice as prevalent in older women as in older men. The progression of osteoarthritis does not follow a systematic, predictable pathway for all individuals afflicted with the disease. Different joints may be involved, which affects the pattern of response of the individual.

The cardinal symptom is pain, which at first occurs after movement of the joint and is relieved by rest. The pain is usually characterized as "aching" and is poorly localized. Stiffness on awakening in the morning or after inactivity is a common complaint, although it is of relatively short duration, rarely persisting for more than 15 minutes.

Medical treatment of osteoarthritis consists of symptomatic relief and minimizing further joint destruction. In addition, some environmental factors can be changed to slow the progress of joint degeneration. Weight-bearing joints such as the knee can be protected from further damage by not engaging in activities that produce large amounts of high impact, such as jogging or aerobic exercise. Swimming is an excellent form of exercise that produces only low impact on weight-bearing joints. Rest is an important aspect of treatment, in combination with exercise that minimizes impact on weight-bearing joints. People who have osteoarthritis and who are overweight should be encouraged to lose weight. Obesity has been found to be associated with some types of osteoarthritis.

A mainstay of treatment is early intervention with physical and occupational therapies. Maintaining muscle strength, improving posture, and protecting joints are invaluable functions that need to be incorporated into the lifestyle of the older adult suffering from osteoarthritis. For appropriate exercises to improve posture, see Figure 12-3. Arthroscopic surgery may produce results for certain older adults with severe knee involvement. If the progression of the disease severely limits mobility and the older person is healthy, surgical joint replacement may be recommended. Hip and knee replacement surgeries are usually very successful and alleviate pain and restore mobility.

Nonsteroidal anti-inflammatory drugs (NSAIDs) provide symptomatic relief because of their analgesic and anti-inflammatory properties, but they do not slow the progression of the osteoarthritis. NSAIDs account for 4% of all prescription drugs used in the United States and for 20% of the drugs used by adults over 60 years of age. This class of drugs has the potential to be life threatening without the ability to be life saving. In spite of the fact that NSAIDs are widely prescribed, it behooves the nurse to understand the potential harm of these drugs. Acetaminophen, a significant pain reliever that does not carry the potential for harm, has been shown to be at least as effective as NSAIDs (Bradley et al., 1991).

The most common adverse effects of NSAIDs are gastrointestinal (GI) symptoms, which have

Stretching Exercises to Improve Posture

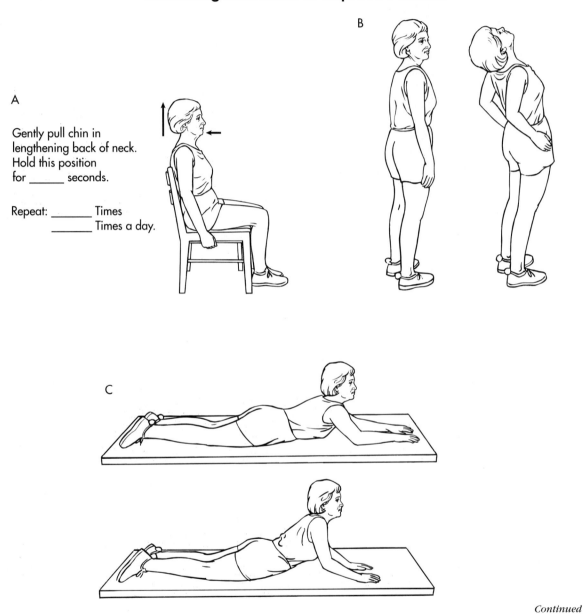

A

Gently pull chin in
lengthening back of neck.
Hold this position
for _____ seconds.

Repeat: _____ Times
         _____ Times a day.

B

C

Continued

FIGURE 12-3 Exercises for improving posture. (From VHI Geriatric Exercise and Rehabilitation Exercise Kit. [1993]. *Visual health/stretching charts.* Tacoma, WA.)

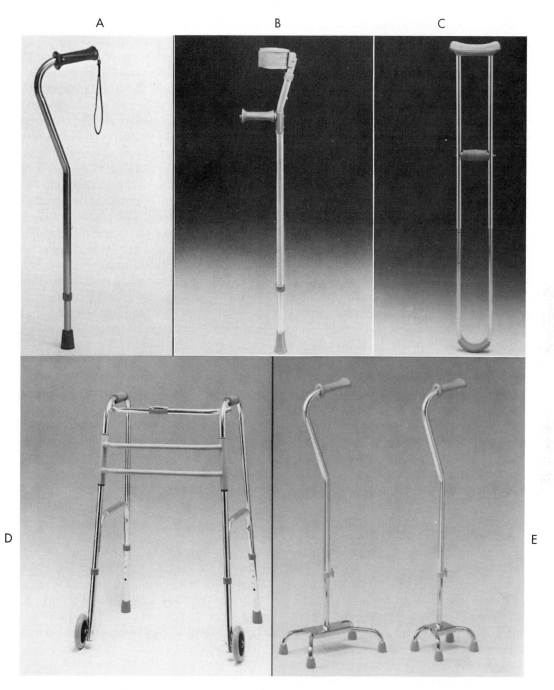

FIGURE 12-5 Assistive devices. *A,* Ortho cane with wrist strap. *B,* A forearm crutch stabilizes your elbow while you walk. *C,* New "rolling" crutch provides smoother contact with the ground. *D,* Walker with front wheels allows constant contact with the ground. *E,* Quad cane offers more support than a single-stem walker. *Courtesy Lumex, Inc., New York.*

as the only form of mobility. This will lead to a decrease in physical strength, and in turn to a loss of the ability to walk. Loss of the strength that is necessary for walking is one of the greatest risks faced by institutionalized older adults.

The nurse must recognize both the risks and the benefits of wheelchair use and be able to arrange a plan of care that maximizes all aspects of the patient's health. A plan that allows an element of choice in activities and freedom of movement is essential to preserving the dignity and well-being of the older adult. The plan should also include time for staff to walk and exercise with the older adult, to ensure that muscle strength will be maintained.

Another feature of the standard wheelchair that presents a potential hazard is the design. Footrests on the wheelchair may cause the older adult to trip and stumble, especially when trying to get out of the chair. The brakes may be difficult for the older adult to lock because of lack of hand strength and the placement of the hand brake. Special care must be taken in teaching the older adult how to dismount from a wheelchair. The position of an older adult resident sitting in a wheelchair needs to be monitored and changed regularly.

It is also critical to verify whether the individual is consistently using the device. Often the older adult considers the cane or walker a stigma and will refuse to use it. Validating the patient's feelings concerning the use of a cane or walker is part of intervening. The nurse respects and tries to understand how the patient perceives the situation. Accepting small gains is one of the principles of care when the patients are older adults who are struggling to maintain positive self-images and self-respect. Allowing the patient to express negative feelings without judging those feelings may help to speed the patient's acceptance of the cane or walker, or it may just make the patient feel better. The nurse can express concern and discuss the reality of a decrease in function and in mobility that results from not using the cane or walker. Over time, allowing expression of feelings and providing a

reality orientation will facilitate an acceptance of the assistive device for most patients.

Some residents who are afflicted with severe dementia still have a high level of mobility; this can be detrimental, as in the case of the older adult with dementia who is agitated and who wanders or paces constantly. Other residents may have limited mobility yet may be cognitively alert, so they may continue to function because of their use of assistive devices and assistance from nursing staff. Still other residents may be immobile and dependent on nursing staff to assist them in many aspects of life, as a result of the sequelae of stroke or other debilitating conditions. Recognition of the wide variations in mobility of nursing home residents is an important consideration in providing individualized nursing care.

Many aspects of care for older adult patients are guided by standards and principles of practice that pertain to all adults or to other selected patient groups. For example, the principles of nursing care for an immobile patient may be highly applicable to the care of many older adult patients. The complexity of nursing care is predicated on the knowledge of the effects of multiple confounding conditions that are so often apparent when caring for older adults. For example, care of the immobile older adult patient may be made more complex by the fact that the patient is hard-of-hearing; this condition interferes with the patient's understanding of the instructions for assisting with movement and transfers.

This level of complexity occurs very often in the care of the nursing home resident who has limited mobility. Nursing care of older adults requires the most sophisticated level of nursing judgment, and nursing interventions in this context demand a high level of interpersonal and technical skill.

In the private or family home

Many older adults living in private or family homes have functional dependencies. Three times as many people who are in the 85-and-older age group as in the 65- to 75-year age group report the need for assistance with activities of daily living (National Center for Health Statistics, 1991). Because of this preponderance of functional dependencies in the older population, many of the patients encountered during home care visits may exhibit limitations in mobility. Sometimes the home visit may be directly related to the physical impairment that results from a loss of mobility, but at other times the limitation in mobility may become evident only after a thorough assessment.

Hazards The nurse caring for the older adult patient in the home must be alert to the potential for home hazards (see Box 12-5). Often, older adults and their family members have been living with these hazards for many years and have difficulty in regarding such things as stairs as a hazard. The addition of a safety mechanism is one way to minimize a hazard—for example, adding a bannister to a staircase or a grab bar in the bathroom. For some older adults, the expense of a safety mechanism may be beyond their financial resources; referral to social services may be an appropriate intervention.

Another nursing intervention to promote the health of the patient is to explain the importance of restoring mobility. The patient can be encouraged to ambulate in a safe manner when it is appropriate. Stretching exercises that improve posture should be part of the nursing interventions for every older adult (Lewis and Campanelli, 1993) (see Figure 12-3). Health practices that protect joints and improve the mobility function should be encouraged.

Foot care The importance of foot care cannot be overemphasized. An assessment of the condition of the patient's feet can be included in the early stage of planning interventions to promote good health practices that contribute to the mobility function (Box 12-6).

During the assessment of the patient's feet, the nurse elicits complaints of any problems (such as itching or pain on walking) that the patient may be experiencing. If shoes do not fit properly, the nurse should determine the ability and the willingness of the patient to buy new

---

BOX 12-6 FOOT ASSESSMENT

1. Appropriateness of types of shoes
2. Condition of shoes
3. Fit of shoes
4. Condition of socks
5. Patient's ability to remove socks and shoes without assistance
6. Condition of feet
   a. Cleanliness
   b. Condition of skin
   c. Edema
   d. Dry, scaly skin
   e. Color
7. Condition of toes
   a. Infection
   b. Fungus
   c. Toenails
   d. Ingrown toenails
   e. Nail thickening
8. Abnormal features
   a. Hammertoe
   b. Bunion
   c. Calluses
   d. Corns
   e. Other

---

shoes. One problem may be transportation to a shopping area where shoes can be purchased. Often, alerting family members to the need may be sufficient to solve the problem; at other times it may be necessary to involve social services.

Medications The nurse reviews with the patient and family members all of the older adult patient's medications and the side effects of each medication. The potential for injury for adults of advanced age who are taking multiple medications and living in private or family homes is high. Two methods of prevention are to increase the patient's awareness of the combined effects of drugs and to teach behaviors that will diminish the risk of injury.

Exercise A program of exercise is an essential interdisciplinary intervention for older adult patients who have limitations in mobility and who are physically able to participate in a prescribed program (Galindo-Ciocon et al., 1995). Many older adults lead a sedentary life that is detrimental to their health. Walking on a regular basis can play an important role in the maintenance of physical and psychologic health. Before suggesting a program of exercise for an older adult home care patient, it is important to consult with the physician to ascertain the type and amount of exercise prescribed.

During the assessment phase, some older adults may be identified as being at high risk for falling. There are times when well-meaning health care professionals restrict mobility because of a perceived need to protect the older adult from the risk of a fall. The paradox in this treatment is that mobility may be lost through the treatment. However, a fractured hip does introduce a significant risk to the life of many older adults, so caution is certainly appropriate. Clinical decisions regarding an older adult's mobility are to be guided by ethical principles of autonomy and beneficence. The clinical dilemma between doing good (beneficence) and providing for choice (autonomy) may be described as a conflict between protection from injury and the risk to the spirit when choice is lost.

Realizing the importance of individualized care and inclusion of the patient in the planning of care is paramount because of the large degree of physical, psychologic, and social variability in the population of older adults.

EVALUATION

The final phase of the nursing process is the evaluation of the results of the plan in terms of accomplishment of the delineated goals. A criterion method that deals with measurable and observable outcomes is employed to validate the effectiveness of the nursing interventions. Also, using qualitative measures to evaluate the patient's perception of outcomes and the acceptance of the nursing care is an important evaluative function. Documentation of evaluation is critical and fundamental to nursing science.

REFERENCES

Baylink, D. & Jennings, J. (1994). Calcium and bone homeostasis and changes with aging. In W.M. Hazzard, E. Bierman, J. Blass, W. Ettinger, & J. Halter (Eds.), *Principles of geriatric medicine and gerontology.* New York: McGraw-Hill.

Bradley, J.D. et al. (1991). Comparison of an antiinflammatory dose of ibuprofen, an analgesic dose of ibuprofen and acetaminophen in the treatment of patients with osteoarthritis of the knee. *New England Journal of Medicine, 325,* 87.

Buchner, et al. (1992). Effects of physical activity on health status in older adults: 2. Intervention studies. *Annual Review Public Health, 13,* 469.

Calkins, E., Reinhard, J., & Vladuitiu. (1994). Rheumatoid arthritis and the autoimmune rheumatic disease in the older patient. In W.M. Hazzard, E. Bierman, J. Blass, W. Ettinger, & J. Halter (Eds.), *Principles of geriatric medicine and gerontology.* New York: McGraw-Hill.

Carlson, J., & Strom, B. (1994). Nonsteroidal antiinflammatory drugs. In W.M. Hazzard, E. Bierman, J. Blass, W. Ettinger, & J. Halter (Eds.), *Principles of geriatric medicine and gerontology.* New York: McGraw-Hill.

Chestnut, C.H. (1992). Osteoporosis and its treatment. *New England Journal of Medicine, 326,* 402.

Chestnut, C.H. (1994). Osteoporosis. In W.M. Hazzard, E. Bierman, J. Blass, W. Ettinger, & J. Halter (Eds.), *Principles of geriatric medicine and gerontology.* New York: McGraw-Hill.

Culliton, B.J. (1987). Osteoporosis reexamined: Complexity of bone biology is a challenge. *Science, 235*(4791), 833-834.

Ettinger, W. (1994). Immobility. In W.M. Hazzard, E. Bierman, J. Blass, W. Ettinger, & J. Halter (Eds.), *Principles of geriatric medicine and gerontology.* New York: McGraw-Hill.

Fiatrone, et al. (1990). High intensity strength training in nonagenarians. *Journal of the American Medical Association, 263*-3029.

Fife, R. (1994). Osteoarthritis. In W.M. Hazzard, E. Bierman, J. Blass, W. Ettinger, & J. Halter (Eds.), *Principles of geriatric medicine and gerontology.* New York: McGraw-Hill.

Gabriel, S.E., et al. (1991). Risk of serious gastrointestinal complications related to use of nonsteroidal antiinflammatory drugs: A meta-analysis. *Annals of Internal Medicine, 115,* 787.

Galindo-Ciocon, D., Ciocon, J., & Galindo, D. (1995). Gait training and falls in the elderly. *Journal of Gerontological Nursing, 21*(6), 10-17.

Glick, O., & Swanson, E. (1995). Motor performance correlates of functional dependence in long term care residents. *Nursing Research, 44*(1), 4-8.

Grisso, J.A., & Kaplan, F. (1994). Hip fractures. In W.M. Hazzard, E. Bierman, J. Blass, W. Ettinger, & J. Halter (Eds.), *Principles of geriatric medicine and gerontology.* New York: McGraw-Hill.

Hunter, G., Treuth, M., Weinsier, R., Kekes-Szabo, T., Kell, S.H., Roth, D.L., & Nicholson, C. (1995). The effects of strength conditioning on older women's ability to perform daily tasks. *Journal of the American Geriatric Society, 43*(7), 756-760.

Kippenbrock, & Soja. (1993). Preventing falls in the elderly: Interviewing patients who have fallen. *Geriatric Nursing, 14,* 205–209.

Lawrence, R.C., et al. (1989). Estimates of the prevalence of selected arthritic and musculoskeletal disease in the United States. *Journal of Rheumatology, 16,* 873.

Lewis, C. & Campanelli, L. (1993). VHI Geriatric Exercise and Rehabilitation Exercise Kit. *Visual health/stretching charts.* Tacoma, WA.

McFarland, G., & McFarlane, E. (1993). *Nursing diagnosis and intervention: Planning for patient care.* St. Louis: Mosby.

Minon, M.A., Hewett, J.E., & Webel, R.R. (1989). Efficacy of physical conditioning exercise in patients with rheumatoid arthritis and osteoarthritis. *Arthritis Rheumatoid, 32,* 1396.

Morey, et al. (1989). Evaluation of a supervised exercise program in a geriatric population. *Journal of the American Geriatric Society, 37,* 348-354.

National Center for Health Statistics. (1987). Preliminary data from the 1985 National Nursing Home Survey (Advance data 135). Washington, DC: Government Printing Office.

National Center for Health Statistics. (1991). *Current estimates from the National Health Interview Survey Series 10: Data from the National Health Survey No. 184* (Vital and Health Statistics, DHHS Pub. No. [PHS] 93-1512). Hyattsville, MD: U.S. Department of Health and Human Services, Public Health Service, Centers for Disease Control, National Center for Health Statistics.

Overgaard, K., et al. (1992). Effect of calcitonin given intranasally on bone mass and fracture rates in established osteoporosis: A close-response study. *British Medicine Journal, 305,* 556.

Peterson, V.S., Solgaard, S., & Simonsen, B. (1989). Total hip replacement in patients aged 80 years and older. *Journal of the American Geriatric Association, 37*(3), 219-222.

Schwartz, R.S., & Buchner, D.M. (1994). Exercise in the elderly: Physiologic and functional effects. In W.M. Hazzard, E. Bierman, J. Blass, W. Ettinger, & J. Halter (Eds.), *Principles of geriatric medicine and gerontology.* New York: McGraw-Hill.

Sorock, G. (1988). Falls among the elderly: Epidemiology and prevention. *American Journal of Preventative Medicine, 4*(5), 282-288.

Taggert, H.M., & Alderice, J.M. (1982). Fatal cholestatic jaundice in elderly patients taking benoxaprofen. *British Medical Journal, 285,* 1372.

Tinetti, M.E. (1994). Falls. In W.M. Hazzard, E. Bierman, J. Blass, W. Ettinger, & J. Halter (Eds.), *Principles of geriatric medicine and gerontology.* New York: McGraw-Hill.

Treuth, M.S., Hunter, G.R., Kekes-Szabo, T., Weinsier, R.L., Goran, M.I., & Berland, L. (1995). Reduction in intra-abdominal adipose tissue after strength training in older women. *Journal of Applied Physiology, 78*(4), 1425-1431.

Vico, L., Pouget, J.F., Calmels, P., Chatard, J.C., Rehailia, M., Minaire, P., Geyssant, A., & Alexandre, C. (1995). The relations between physical ability and bone mass in women aged over 65 years. *Journal of Bone Mineral Research, 10*(3), 374-383.

World Health Organization. (1976). *International classification of impairment, disabilities, and handicaps* (WHA 29, 35). Geneva, Switzerland: Author.

Young, D.R., Masaki, K.H., & Curb, J.D. (1995). Associations of physical activity with performance-based and self-reported physical functioning in older men: The Honolulu Heart Program. *Journal of the American Geriatric Society, 43*(8), 845-854.

Yura, H., & Walsh, M.B. (1988). *The nursing process.* East Norwalk, CT: Appleton and Lange.

BIBLIOGRAPHY

Arnett, F.C. (1989). The 1987 revised American Rheumatism Association criteria for classification of rheumatoid arthritis. In D.J. McCarthy (Ed.), *Arthritis and allied conditions: A textbook of rheumatology* (p. 20). Philadelphia: Lea and Febiger.

Grob, D. (1989). Common disorders of muscles in the aged. In W. Reichel (Ed.), *Clinical aspects of aging* (pp. 296-313). Baltimore: Williams & Wilkins.

Tinetti, M.E. (1987). Factors associated with serious injury during falls by ambulatory nursing home residents. *Journal of the American Geriatric Society, 35*(3), 644-648.

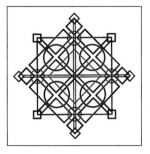

C H A P T E R   13

Aging is not for sissies.
TERRY SCHUCKMAN, 1975

Urinary Incontinence

■ Learning Objectives

On completion of this chapter, the reader will be able to do the following:

1. Identify and describe the types and causes of urinary incontinence experienced by older adults.
2. Describe and/or perform history taking, and physical and functional assessments for patients with urinary incontinence.
3. Describe urodynamic assessment.
4. Recognize the psychosocial consequences of urinary incontinence for older adults and their families.
5. Identify and describe behavioral therapies for urinary incontinence.
6. Provide appropriate nursing interventions, patient education, and advocacy for older adults with urinary incontinence.

Urinary incontinence (UI), the involuntary loss of urine, is a troublesome health problem among older adults, with an incidence of 37.7% in women and 18.9% in men who reside in private or family homes (Diokno et al., 1986). It is more common in nursing homes, where approximately 50% of the residents experience incontinence (Mohide, 1986; Ouslander, 1992). Research indicates that this condition often contributes to the decision to place homebound individuals in long-term care facilities (Johnson & Warner, 1982; Noelker, 1987; Smallegan, 1985). In acute care settings the rate of incontinence in older patients is estimated to range from 15% to 35%,

although these episodes may be transitory and related to acute illnesses (Mohide, 1986; Ouslander, 1992).

Although incontinence increases with age, it is not a part of the normal aging process; neither is it untreatable. During the past decade, advances in the assessment and treatment of urinary incontinence have shown that urinary incontinence can be successfully diagnosed and treated in even the oldest of individuals (Ouslander, 1986; Ouslander, 1992; Resnick et al., 1989). Still, a large number of older people do not seek help for this condition (National Institutes of Health [NIH], 1988). Some fear surgical intervention and are not aware that nonsurgical approaches are available. Others are unaware that treatment of any form is available. Many health care providers lack information about incontinence and hold negative attitudes about the problem. Too often, patients are told, "It is something you will have to learn to live with," when in fact, incontinence can be significantly improved or cured in nine out of ten (NIH, 1988). In many communities there is a scarcity of nurses, physicians, and other health care providers who have the knowledge and skills to apply nonsurgical approaches to the problem of incontinence. As more health care providers become educated in this specialty, the problem of incontinence in older people should decrease considerably.

■ Normal Structure and Function

Normal micturition is a complex process that involves the lower urinary tract, the spinal cord (T11 to S4), the brain, and the autonomic and somatic nervous systems. The bladder, the detrusor muscles surrounding the bladder, the urethra, and the internal and external sphincters make up the lower urinary tract (Figure 13-1). Bladder relaxation and urethral contraction,

which are important in the maintenance of continence, are controlled by the sympathetic nervous system. Bladder contraction, essential for the expulsion of urine, is stimulated by the parasympathetic nervous system. The bladder and the urethra are supported by pelvic floor muscles, which are important in bladder control. The pelvic floor, including the external sphincter, is controlled by the somatic nervous system, specifically the pudendal nerve.

Micturition is mediated by the brain. The cerebral cortex appears to inhibit the loss of urine, whereas the brainstem facilitates urination (Ouslander, 1994a, 1994b). Maintenance of continence requires the coordination of all these systems. During bladder filling, stretch receptors in the bladder wall signal the sacral spinal cord. Once a critical volume is reached, approximately 300 ml, a spinal reflex stimulates the bladder to empty. At the same time, bladder sensory nerves transmit signals via the spinal cord to the brain. Although the neurophysiology of urination is still under investigation, it appears that the cerebral cortex sends inhibitory messages to delay urination. Thus continence is maintained. Any disorder that affects the normal physiologic function of any of these systems may cause incontinence to occur.

■ Age-Related Changes

A variety of pathologic and functional factors that are frequently seen in older adults may predispose them to loss of bladder control. For example, benign prostatic hypertrophy (BPH) increases with age in men and often leads to urinary incontinence, urinary frequency, urgency, decreased force of the urinary system, and hesitancy in initiating urine flow. Similarly, normal age-related estrogen loss in women causes changes in the squamous epithelium of the distal urethral and vaginal wall, a decrease in vaginal muscular tone, and vascular profusion. These physiologic and anatomic changes contribute to urinary incontinence in older women and may be accompanied by urgency or frequency of urination.

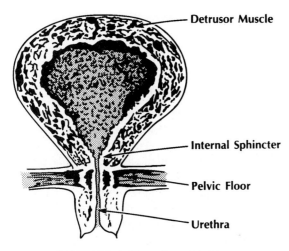

— Detrusor Muscle

— Internal Sphincter

— Pelvic Floor

— Urethra

FIGURE 13-1 The urinary bladder.

Increasing age is also associated with an increase in involuntary bladder contractions, a reduction in bladder capacity, and an increase in residual volume (Leach & Yip, 1986; Staskin, 1986). These alterations in bladder function, especially involuntary contractions, may contribute to the development of urinary incontinence in older adults.

The complex nature of urination, combined with age-related physiologic changes, underscores the importance of comprehensive assessment to discover the underlying cause of urinary incontinence in older adults. Only after the mechanism of the incontinence has been identified can appropriate treatments be applied with success.

■ Types of Urinary Incontinence

Urinary incontinence (UI) is typically categorized as acute (transient) or persistent (established) (Box 13-1). Acute alterations in urinary elimination are associated with acute illness, which may either be systemic or involve the urinary tract specifically. Many illnesses, such as hip fracture, congestive heart failure, pneumonia, and delirium, can upset the homeostatic balance of the older adult sufficiently to affect urinary control. Factors associated with acute health breakdown, such as bed rest, inability to toilet independently, or lack of staff or caregivers to assist in toileting, also affect the patient's ability to maintain urinary control. Continence is usually restored once the acute illness, immobility, and resulting dependency are resolved. Conditions such as acute urinary tract infection, urethritis, or vaginitis cause irritation and inflammation of the bladder and urethral squamous epithelium, resulting in involuntary urine loss. Appropriate treatment of these conditions will result in a return to normal bladder function in most instances. Fecal impaction can result in urinary incontinence, either by causing obstruction of the urethra and occluding urine flow or by inducing bladder spasms by means of pressure from the distended bowel. Removal of fecal impaction and institution of a bowel regimen

BOX 13-1 TYPES OF URINARY INCONTINENCE

Acute (transient)
Persistent (established)
   Stress
   Urge
   Overflow
   Functional

often result in a reduction or elimination of urinary incontinence in affected individuals.

Medications often result in underreported side effects in older adults. Antidepressants, antipsychotics, and narcotic analgesics have an anticholinergic effect, which can inhibit or diminish bladder contractions, resulting in inadequate bladder emptying and overflow incontinence. Alpha- and beta-adrenergic agonists and calcium channel blocker agents are used in the treatment of cardiovascular disease and have also been implicated in causing urinary retention, with resulting overflow incontinence (Ouslander, 1994a, 1994b).

Incontinence that has been present over a period of months and is not the result of acute illness or effects of medication is called persistent incontinence. Major types of persistent incontinence include stress, urge, overflow, and functional incontinence (NIH, 1988).

STRESS INCONTINENCE

Stress incontinence, one of the most common forms of incontinence in women, is the involuntary leakage of urine that occurs with physical exertion, such as coughing, sneezing, laughing, lifting, or exercising. These activities cause a rise in intraabdominal pressure, which results in increased bladder pressure. If the urethra is competent and pelvic floor muscle tone is adequate, continence is maintained. However, increased intra-abdominal pressure in people with incompetent urethras or weak pelvic floor muscles can result in accidental urine loss. Stress incontinence in women is associated with damage to the pelvic musculature during pregnancy, vaginal delivery, or trauma during gynecologic or urologic surgery. Men rarely experience stress incontinence, except as the result of urethral injury, such as injury that occurs during prostatectomy (Hadley et al., 1986).

URGE INCONTINENCE

Urge incontinence is also seen frequently in older adults. In this condition the bladder escapes central nervous system inhibition and contracts spontaneously, resulting in leakage of small to large amounts of urine. Uninhibited detrusor spasms are commonly referred to as "bladder instability" or "detrusor instability." Typically, patients experience an urgent sensation to void followed quickly by involuntary loss of urine. Frequent urination and nocturia are commonly associated with this condition. Patients often complain of not being able to get to the bathroom in time, or of inability to control the bladder when putting the key in the door to a locked bathroom or when washing their hands. Urge incontinence is seen in patients with spinal cord damage or central nervous system problems—for example, Parkinson's disease, strokes, dementia, bladder or urethral irritation and/or infection, fecal impaction, uterine prolapse, prostatic hypertrophy, or radiation damage to the bladder or urethra (Ouslander, 1994a, 1994b). It has also been asserted that the habit of frequent urination can contribute to development of bladder instability and incontinence (Frewen, 1978, 1980). Frequently, however, none of these conditions exists in patients experiencing this form of incontinence. Urge incontinence often coexists with stress incontinence in older adults. In such mixed cases of incontinence, one form usually predominates.

OVERFLOW INCONTINENCE

Overflow incontinence is caused by incomplete bladder emptying that results in urinary reten-

tion. Leakage of urine occurs when pressure resulting from a chronically full bladder exceeds urethral pressure. Frequent leakage of small amounts of urine, with or without urgency, is noted. Patients may also describe an inability to empty the bladder. Causative factors include atonic bladder, side effects of medication, mechanical obstruction, detrusor hyperactivity with incomplete bladder contraction (DHIC), and dyssynergia of sphincter and bladder contraction.

Atonic bladder is characterized by failure of the detrusor muscle to contract adequately and to expel the total volume of urine. This condition typically results from spinal cord injury or diabetes mellitus. Also, side effects of medications, such as muscle relaxants, antidepressants, or antipsychotics, can reduce the force of detrusor muscle contraction, resulting in incomplete bladder emptying.

Mechanical obstruction caused by an enlarged prostate, uterine prolapse, a large cystocele, or fecal impaction can cause urinary retention through partial or complete occlusion of the urethra. Dyssynergia and DHIC are more complex and less common. In dyssynergia, the urinary sphincter and bladder contract simultaneously. Normally the muscles surrounding the urethra relax as the bladder contracts, permitting micturition to occur. Dyssynergia is most often seen in patients with suprasacral neurologic impairment.

FUNCTIONAL INCONTINENCE

Functional incontinence is caused not by bladder or sphincter dysfunction, but by physical, mental, psychologic, or environmental factors. Physical disabilities that interfere with gait and ambulation can impair a patient's ability to reach the toilet in a timely fashion. Patients with cognitive disabilities have difficulty remembering the location of the bathroom or recognizing the need to void. Other patients may be acutely depressed and lack motivation to attend to personal habits. Environmental barriers can also play an important role in the inability to toilet properly. People confined to bed or physically restrained cannot be expected to remain continent if regular toileting is not provided by their caregivers. Bathrooms located at a great distance from the patient with gait problems and slowed ambulation can create an obstacle beyond the person's ability to overcome. Similarly, inadequate toilet facilities in public or private buildings put even the most agile and continent older individuals to the test.

■ Nursing Process

ASSESSMENT

The purpose of assessing the patient who is experiencing urinary incontinence is to discover any altered mechanism that underlies the condition, so that appropriate therapies can be initiated. The assessment includes a history; physical examination; psychosocial, functional, and environmental assessments; urodynamic evaluation; and a daily diary of bladder habits and incontinent episodes. The subjective reports and objective observations are important data that assist the nurse in arriving at an accurate nursing diagnosis.

History

The incontinence history covers the onset, progression, characteristics, and circumstances of the patient's urinary incontinence. It also contains information regarding the patient's bladder habits, and the signs and symptoms of urinary pathology (Box 13-2). The patient's description of the problem is one of the most important aspects of the assessment. Ideally this information will be provided by the patient. However, if the patient is cognitively impaired, family care providers and nursing records are valuable resources that the nurse can utilize to obtain relevant data.

Through a comprehensive health history (Box 13-3), the nurse seeks to discover the patient's perceptions of the continence problem, and to determine general health and functional

---

BOX 13-2
HISTORY OF INCONTINENCE

1. Characteristics of incontinence: onset, clinical course, frequency and volume of urine loss
2. Circumstances associated with urine loss: coughing, sneezing, laughing, lifting, stooping, walking, climbing stairs, sleeping, urgency, running water, cold weather, caffeine, alcohol, fluid intake, medications, postvoid dribbling, urine loss without sensation, continual leakage
3. Bladder habits: frequency and volume of daytime urination, frequency and volume of nocturia, methods of management (e.g., frequent voiding, pads, diapers, or urine collection device), fluid intake
4. Other signs and symptoms: urgency, burning, pain, hematuria, weakness of urinary stream, hesitancy, intermittent stream, constipation, bowel incontinence

---

status. Careful history taking should reveal current medical problems, current medications, and past medical, surgical, urologic, and obstetric events that may impinge on the current situation.

The nurse should always ask specifically about current or past diagnoses of diabetes mellitus, congestive heart failure, bladder infections, kidney infections, stroke, Parkinson's disease, depression, memory problems, and other neurologic conditions or injuries, because any of these conditions can affect bladder function. (Box 13-3 lists general areas of health history that should be included as part of the assessment of urinary incontinence.) The history taking should determine whether the patient has undergone urologic evaluation, urologic surgery, or other treatments for incontinence. Women should be asked

The focus of evaluation centers around the stated short- and long-term patient-centered goals. The patient's stated satisfaction with care is of paramount importance to the process of evaluation. Documentation of all parameters of the evaluative process must be recorded in formal health care records.

REFERENCES

Brink, C., Wells, T., & Diokno, A. (1983). A continence clinic for the aged. *Journal of Gerontological Nursing, 9*(12), 651-655.

Burgio, K.L., & Burgio, L.D. (1986). Behavior therapies for urinary incontinence in the elderly. *Clinics in Geriatric Medicine, 2*(4), 809-827.

Burgio, K.L., Robinson, J.C., & Engel, B.T. (1986). The role of biofeedback in Kegel exercise training for stress urinary incontinence. *American Journal of Obstetrics and Gynecology, 154*, 58-64.

Burgio, K.L., Whitehead, W.E., & Engel, B.T. (1985). Urinary incontinence in the elderly: Bladder-sphincter biofeedback and toileting skills training. *Annals of Internal Medicine, 103*(4), 507-515.

Burgio, L., Engel, B.T., McCormick, K., Hawkins, A., & Scheve, A. (1988). Behavioral treatment for urinary incontinence in elderly inpatients: Initial attempts to modify prompted voiding and toileting procedures. *Behavior Therapy, 19*(3), 345-357.

Creason, N.S., Glybowski, J.A., Burgene, L.S., Whippo, C., Yeo, S., & Richardson, B. (1989). Prompted voiding therapy for urinary incontinence in aged female nursing home residents. *Journal of Advanced Nursing, 14*, 120-126.

Diokno, A.C., Brock, B.M., Brown, M.B., & Herzog, A.R. (1986). Prevalence of urinary incontinence and other urological symptoms in the non-institutionalized elderly. *Journal of Urology, 136*, 1022-1025.

Dougherty, M., Bishop, K., Mooney, R., & Gimotty, P. (1989). The effect of circumvaginal muscle (CVM) exercise. *Nursing Research, 38*(6), 331-335.

Duke University Center for the Study of Aging and Human Development. (1978). *Multidimensional functional assessment: The OARS methodology.* Durham, NC: Duke University.

Fantl, J.A., Wyman, J.F., Harkins, S.W., & Hadely, E.C. (1990). Bladder training in the management of lower urinary tract dysfunction in women: A review. *Journal of the American Geriatric Society, 38*(3), 329-332.

Folstein, M.F., Folstein, S., & McHugh, P.R. (1975). Minimental state: A practical method for grading the cognitive state of patients for the clinician. *Journal of Psychiatric Research, 12*, 189-198.

Frewen, W.K. (1978). An objective assessment of the unstable bladder of psychosomatic origin. *British Journal of Urology, 50*, 246-249.

Frewen, W.K. (1980). The management of urgency and frequency of micturition. *British Journal of Urology, 52*, 367-369.

Hadley, H.R., Zimmern, P.E., & Raz, S. (1986). The treatment of male urinary incontinence. In P.C. Walsh, R.F. Gittes, A.D. Perlmutter, & T.A. Stamey (Eds.), *Campbell's urology* (5th ed., pp. 2658-2679).

Johnson, M.J., & Warner, C. (1982). We had no choice—A study of familial guilt feelings surrounding nursing home care. *Journal of Gerontological Nursing, 8*, 641-645, 654.

Kaltreider, D.L., Wei, H., Iqou, J.F., Yu, L.C., & Craighead, W.E. (1990, January-February). Can reminders curb incontinence? *Geriatric Nursing*, pp. 17-19.

Katz, S., Ford, A.B., Moskowitz, R.W., Jackson, B.A., & Jaffee, M.W. (1963). Studies of illness in the aged: The index of ADL—A standardized measure of biological and psychosocial function. *Journal of the American Medical Association, 185*, 94ff.

Kegel, A.H. (1948). Progressive resistance exercise in the functional restoration of the perineal muscles. *American Journal of Obstetrics and Gynecology, 56*(2), 242-245.

Leach, G.E., & Yip, C.M. (1986). Urologic and urodynamic evaluation of the elderly population. *Clinics in Geriatric Medicine, 2*(4), 731-756.

McDowell, B.J., & Burgio, K.L. (1990). Urinary incontinence. In A.S. Staab & M.F. Lyles (Eds.), *Manual of geriatric nursing* (pp. 432-456). Glenview, IL: Scott, Foresman/Little Brown Higher Education.

McDowell, B.J., Burgio, K.L., & Candib, D. (1989). Assessment of urinary incontinence in the elderly. *Journal of the American Academy of Nurse Practitioners, 1*(1), 24-29.

McDowell, B.J., Burgio, K.L., & Candib, D. (1990). Behavioral and pharmacological treatment of persistent urinary incontinence in the elderly. *Journal of the American Academy of Nurse Practitioners, 2*(1), 17-23.

McDowell, B.J., Burgio, K.L., Dombrowski, M., Locher, J., & Rodriguez, E. (1992). An interdisciplinary approach to the assessment and behavioral treatment of urinary incontinence in geriatric outpatients. *Journal of the American Geriatric Society, 40*, 370-374.

McDowell, B.J., Engberg, S., Weber, E., Brodak, I., & Engberg, R. (1994). Successful treatment using behavioral interventions for urinary incontinence for homebound older adults. *Geriatric Nursing, 15*(6), 303-307.

Mohide, E.A. (1986). The prevalence and scope of urinary incontinence. *Clinics in Geriatric Medicine, 2*(4), 639-655.

Morishita, L. (1988). Nursing evaluation and treatment of geriatric outpatients with urinary incontinence. *Nursing Clinics of North America, 23*(1), 189-206.

National Institutes of Health. (1988). *Urinary incontinence in adults: Consensus development conference* (Office of Medical Applications of Research, NIH Vol. 7, No. 5). Bethesda, MD: Author.

Newman, D.K., & Smith, D.A. (1989). Incontinence in elderly homebound patients. *Holistic Nursing Practice, 4*(1), 52-60.

Noelker, L.S. (1987). Incontinence in elderly cared for by family. *Gerontologist, 27,* 194-200.

Ouslander, J.G. (1986). Diagnostic evaluation of geriatric urinary incontinence. *Clinics in Geriatric Medicine, 2*(4), 715-730.

Ouslander, J.G. (1992). Geriatric urinary incontinence. *Disease of the Month, 38*(2), 71-149.

Ouslander, J.G. (1994a). Incontinence. In R.L. Kane, J.G. Ouslander, & I.B. Abrass (Eds.), *Essentials of clinical geriatrics* (2nd ed., pp. 139-189). New York: McGraw-Hill Health Professions Division.

Ouslander, J.G. (1994b). Urinary incontinence. In W.R. Hazzard, R. Andres, E.L. Bierman, & J.P. Blass (Eds.), *Principles of geriatric medicine and gerontology* (pp. 1123-1142). New York: McGraw-Hill.

Ouslander, J.G., Greengold, B., & Chen, S. (1987). Complications of chronic indwelling urinary catheters among male nursing home patients: A prospective study. *Journal of Urology, 138,* 1191-1195.

Pannill, F.C., Williams, F.T., & Davis, R. (1988). Evaluation and treatment of urinary incontinence in long-term care. *Journal of the American Geriatric Society, 36,* 902-910.

Platt, R., Polk, B.F., & Murdock, B. (1983). Reduction of mortality associated with nosocomial urinary infections. *Lancet, 1,* 893-897.

Resnick, N.M., Yalla, S.V., & Lawrence, E. (1989). The pathophysiology of urinary incontinence among institutionalized elderly persons. *New England Journal of Medicine, 320,* 1-7.

Rose, M.A., Smith, J.B., Smith, D., & Newman, D. (1990). Behavioral management of urinary incontinence in homebound older adults. *Home Health Care Nurse, 8* (5), 10-15.

Sier, H., Ouslander, J., & Orzek, S. (1987). Urinary incontinence among geriatric patients in an acute-care hospital. *Journal of the American Medical Association, 257*(13), 1767-1771.

Smallegan, M. (1985). There is nothing else to do: Needs for care before nursing home admission. *Journal of Gerontology, 25*(4), 364-369.

Smith, D.A. (1988). Continence restoration in the homebound patient. *Nursing Clinics of North America, 23*(1), 207-218.

Smith, J.B., Smith, D.A., Rose, M., & Newman, D.K. (1989). Managing urinary incontinence in community-residing elderly persons. *Gerontologist, 29*(2), 229-233.

Staskin, D.R. (1986). Age-related physiologic and pathological changes affecting lower urinary tract function. *Clinics in Geriatric Medicine, 2*(4), 701-710.

Warren, J.W., Muncel, H.L., & Berquist, E.J. (1981). Sequelae and management of urinary infection in the patient requiring chronic catheterization. *Journal of Urology, 125,* 1-7.

Wyman, J.F., Choi Sung, C., Harkins, S.W., Walson, M., & Fantl, A. (1988). The urinary diary in evaluation of incontinent women: A test-retest analysis. *Obstetrics and Gynecology, 71*(6), 812-817.

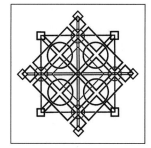

C H A P T E R   14

So here I sit in the early candle-light of old age—I and my book—casting backward glances over our travel'd road.

WALT WHITMAN

Bowel Elimination

■ Learning Objectives

On completion of this chapter, the reader will be able to do the following:

1. Explain the normal structure and function of the gastrointestinal (GI) system and identify age-related changes that influence bowel elimination.
2. Recognize the significance and prevalence of constipation in older adults.
3. Identify the contributing factors that cause constipation.
4. Assess patients for actual or potential constipation.
5. Develop a plan of care to manage constipation.
6. Discuss appropriate nursing interventions for patients with constipation.
7. Promote normal bowel elimination for older adults.
8. Evaluate the effectiveness of a plan of care for constipation.

■ Constipation

Constipation is the most common chronic digestive complaint among all age groups in the United States, affecting approximately 4.5 million people per year and causing considerable morbidity, physical discomfort, and emotional distress (Donatelle, 1990). Two and one-half million physician visits per year are made to manage this common complaint. As people age, the prevalence of constipation increases, with 4% of those age 65 to 74 years old experiencing constipation, and 10.2% of those over 75 years of age experiencing constipation. Women are twice as likely as men to complain of constipation, and

it is 1.3 times more common in nonwhite people than in white people (Goldstein & Oliveira, 1993).

Bowel elimination is highly subjective, and individuals have differing ideas about what constitutes normalcy. A standard definition of constipation is difficult to apply to all individuals, however, the literature for the United States demonstrates an objective consensus as to when constipation can be diagnosed. It is defined as being present when any of the following are described or observed in relation to the individual's elimination pattern: passage of stools fewer than 3 to 5 times per week; deficient quantity of stool; incomplete passage of stool; abnormally hard and dry stool; or straining at stools more than 25% of the time (Camilleri et al., 1994; Chenitz et al., 1991; Donatelle, 1990; Merkel et al., 1993). Constipation is considered a chronic condition when these characteristics last longer than 6 weeks (Castle, 1989). However, it must be noted that the preceding definitions are not accepted worldwide. In many different cultures and in different parts of the world, a normal elimination pattern of passage of stool 3 times a day is common.

Constipation can be classified into three broad categories according to its causes: (1) constipation that is caused by physiologic changes at a level that affects bowel function, including colorectal diseases (e.g. tumors and diverticular disease), metabolic and endocrine disorders, and neurologic disorders; (2) constipation that is caused by the administration of pharmacologic agents or other medical therapeutics; and (3) constipation resulting from extrinsic factors such as age-related changes in physical activity, the inadequate ingestion of fluids and fiber, and unfavorable environmental conditions such as lack of privacy or access to a toilet (Cameron, 1992; Donatelle, 1990; McMillan & Williams, 1989). Over 90% of complaints of constipation are attributed to nonpathologic factors (Camilleri et al., 1994). The patient and/or family members need to be educated about the contributing factors for constipation and therapeutic interventions that will enhance a routine bowel elimination pattern. The purpose of this chapter is to focus on the management of the clinical problem of constipation in older adults.

■ Normal Structure and Function

Bowel elimination is achieved as a result of the physiologic functions of motility and innervation of the gastrointestinal tract. The digestive tract is a muscular tube that extends from the mouth to the anus with the primary functions of storing, digesting, and absorbing nutrients, and eliminating waste (Figure 14-1). The primary areas re-

lated to bowel elimination are the small and large intestines, the rectum, and the anus. The structure of the intestinal wall is similar in both the large and small intestine and consists of five layers: the serosa, a longitudinal muscle layer, a circular muscle layer, the submucosa, and the mucosa. The motor functions of the gut are performed by layers of smooth muscle that lie in the deep layers of the mucosa (Guyton, 1991; Luckman & Sorensen, 1993).

There are two types of movement in the GI tract: mixing and propulsive. These movements are produced by rhythmic contractions of the smooth muscle fibers. Mixing movements occur when a portion of the small intestine becomes distended with gastric content, followed by contractions spaced at intervals along the intestine. As one set of contractions relaxes, a new set begins. Peristalsis is a propulsive contraction that forces the contents of the GI tract to move forward. Peristaltic waves occur much faster in the proximal intestine and much slower in the large intestine, and are greatly increased after meals (Guyton, 1991; Luckman & Sorensen, 1993). The gastrointestinal tract has an intrinsic nervous system that begins at the esophagus and extends all the way to the anus. This system is composed of two layers of neurons, the myenteric plexus and the submucosal plexus, and is responsible for coordination of movements of the intestine. The parasympathetic nervous system stimulates the plexuses, resulting in increased tone of the gut, decreased tone of the sphincters, and increased frequency, volume, and velocity of gut contractions. The actual urge to defecate results when feces enter the rectum. Distention of the rectal wall sends signals throughout the neural plexuses, initiating peristaltic waves in the descending colon, sigmoid, and rectum and forcing fecal matter toward the anus. The internal and external sphincters, via the defecation reflex, become relaxed, and fecal matter may then be passed. The individual may voluntarily suppress this urge by contracting the muscles of the pelvic floor (Guyton, 1991).

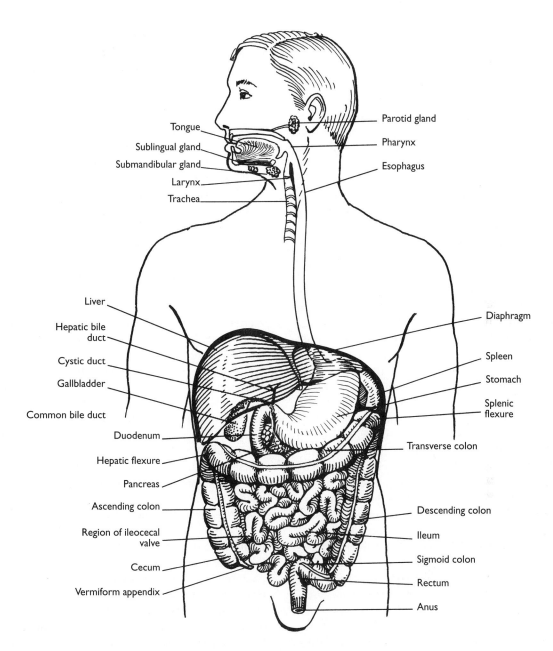

FIGURE 14-1 The organs of the GI system and related structures. (From Phipps, W.J. et al. [1995]. *Medical-surgical nursing: Concepts and clinical practice* [5th ed.]. St. Louis: Mosby.)

■ Physical Age-Related Changes Affecting Bowel Elimination

A variety of structural and functional changes in the GI system can be seen in older adults, although the incidence and significance of GI changes are not universal among them. Changes of the GI system begin with decreased saliva production after the age of 50, and altered taste and smell. These changes, combined with impaired mastication or swallowing, can affect the ability to eat foods high in fiber and roughage or to consume adequate fluid intake (Kallman, 1983). Throughout the small intestine there is little change in structure or transit time. In the large intestine there is a weakening of the colonic wall, which, in association with high lumenal pressures, leads to the development of muscular atrophy, abnormalities of the mucosal glands, and hypertrophy of the muscularis mucosa. A significant effect of aging on the GI tract is the loss of neurons from the intrinsic nervous system (Kenney, 1989). Colonic transit time can be decreased because of a deficit in innervation and decreased responsiveness of neurotransmitters (Hazzard et al., 1990; Kenney, 1989).

Changes in sensory mechanisms related to the urge to defecate may also occur. The inability to recognize the urge to defecate, repeatedly ignoring the call to defecate, and/or having physical limitations in toileting oneself appropriately can lead to a deterioration of the sensory mechanisms that stimulate the urge to have a bowel movement. When this occurs, as more stool arrives in the rectum, a reverse peristalsis occurs into the proximal parts of the colon, which may result in constipation and megarectum (Barnes, 1987). Constipation occurs when stool is delayed in the colon and water continues to be absorbed from the fecal matter. Stool becomes harder and drier and subsequently more difficult to pass (Guyton, 1991).

Constipation can lead to abdominal distention, which in turn can result in decreased oral intake, further resulting in dehydration and malnutrition. Hemorrhoids and anal fissures may result when excessive straining at stool produces

Aging Alert
Change in bowel habits

A sudden change in bowel habits could indicate an acute functional, metabolic, or neurologic condition that warrants referral to a gastroenterologist for a full medical physical examination and GI workup.

From Wong, R.D., Gold, S., & Blanchette, P.A. (1991, January-February). Correcting constipation: A regimen that works. *Senior Patient*, pp. 37-41.

tears or passive congestion of tissues near the rectum (Cheskin & Schuster, 1994). Hemorrhoids themselves cause pain, bleeding, and possible need for surgery (Chenitz et al., 1991).

A serious result of constipation is fecal impaction (Wrenn, 1989). Typical symptoms associated with impaction are anorexia, nausea, vomiting, abdominal distention, and abdominal pain. Paradoxic diarrhea and incontinence of urine and stool may be present. Continuous seepage of moist bacteria-laden mucus and stool may cause the development of decubitus. In the bowel itself, obstruction of the large bowel can occur. Continued pressure and ischemic necrosis on the wall of the colon may cause stercoral ulceration. Perforation of diverticula caused by increased intralumenal pressure may also occur. Fecal impactions need to be removed either with an enema or by gentle digital removal (Wrenn, 1989). Bladder elimination may also become affected when an impaction exists. Urinary problems of frequency, retention, overflow incontinence, and urinary tract infection are conditions commonly caused by impaction (Wrenn, 1989).

The complexity and sequelae of constipation, which occur as a result of the many associated physical and environmental factors, may be prevented through early detection and management of the problem.

■ Factors Influencing Bowel Elimination

The factors that contribute to the development of constipation in older adults are the following: (1) structural and functional changes of the GI tract resulting from aging; (2) diet; (3) activity; (4) medical conditions; (5) common medications taken by older adults; and (6) the environment. Many of these factors may overlap and contribute to the development or severity of constipation.

DIET

The two dietary factors that influence bowel elimination the most are fiber and fluid consumption.

Fiber

Dietary fiber is a term used for a diverse group of complex carbohydrates, found in plant structure, of differing chemical structure and physical properties that are not digestible by human intestinal enzymes (Taylor, 1990). In the colon, fiber increases stool bulk by holding water and acting as a substrate for colonic microflora. This process further increases stool bulk by increasing bacterial, water, and salt content and producing gases that augment the bulking effect. As a result of these properties, fiber exerts a laxative effect, accelerates intestinal transit, increases fecal weight, and reduces gastrointestinal pressure (Gorman & Bowman, 1993).

Over the last century in most Western countries there has been a steady decline in the consumption of fiber, from about 40 gm per day 100 years ago to a current value of 15 to 20 gm per day (Taylor, 1990; Cheskin & Schuster, 1990). The decreased intake can be attributed to the refinement of food that began in the industrial revolution. Since then, there has been a steady fall in the consumption of fiber, with a corresponding increase in the intake of sugar, fat, and protein (Taylor, 1990).

Consumption of fiber by older adults may be limited by the following:

1. Lack of knowledge of foods high in fiber
2. Inability to read food labels for fiber content

3. Intolerance of foods high in fiber as a result of dental or digestive disorders
4. Inability to purchase and prepare their own food
5. Institutional diets low in fiber
6. Poor appetite
7. Lack of interest in eating

Fluid

Fluid is needed in the gut to keep fecal matter soft and moving. An average of eight glasses of fluid per day should be consumed to promote normal bowel absorption in the small intestine and colon (Cameron, 1992). Absorption through the GI tract decreases this amount resulting in a daily stool volume of approximately 150 cc. A change of intake or absorption of even 100 cc can lead to harder, drier stools (Canty, 1994; Castle, 1989).

Consumption of fluid by older adults may be limited by the following:

1. Decreased thirst mechanism
2. Limited access to fluids
3. Therapeutic fluid restriction
4. Difficulty swallowing
5. Increased voiding

ACTIVITY

Propulsion of mass in the colon is correlated with physical activity. GI motility increases during and after ingestion of food; however, this propulsive movement is found only in physically active people. With inactivity there is slowed movement of feces into the descending colon and rectum (Harper & Lyles, 1988). The lack of propulsive movement in resting individuals has been shown to increase the occurrence of constipation (Barnes, 1987).

Physical activity in older adults may be limited by the following:

1. Decreased cognition and lack of motivation
2. Poor vision
3. Skeletal changes
4. Neuromuscular impairments
5. Poor environment

6. Lack of available assistance or assistive devices
7. Fear of personal safety in the neighborhood

MEDICAL CONDITIONS

Many older adults have at least one chronic medical condition, often treated with medication. Disease processes may directly alter bowel elimination, and the GI system is vulnerable to the effects of medication because of the nervous system control of GI motility. The effects of the medical condition and its treatment, and the impact on lifestyle need to be analyzed for factors that increase the risk for development of constipation (Chenitz et al., 1991; Donatelle, 1990; Kopac, 1993; Merkel et al., 1993; Wrenn, 1989).

Medical conditions that can affect bowel elimination in older adults include the following:

1. GI disorders
2. Endocrine and metabolic disorders (hypothyroidism, diabetes mellitus)
3. Neurologic impairments (Parkinson's disease, stroke)
4. Depression
5. Dementia
6. Anxiety

LAXATIVE USE

In the United States, cathartics are prescribed for more than 3 million people annually, and as many as 78% of patients in long-term care are dependent on laxatives for routine bowel evacuation (Donatelle, 1990; Rodrigues-Fisher et al., 1993). There are over 700 different laxative products on the market—the majority of which are available without a prescription. Annual expenditures on laxatives are between $250 and $400 million per year (Cerrato, 1989).

A review of commonly used laxatives follows.

Bulk-forming products

Bulk-forming products (e.g., bran and psyllium mucilloid [Metamucil]) provide a more concentrated form of fiber than can be obtained from most food sources. The dose needs to be adjusted so that the patient is ingesting up to 15 gm of dietary fiber a day. Each dose must be taken with 8 oz of fluids. Bulk laxatives usually work within 24 hours by absorbing water, swelling, and then stimulating peristalsis (Cerrato, 1989). Side effects include flatus, cramping, bloating, and obstruction if the laxatives are taken without adequate fluid (Allison et al., 1994; Tedesco, 1985). A positive effect can be the lowering of serum lipid levels (Melmon et al. 1992).

Stool softeners

Stool softeners (e.g., dioctyl sodium succinate, or docusate) facilitate the mixture of aqueous and fatty substances in the fecal mass. This mechanism softens the stool and increases water secretion in the small and large intestines. Peristalsis is not promoted, but the process makes hard stools easier to pass, either by breaking the fecal mass into smaller particles or by lubricating a dry stool. Stool softeners may take up to 72 hours to work (Cerrato, 1989) and are useful for short-term therapy, but have little value for the treatment of long-term constipation. They will not prevent constipation caused by major contributing factors (Tedesco, 1985).

Lubricants

Lubricants (a major lubricating laxative is mineral oil [Haley's M-O]) coat fecal contents and decrease colonic absorption of water, thus making stools easier to pass within 8 hours. Use of mineral oil should be avoided in debilitated patients or those at risk for aspiration pneumonia because toxic effects can occur in lung tissue if the mineral oil is aspirated (Castle, 1989; Tedesco, 1985).

Osmotic laxatives

Osmotic laxatives (e.g., Golytely and Colyte) pull fluids into the intestinal lumen, producing increased intralumenal volume that stimulates intestinal motility. They usually act within ½ hour to 3 hours when taken orally or within 15 to 30 minutes when taken rectally and can be given on a scheduled basis 2 to 3 times a week when all other measures have failed. Active agents in these laxatives include magnesium citrate, magnesium hydroxide, magnesium sulfate, and sodium phosphates (Tedesco, 1985). These laxatives are rarely used for treatment of common constipation; rather, they are used frequently in preparation for GI diagnostic testing.

Lactulose, sorbitol, and glycerin suppositories are sometimes used for treating constipation in older adults. Glycerin has an irritant, as well as osmotic, effect on the distal portion of the colon and on the rectum, and usually works in 30 to 60 minutes. Lactulose has an osmotic effect and is metabolized by bacteria in the colon, thus lowering the pH of the colon and increasing peristalsis. Lactulose usually requires 24 to 48 hours to work, and may cause flatulence, cramps, diarrhea, and electrolyte imbalances (Allison et al., 1994).

Stimulant laxatives

Stimulant laxatives (e.g., cascara or senna, castor oil, and bisacodyl) promote peristalsis by irritating the colon wall and nerves that feed it. They are more likely to work by increasing fluid secretion in the small intestine and colon (Melmon et al., 1992). A bowel movement can be anticipated within 6 to 8 hours after administration of an oral preparation and within 15 to 60 minutes after rectal insertion. These drugs should not be used over a long period because of potential severe abdominal cramping, nerve damage to the myenteric plexus, acid base disorders, and chronic long-term effects (atonic colon) (Cerrato, 1989; Melmon et al., 1992).

Laxative use should be discouraged, because many toxic effects are related to long-term use. Health-promoting behaviors such as appropriate food and fluid intake and regular exercise will help many older adults to develop regular patterns of bowel elimination without reliance on laxatives.

Aging Alert
Laxative abuse

Laxatives can contribute to constipation when abused or used on a long-term basis. Stimulant laxatives such as bisacodyl are the most commonly abused. Long-term use can cause damage to the neural fibers that regulate the movements of the colon, thereby causing motility dysfunction. Bulk-forming laxatives or fiber supplements taken without adequate hydration cause hard stools and may lead to development of fecal impaction.

From Castle, S.C. (1989). Constipation: Endemic in the elderly? Gerontopathophysiology, evaluation, and management. *Medical Clinics of North America, 73* (6), 1497-1509. Wrenn, K. (1989). Fecal impaction. *New England Journal of Medicine, 321*(10), 658-662.

MEDICATION USE

Common potentially constipating drugs taken by older adults include the following (Castle, 1989; Wrenn, 1989):

1. Minerals (aluminum-containing antacids)
2. Narcotics and opiates
3. Antihypertensives
4. Antiarrhythmics
5. Anticholinergics
6. Sympathomimetics
7. Nonsteroidal anti-inflammatory agents
8. Diuretics

ENVIRONMENT

Older adults are faced daily with multiple factors in the environment that may adversely affect their ability to maintain a regular bowel elimination pattern. The physical layout for toileting may be a huge deterrent in that the bathroom may be too small to accommodate a wheelchair. Older adults may be unable to lift their own weight off the toilet, and there may be a lack of assistive devices such as side bars. Shared bathrooms in institutions may be the cause of constipation because the need for privacy is not met. Other environmental constraints exist in all types of settings—home, acute care, and long-term care.

Environmental factors that may influence bowel elimination include the following:

1. Access to a toilet
2. Privacy
3. Available assistance for toileting
4. Caregiver embarrassment or repulsion regarding bowel elimination
5. Ability to maintain physical activity

■ Nursing Process

The literature presents strong evidence that most cases of constipation are not caused by underlying pathologic conditions of the GI system; thus constipation is primarily an issue that nursing can manage independently (Camilleri et al., 1994). In all settings of practice, the focus of management should be on *screening* and *prevention of constipation*. Promotion of routine bowel elimination should be the goal of those who are working with older patients in any setting or through community-based health promotion programs for independent older adults. Identification of those at risk for becoming constipated and prevention of constipation should be the focus of the health care provider. A thorough screening for the contributing factors for constipation provides the base from which the health care provider delivers care and teaches the patient and family healthy bowel elimination habits.

ASSESSMENT

The purpose of assessment is to discover contributing factors that cause or may cause constipation. The assessment should include the following areas: health history, bowel history, dietary history, medications, environment, and a physical examination. The patient, family member, caregiver, and medical record are all sources of data

---

BOX 14-1 BOWEL HISTORY

1. Do you have a set time for bowel elimination?
2. How many times a week do you have a bowel movement?
3. What is the consistency of your stool?
4. Do you have to strain to have a bowel movement?
5. Have you ever had a fecal impaction?
6. Do you ever delay having a bowel movement after you feel the urge to defecate?
7. Do you have a current ritual, including laxative use, for moving your bowels?
8. Are you able to get to a toilet when you feel the urge to defecate?
9. Do you ever have diarrhea accompanied by the feeling of incomplete evacuation?

---

utilized to complete the assessment of bowel elimination.

Health history

Begin the health history with a review of systems and include any surgical procedures, particularly oral and abdominal procedures. Recent weight gain or loss should also be documented.

Bowel history

The bowel history includes the patient's definition of normalcy and constipation. The terminology for bowel elimination may vary with patients. It is important for the nurse to speak in terms with which the patient is familiar regarding bowel elimination. If the patient is cognitively impaired or unable to give information, data are gathered from other sources. Specific questions about bowel elimination are listed in Box 14-1.

Diet history

Diet history is an important component of the assessment and is especially pertinent when a patient has a complaint of constipation. Begin the diet history with the type of diet, including any restrictions currently prescribed for the patient. An average 24-hour recall of food consumed is reviewed and analyzed for fiber content. Food frequently eaten, as well as food likes and dislikes, should also be reviewed. Other considerations in the diet history are religious or ethnic food restrictions and the effects of lifestyle variables such as food purchasing, preparation, and consumption habits (Seidel et al., 1995). A review of fluid intake must also be conducted, including type, frequency, quantity of fluid consumed per serving, and total 24-hour intake.

Medications

A review of medications must include prescribed medications, all over-the-counter medications, laxatives, and nondietary fiber supplements. It is important to ascertain the amount of liquids that the older adult takes with the medications and throughout the day. The use of any alternative cultural or herbal remedy for constipation should be assessed. The nurse should be sensitive to the cultural importance that the patient places on bowel elimination. This will ensure that the physical and cultural needs of the older adult are respected.

Environment and functional ability

Assessment of the environment includes the patient's ability to function in the environment to meet toileting needs, and the assistance of a caregiver if the patient is unable to meet these needs alone. Questions to include in assessing the environment are listed in Box 14-2.

Physical examination

For the physical examination, see Box 14-3.

Conclusion

A comprehensive assessment form is presented in Figure 14-2. The assessment form can be used in any setting of practice to determine the risk factors a patient has for potential or actual constipation.

BOX 14-2 ENVIRONMENTAL AND FUNCTIONAL ABILITY ASSESSMENT

1. What is the layout of your living arrangement?
2. Do you have access to a toilet when the urge to defecate is felt?
3. What type of device do you usually use for bowel elimination—toilet, bedside commode, bedpan, or incontinence brief?
4. Are you able to remove your clothing in time to have a bowel movement?
5. Is there a caregiver present who is able and willing to assist with toileting for bowel elimination?
6. Is there enough privacy to provide a relaxed atmosphere for elimination?
7. Is there enough time provided to have a bowel movement?

NURSING DIAGNOSIS

After a comprehensive assessment of the patient is completed, a diagnosis can be made based on the subjective and objective data that have been collected through the process of history taking and physical examination. In the case of constipation, the individual is experiencing inadequate bowel elimination. The defining characteristics associated with this diagnosis are the following:

1. Passage of stool less than 3 to 5 times per week
2. Insufficient quantity of stool to cause feeling of complete evacuation
3. Incomplete passage of stool
4. Passage of hard and dry stool
5. Straining at evacuation more than 25% of the time

The major factors contributing to constipation in older adults are the following:

1. Inadequate intake of dietary fiber and/or fluid
2. Limited physical mobility

BOX 14-3 PHYSICAL EXAMINATION

1. Cognition assessment—Mental status must be assessed, with attention focused on the older adult's ability to recognize the urge to defecate, the ability to request assistance if needed, the ability to find a toilet when the urge to defecate is felt, and memory retention of instructions on how to call for assistance.
2. Functional status assessment—Functional status includes the older person's ability to perform self-toileting. Older adults with arthritis or debilitating diseases may recognize the urge to defecate, but may move too slowly to toilet independently. One way to collect this data is to directly observe the patients toileting.
3. Physical endurance assessment—It is important to observe gait and strength, and to discuss with the patient average daily exercise and endurance for physical activity. It is important to assess the minimum activity level a patient can tolerate. This would include amount of exercise, distance for walking, ability to get up independently, ability to get up with assistance, or the inability to get out of bed.
4. Oral examination—The oral examination should include evaluation of dentition; mucous membranes; presence of lesions, sores, or tumors; gag reflex; swallowing; and taste sensation.
5. Abdominal examination—The abdominal examination should include the following: inspection—for contour, visible peristalsis, or visible bulges; auscultation—frequency and character of bowel sounds; percussion—for tympanic or dull sounds; palpation—tenderness or firmness over lower abdomen.
6. Rectal examination—A rectal examination should be done at the conclusion of the assessment. The following should be noted: hemorrhoids (external and/or internal), anal sphincter tone, presence of stool in the rectal vault, or presence of an impaction indicated by dry, hard stool.

From Allison, O.C., Porter, M.E., & Briggs, G.C. (1994). Chronic constipation: Assessment and management in the elderly. *Journal of the American Academy of Nurse Practitioners,* 6(7), 311-317; Bates, B. (1995). *A guide to physical examination* (6th ed.). Philadelphia: J.B. Lippincott; Seidel, H., et al. (1995). *Mosby's guide to physical examination* (3rd ed.). St. Louis: Mosby.

3. Environmental impediments to toileting
4. Medications that affect GI motility, hydration, or appetite
5. Cognitive impairment that affects independence in relation to defecation
6. Medical illness

The defining characteristics and contributing factors may vary from patient to patient; however, both components need to be included in the diagnosis. For example, the diagnosis might be as follows: alteration in bowel elimination: constipation—as defined by bowel movement less than 3 times a week associated with straining at stool 25% of the time; related to activity intolerance (arthritis) and pain medication.

PLANNING AND GOAL IDENTIFICATION

The goal is to establish a bowel elimination regimen that facilitates normal bowel function that is appropriate and adequate for the patient's physical and emotional well-being. The patient's definition of normalcy must be considered when establishing the desired outcome. Intervention for maintaining bowel elimination must be based on the assessment data collected.

A common goal for bowel elimination can be stated as follows: *a soft-formed bowel movement*

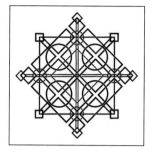

CHAPTER 15

There is an appointed time for every thing,
and a time for every affair under the heavens.
A time to be born, and a time to die;
a time to plant, and a time to uproot.

ECCLESIASTES 3:2-3

Nutrition and Digestive Function

■ Learning Objectives

On completion of this chapter, the reader will be able to do the following:

1. Discuss nutritional requirements for the older adult.
2. Explain the use of the food guide pyramid and food labels.
3. Describe age-related changes in the digestive system of the older adult.
4. Recognize the physiologic, psychosocial, and environmental factors that influence the maintenance of the nutritional status of the older adult.
5. Discuss drug-nutrient interactions and their effect on older adults.
6. Discuss pathologic conditions that affect the nutritional status of the older adult.
7. Describe the components of nutritional assessment for the older adult.
8. Develop a plan of care for the older adult with an alteration in nutrition.
9. Design appropriate nursing interventions for older adults with alterations in nutrition.
10. Describe strategies for promoting optimum nutrition in the older adult.

As people go about their daily activities, whether at play, work, or rest, or even in sleep, their bodies need energy. Nutrition is one of the basic human needs that supplies this energy and sustains life. "Nutrition thus concerns the food people eat and how their bodies use it. Nutritional science comprises the body of scientific knowledge governing the nutritional requirements of humans for maintenance, growth, activity, and reproduction" (Williams, 1989). Sound nutrition is considered to be a primary basis for promoting health and preventing disease throughout the life span.

Food provides the essential nutrients the body requires for its vital processes. A wide variety of foods provide important ingredients that sustain physiologic processes. Personal choice and food availability govern the selection of nutrients. The major nutrients essential for healthy aging include protein, carbohydrates, fat, minerals, vitamins, and water.

Food plays a vital role in family life and is a part of many rituals and ceremonies in the larger society. Thus motivation for eating may spring from the need for love, belonging, or meeting the expectations of others. Furthermore, religious practices, as well as personal preferences, may dictate what older adults will eat and what they will refuse to eat. As with all of the important processes of life, meeting the nutritional requirements for a healthy life is neither simple nor easy.

■ Nutritional Requirements in Older Adults

The nutrient needs and nutrition status of older adults are becoming increasingly important, not only because of the unprecedented increase in the number of older people in the population, but also because of the high cost of nutrition-related chronic diseases. Good nutrition and adequate exercise can improve the quality of life and the health of older adults. Concern has been expressed in the literature regarding the adequacy of the available research data for guiding accurate recommendations for dietary intake, especially for older adults over 75 to 80 years of age (Brookbank, 1990). Many of the studies group all people age 65 and older in one category and do not differentiate among those in their later years.

The National Health and Nutrition Examination Survey provides needed information about the diet of Americans and is of major importance in establishing specific nutrient recommendations for groups of people over 50 years of age (1989). The tenth and most current edition of the recommended dietary allowances (RDAs) continues to use a category of 51+ years because the subcommittee of the National Research Council did not consider the data adequate to establish separate RDAs for people 70 years and older (National Research Council, 1989) (Table 15-1).

TABLE 15-1 Recommended dietary allowances for older adults (1989)

Characteristic or dietary element	Value	
	Male	Female
Age	51+	51+
Weight (kg)	77	65
Weight (lb)	170	143
Height (cm)	173	160
Height (in)	68	63
Protein (gm)	63	50
Vitamin A (µg, RE*)	1000	600
Vitamin D (µg)	5	5
Vitamin E (mg)	10	8
Vitamin K (µg)	80	65
Vitamin C (mg)	60	60
Thiamin (mg)	1.2	1.0
Riboflavin (mg)	1.4	1.2
Niacin (mg)	15	13
Vitamin B_6 (mg)	2.0	1.6
Folate (µg)	200	180
Vitamin B_{12} (µg)	2.0	2.0
Calcium (mg)	800	800
Phosphorus (mg)	800	800
Magnesium (mg)	350	280
Iron (mg)	10	10
Zinc (mg)	15	12
Iodine (µg)	150	150
Selenium (µg)	70	55
Copper (mg)	1.5-3.0	1.5-3.0
Manganese (mg)	2.0-5.0	2.0-5.0
Fluoride (mg)	1.5-4	1.5-4
Chromium (µg)	50-200	50-200
Molybdenum (µg)	75-250	75-250
Sodium (mg) minimum	500	500
Chloride (mg) minimum	750	750
Potassium (mg) minimum	2000	2000

Adapted from National Research Council. (1989). *Recommended dietary allowances.* Washington, DC: National Academy of Sciences.
*µg = microgram, one millionth of a gram. RE = retinol equivalent, which is the vitamin A activity in foods.

The RDAs have been called "the Gold Standard for evaluating nutritional adequacy in the United States" (Sutnick, 1988, p. 193). They are defined as "the levels of intake of essential nutrients that, on the basis of scientific knowledge, are judged by the Food and Nutrition Board to be adequate to meet the known needs of practically all healthy persons" (National Research Council, 1989, p. 1). The RDAs are extrapolated from the measurements made on young adults. The National Research Council (1989) has noted the wide variations in health with advancing age and stated, "there is some evidence that the elderly have altered requirements for some nutrients" (p. 19). It must be stressed that the RDAs are not designed to account for changes resulting from disease, drug interactions, or psychosocial factors that affect food intake.

Data from the National Council of Aging indicate that undernutrition and malnutrition affect between 15% and 50% of the population of older adults, with signs and symptoms that are not always recognized by health care givers.

OVERVIEW OF BASIC NUTRIENTS
Protein

Protein is an essential nutrient for growth and tissue repair. Proteins are made up of carbon, hydrogen, oxygen, and nitrogen. When protein is used for energy, most of the nitrogen becomes a waste product and must be converted to urea and excreted. All living cells, including muscle, bone, lymph, blood, enzymes, and brain tissue, contain protein. For cellular synthesis to occur, protein must first be broken down to amino acids. These amino acids are classified as essential and nonessential.

Nonessential amino acids are synthesized by the liver from other amino acids, whereas the body relies on dietary sources for the essential amino acids. It is generally believed that essential amino acids must all be present in the right quantity and at the right time in order to facilitate their maximum efficient use for cellular metabolism. A food that contains adequate amounts of essential amino acids is classified as a complete protein of high biologic value. Animal proteins

such as eggs, milk and milk products, meats, poultry, and fish fall into this category. An incomplete protein of low biologic value is a food that is lacking in one or more of the essential amino acids. These foods (cereal, vegetables, and legumes), although lacking in some essential amino acids, may be combined with other non-animal proteins. If the right combination of non-animal proteins is consumed at the same meal, it will provide a protein quality equal to that of an animal protein.

Many older adults may have an inadequate intake of protein; attention should be given to encouraging them to eat foods that are good sources of protein. In spite of the wide acceptance of the RDAs as the standard of diet adequacy, there has been considerable discussion and disagreement in the literature concerning the recommended levels of protein for older adults.

The National Research Council (1989) continues to recommend the same level of protein for older adults as for young adults (0.8 gm/kg body weight). The council explains that because of the difference in body composition, this is actually a higher allowance per unit of lean body mass and should compensate for the lessened efficiency of older adults in utilizing protein. The daily requirement of protein for women can be met with 4 oz of fish, meat, or poultry, plus 2 oz of milk or 3 oz of cheese. For men, an additional 2 oz of meat will provide the required daily supply of protein. Usually, if 12% to 15% of total calories come from protein, this is enough to meet daily needs.

Carbohydrates

There are indications that carbohydrate absorption may be slightly decreased in older adults (Ausman & Russell, 1990). There are no RDAs for carbohydrate intake in older adults, but the U.S. Department of Agriculture, the American Cancer Society, and the American Heart Association have endorsed the suggestion that 55% to 60% of total calories be composed of carbohydrates. The carbohydrates in the diet should be primarily complex, with few simple sugars. Four or more servings of fresh or cooked fruits and vegetables incorporated into the diet will meet the standard recommended percentage.

Complex carbohydrate foods rich in fiber should make up at least 55% of the total intake of calories. When eating breads, pasta, and potatoes, the older adult must limit the amount of fats in the form of butter, margarine, and sour cream used to complement foods high in complex carbohydrates. Simple carbohydrates come mainly from sugars in fresh fruit and from low-fat milk and milk products.

Lipids

Lipids include fats and oils and are made up of carbon, hydrogen, and oxygen. They provide 9 calories per gram, with excesses stored mainly in adipose tissue. Lipids (1) provide linoleic and linolenic acids, essential fatty acids; (2) add taste and satiety value to foods; and (3) aid in the absorption of fat-soluble vitamins. The classification system for lipids contains three major branches: simple, compound, and derived. Simple lipids are made up of glycerol and fatty acids, which are further designated as monoglycerides, diglycerides, and triglycerides. The triglycerides make up over 90% of the lipids in food and in the body. Compound lipids are simple lipids with the addition of a nonlipid fraction like protein (lipoprotein), phospholipids, and glycolipids (glucose and lipid). Derived lipids such as cholesterol result from the breakdown of compound and simple lipids.

Saturated fats are found mostly in animal fats and in coconut and palm oil. These fats are thought to raise cholesterol levels and to contribute to the development of atherosclerosis. Unsaturated fats are classified as monosaturated or polyunsaturated fat. Hydrogenated fats, created by a commercial process with polyunsaturated fats, are saturated fats that seem to be as atherogenic as the naturally occurring saturated fat. Examples of hydrogenated fats are margarine and

vegetable shortening, with the soft, tub margarine being less saturated than the hard, stick margarine. Plant lipids are mostly polyunsaturated. Olive oil, a monosaturated lipid, is thought to lower serum cholesterol.

Most lipid metabolism occurs in the liver, where lipids are released into the bloodstream as very low-, low-, and high-density lipoprotein (VLDL, LDL, and HDL) cholesterol. HDLs carry a higher proportion of protein to lipid than do the LDLs, and are believed to have a serum cholesterol lowering effect. The VLDLs have a higher proportion of triglycerides, which the cells use for energy.

The guidelines recommend that dietary fat should make up no more than 30% of the total caloric intake, with a daily cholesterol intake not to exceed 300 mg. The diet health guidelines also suggest limiting saturated fat intake to no more than 10% of the total fat intake, with 10% of the total fat intake being from monosaturated and the remaining from polyunsaturated fatty acid (National Research Council, 1989). This can be done by avoiding fried and fatty foods, trimming visible fat from meat, using low-fat milk, and reducing the amount of fats used as salad dressings and spreads. The amount of fat in the average American diet has usually exceeded the recommended percentage of 20% to 30% and is estimated to be in the range of 38% to 42% of total calories.

Minerals

Calcium, iron, and zinc are three of the minerals that are important dietary elements.

Calcium Discussions regarding calcium intake in older people, particularly in women, center around a concern about the prevention and treatment of osteoporosis, a condition of reduced bone mass that occurs after menopause. As they age, both men and women experience a reduction in bone mass, which is much more pronounced in women. The 1994 National Institutes of Health (NIH) consensus conference reported that both older men and older women average a daily intake of only 600 mg of calcium. The National Research Council (1989) recommends for older adults a daily intake of 800 mg of calcium, usually obtained in a balanced diet. This is the level recommended for healthy people and does not address the special needs of people with osteoporosis. Based on the high incidence of osteoporosis in women, the NIH conference recommended that postmenopausal women on estrogen consume 1000 mg/day and those not on estrogen consume 1500 mg/day. It was also recommended that the increases should come from dietary sources rather than from calcium supplements. The National Research Council emphasized that, besides calcium, other nutrients are necessary for bone health.

Some of the risks of a high intake of calcium were noted by the National Research Council, such as increased risk of urinary tract stones, especially in hypercalciuric men, and potential decreased absorption of iron, zinc, and other essential minerals. Constipation may also result. In addition to hypercalciuria, amounts of calcium higher than those recommended may cause hypercalcemia and deterioration in renal function. Because of the antacid effects of calcium, calcium supplementation at mealtimes can cause a reduction in dietary folate and iron absorption (Roe, 1987). For these reasons the National Research Council (1989) does not recommend supplementing calcium to a level much above the RDA for the average person.

Besides their calcium intake in later years, other factors that influence the rate and amount of bone mass loss in older women are exercise and the adequacy of calcium taken in during the peak years of bone mass development—the late teens and early 20s. For women ages 80 years and older, the RDA of 800 mg appears to be adequate (Anderson, 1990).

An increase in calcium intake for postmenopausal women needs to be encouraged. The best way to achieve this increase is through dietary means, such as low-fat milk, cheese, and yogurt. Some experts recommend calcium supplement

---

BOX 15-1 CALCIUM-RICH FOODS AND CALCIUM SUPPLEMENTS

CALCIUM IN THE KITCHEN

Tofu (8 oz): 280 mg calcium
Canned salmon, with bones (1 oz): 60 mg
Canned sardines, with bones (1 oz): 125 mg
Whole milk (8 oz): 290 mg
Low-fat milk (8 oz): 298 mg
Skim milk (8 oz): 300 mg
Yogurt (8 oz): 400 mg
Cottage cheese (8 oz): 170 mg
Mozzarella cheese, skim (1 oz): 183 mg
American cheese (1 oz): 170 mg
Parmesan cheese (2 tbsp): 140 mg
Green leafy vegetables (8 oz): 400 mg
Ice cream, vanilla (8 oz): 208 mg

. . . IN THE MEDICINE CHEST

Calcium carbonate (40% calcium)
Calcium sulfate (36.1%)
Dibasic calcium phosphate (29.5%)
Tribasic calcium phosphate (38.8%)
Calcium lactate (13%)
Calcium citrate (21%)
Calcium gluconate (9.3%)
Calcium glubionate (6.5%)

From Holm, K., & Walker, J. (1990). Osteoporosis: Treatment and prevention update. *Geriatric Nursing*, *11*(3), 142.

---

administration with food. The addition of calcium supplements to the normal diet can be suggested along with dietary recommendations (see Box 15-1 for typical calcium supplements).

Iron There may be impaired iron absorption in older adults as a result of decreased secretion of hydrochloric acid, which is needed to convert the iron into a usable form for the body. Although this represents a potential risk of iron deficiency, there has been little evidence that decreased iron intake or absorption is a frequent cause of anemia in older adults. When iron deficiency does occur in older people, it is more often the result of bleeding from a variety of causes, such as chronic use of aspirin or similar drugs, peptic ulcer, esophageal varices, cancer, or inflammatory disease of the bowel (National Research Council, 1989).

There is a tendency for iron stores to increase with age, and the American diet, including that of older men and women, usually supplies more than the current RDA of 10 mg/day (Roe, 1987). Nonetheless, there is a risk of iron deficiency among poor older adults and those with mobility problems who are unable to acquire or prepare foods, such as meat and green leafy vegetables, that contain adequate sources of iron.

Zinc There is some evidence that the daily intake of zinc by older people is less than the recommended amounts of 15 mg for men and 12 mg for women. However, it is difficult to determine anyone's exact zinc status because of a lack of sensitive indicators (National Research Council, 1989). Suggestions have been made that deficiency of zinc may be responsible for the delay in wound healing and the decline in immune function that have been noted in older adults (National Research Council, 1989; Roe, 1987). There is also some suggestion that the loss of taste and smell may be related to low zinc levels. There is a need to reexamine the zinc requirements of older adults and to inform older adults regarding good dietary sources of zinc, such as selected seafoods and meats.

Vitamins

Vitamins are essential nutrients that perform special metabolic functions. Most vitamins are not produced by the body and must be obtained from dietary sources. They are required in small amounts for various physiologic functions including regulating metabolism and functioning as catalysts. They are generally classified as being either fat soluble or water soluble. The RDAs of vitamins for people over 50 years of age do not differ greatly from the RDAs for 25- to 50-year-

olds. Niacin, riboflavin, and thiamin requirements are slightly reduced. A number of studies indicate that the vitamin levels most likely to be low in older men and women are those of vitamin A, thiamin, riboflavin, and pyridoxine (vitamin B_6) (Yearick et al., 1980). Factors influencing adequate intake of vitamins are nutrient quality of the diet in view of reduced caloric intake; medication and alcohol use that could interfere with absorption; and socioeconomic and cultural factors.

The recommended adult dietary allowance of vitamin C is 60 mg/day. Adequate dietary intake of vitamin C is essential for the healthy nutrition of the aging person. Because vitamin C, along with the B-complex vitamins, is water soluble, it is not stored in the body's tissues as are fat-soluble vitamins. This storage incapability makes the water-soluble vitamins less apt to become toxic but more likely to be deficient.

Studies have shown that levels of vitamin C are lower in older men than in older women who eat the same diet (VanderJagt et al., 1987). Studies also indicate that smokers need a higher intake of vitamin C to reach required levels (Viteri, 1988).

There is some evidence that the onset of cataracts can be retarded with behavioral and nutritional modifications (Rosenberg, 1994). There seems to be a protective effect with increasing levels of vitamin C, vitamin E, and beta-carotene. This is an area in which health care professionals need to be involved, in research and in advancing sound, evidence-based health promotion activities.

Supplemental use of vitamin C and the clinical significance of high doses are controversial. No clinical benefits have been reported from taking high doses of vitamin C. In the 1970s, Nobel Laureate Linus Pauling popularized the notion that large doses of vitamin C would prevent or cure colds; this claim has not been substantiated (Dykes & Meier, 1975; Levine, 1986). (See Tables 15-2 and 15-3 for a summary of water- and fat-soluble vitamins.)

Water

Water functions as a medium for cell metabolism; it provides structure and form to the body by the turgor it gives to the tissue; and it helps to maintain body temperature. Water provides the aqueous medium necessary for many chemical and physical processes to take place. It helps to dilute water-soluble medications, aids in excretion of body wastes, and provides for the transport of nutrients. There is general agreement that the water content of the body decreases with age. The body of a mature adult is composed of about 70% water; at age 65, water content is about 60%. Recent findings indicate that people older than 80 years of age (late senescence) have body water content of less than 60% (Reif, 1987). The physiologic consequences of the decrease in body water in older adults can be far reaching. Concentrations of water-soluble drugs in the body are higher, and thermoregulation is less stable. There is an increased susceptibility to both dehydration and overhydration with a reduced water compartment. This risk of dehydration or overhydration is a significant physiologic threat to the health of the older adult. (For a summary of water and other minerals, see Table 15-4.)

DIETARY RECOMMENDATIONS

The food guide pyramid replaces the basic four food groups and reflects the current health recommendations with respect to food groupings and numbers of servings (U.S. Department of Health and Human Services [USDHHS], 1992). These recommendations, in turn, achieve the recommended dietary allowances when a variety of foods are selected from the groups with serving sizes adjusted according to individual caloric needs. (Recommendations for daily intake are seen in Figure 15-1.)

New food labels, legislated by the Food and Drug Administration (FDA), allow older adults to make informed, healthier food choices. The new food labels must follow strict guidelines in regard to serving sizes, nutritional content, and health claims. The daily values (DVs) replace the RDAs for protein, vitamins, and minerals and provide recommendations for total fat, saturated fat, cholesterol, and sodium. Maximum DVs are established for nutrients of fat, sodium, and cholesterol because of their linkages to the development of chronic diseases. However, maximum DVs for fiber, calcium, iron, and vitamins A and C are included because surveys reflect inadequate intake. The percent daily values show how the nutritional content of a particular food fits into a 2000-calorie diet. For an explanation of food labels, refer to Figure 15-2.

■ Age-Related Changes That Affect Nutrient Needs

METABOLISM

Total energy expenditure is composed of energy used at rest, in activity, and in thermogenesis. These components are affected by age, body size and composition, intake of energy, genetics, physiologic and pathologic conditions, and ambient temperature. Lean body mass declines, and as the muscle mass of the older person declines, energy requirements diminish. This makes it a challenge for older people to satisfy all of their micronutrient requirements through diet alone. Most health care providers ask older people to supplement their diet with at least one multivitamin on a daily basis.

Peripheral tissues of older people take up fat-soluble vitamins at slower rates; thus vitamin A and vitamin E intake results in higher circulating levels of vitamins A and E.

There is a decline in the immune function with age that may be responsible in part for the increased susceptibility to conditions such as infection and malignancy. There is some evidence that increased vitamin and mineral intake, including that of zinc, may counteract this age-related change (Chandra, 1992).

Metabolic utilization of vitamin B_6 is less efficient in older people. This in turn affects the immune system. Twenty percent of the older

TABLE 15-2 Summary of water-soluble vitamins

Name and coenzyme	Major functions	Deficiency symptoms
Thiamin; TPP	Glycolysis, citric acid cycle, and hexosemonophosphate shunt activity; nerve function	Beriberi: nervous tingling, poor coordination, edema, heart changes, weakness
Riboflavin; FAD and FMN	Citric acid cycle and electron transport chain activity; fat breakdown	Ariboflavinosis: inflammation of mouth and tongue, cracks at corners of mouth, eye disorders
Niacin; NAD and NADP	Glycolysis, citric acid cycle, and electron transport chain activity; fat synthesis, fat breakdown	Pellagra: diarrhea, bilateral dermatitis, dementia
Pantothenic acid; coenzyme A, acyl carrier protein	Citric acid cycle; fat synthesis, fat breakdown	Tingling in hands, fatigue, headache, nausea
Biotin; biocytin	Glucose production; fat synthesis; purine (part of DNA, RNA) synthesis	Dermatitis, tongue soreness, anemia, depression
Vitamin B_6, pyridoxine and other forms; PLP	Protein metabolism; neurotransmitter synthesis; many other functions	Headache, anemia, convulsions, nausea, vomiting, dermatitis, sore tongue
Folate; THFA	DNA and RNA synthesis; amino acid synthesis; red blood cell maturation	Megaloblastic anemia, inflammation of tongue, diarrhea, poor growth, mental disorders, birth defects
Vitamin B_{12} (cobalamin, methylcobalamin)	Folate metabolism; nerve function	Megaloblastic anemia, poor nerve function
Vitamin C (ascorbic acid)	Collagen synthesis; hormone and neurotransmitter synthesis	Scurvy: poor wound healing, pinpoint hemorrhages, bleeding gums

From Wardlaw, G.M., & Insel, P.M. (1996). *Perspectives in nutrition* (3rd ed.). St. Louis: Mosby.

TABLE 15-2 Summary of water-soluble vitamins—cont'd

Deficiency risk conditions	Adult RDA or ESADDI	Dietary sources	Toxicity
Alcoholism, poverty	1.1-1.5 mg	Sunflower seeds, pork, whole and enriched grains, dried beans, peas, brewer's yeast	None possible from food
Possibly use of certain medications if no dairy products consumed	1.2-1.7 mg	Milk, mushrooms, spinach, liver, enriched grains	None reported
Severe poverty where corn is the dominant food; alcoholism	15-19 mg NE	Mushrooms, bran, tuna, salmon, chicken, beef, liver, peanuts, enriched grains	Flushing of skin at intake levels >100 mg
Alcoholism	4-7 mg	Mushrooms, liver, broccoli, eggs (most foods have some)	None
Alcoholism	30-100 µg	Cheese, egg yolks, cauliflower, peanuts, liver	Unknown
Being female adolescent or adult; use of certain medications; alcoholism	1.6-2 mg	Animal protein foods, spinach, broccoli, bananas, salmon, sunflower seeds	Nerve destruction at doses of 2 gm/day or more for a few months or 500 mg/day for long-term use
Alcoholism; pregnancy; use of certain medications	180-200 µg	Green leafy vegetables, orange juice, organ meats, sprouts, sunflower seeds	None; nonprescription vitamin dosage is controlled by FDA
Being older, because of poor absorption; veganism	2 µg	Animal foods, especially organ meats; oysters; clams (not natural in plants)	None
Alcoholism; being older, male, and living alone	60 mg	Citrus fruits, strawberries, broccoli, greens	Doses >1-2 gm cause diarrhea and can alter some diagnostic tests; increased iron absorption can induce iron toxicity in some people

TABLE 15-3 Summary of fat-soluble vitamins

Vitamin	Major functions	Deficiency symptoms
A (retinoids) and provitamin A (carotenoids)	Promote vision, night and color; promote growth; prevent drying of skin and eyes; promote resistance to bacterial infection	Night blindness; xerophthalmia; poor growth; dry skin (keratinization)
D (cholecalciferol and ergocalciferol)	Facilitate absorption of calcium and phosphorus; maintain optimum calcification of bone	Rickets; osteomalacia
E (tocopherols, tocotrienols)	Antioxidant: prevent breakdown of vitamin A and unsaturated fatty acids	Destruction of red blood cells (hemolysis): nerve destruction
K (phylloquinone and menaquinone)	Help form prothrombin and other blood-clotting factors	Hemorrhage

Americans most at risk	Dietary sources	RDA	Toxicity symptoms
People in poverty, especially preschool children (still very rare)	Vitamin A: liver, fortified milk; provitamin A: sweet potatoes, spinach, greens, carrots, cantaloupe, apricots, broccoli	Women: 800 RE (4000 IU); men: 1000 RE (5000 IU)	Fetal malformations, hair loss, skin changes, pain in bones
Breastfed infants, older shut-ins	Fortified milk, fish oils, sardines, salmon	5-10 µg (200-400 IU)	Growth retardation, kidney damage, calcium deposits in soft tissue
People with poor fat absorption (still very rare)	Vegetable oils, some greens, some fruits	Women: 8 mg (alpha-tocopherol equivalents); men: 10 mg (alpha-tocopherol equivalents)	Muscle weakness, headaches, fatigue, nausea, inhibition of vitamin K metabolism
People taking antibiotics for months at a time (still quite rare)	Green vegetables, liver	60-80 µg	Anemia, jaundice

From Wardlaw, G.M., & Insel, P.M. (1996). *Perspectives in nutrition* (3rd ed.). St. Louis: Mosby.

TABLE 15-4 Summary of water and the major minerals

Name	Major functions	Deficiency symptoms	People most at risk
Water	Medium for chemical reactions, removal of waste products, perspiration to cool the body	Thirst, muscle weakness, poor endurance	Infants with fever; older persons especially those in nursing homes; endurance athletes
Sodium	A major electrolyte of extracellular fluid; nerve impulse conduction	Muscle cramps	People who severely restrict sodium to lower blood pressure (250-500 mg/day)
Potassium	A major electrolyte of intracellular fluid; nerve impulse conduction	Irregular heartbeat, loss of appetite, muscle cramps	People who use potassium-wasting diuretics or have poor diets, as seen in poverty and alcoholism
Chloride	A major electrolyte of extracellular fluid; acid production in stomach; nerve impulse conduction	Convulsions in infants	No one probably, as long as infant formula manufacturers control product quality adequately
Calcium	Bone and tooth strength; blood clotting; nerve impulse transmission; muscle contraction; cell regulation	Increased risk of osteoporosis	Women in general, especially those who constantly restrict their energy intake and consume few dairy products
Phosphorus	Bone and tooth strength; part of various metabolic compounds; major ion of intracellular fluid	Probably none; poor bone maintenance is a possibility	Older persons consuming very nutrient-poor diets; possibly vegans and people with alcoholism
Magnesium	Bone strength; enzyme function; nerve and heart function	Weakness, muscle pain, poor heart function	Women in general; people on thiazide diuretics
Sulfur	Part of vitamins and amino acids; drug detoxification; acid base balance	None has been described	No one who meets his or her protein needs

Continued

From Wardlaw, G.M., & Insel, P.M. (1996). *Perspectives in nutrition* (3rd ed.). St. Louis: Mosby.
*Values for calcium, potassium, and magnesium are RDAs. Values for other minerals are minimum requirements for health in adults.
†Just an approximation. It is best to keep urine volume greater than 1 L (4 cups) per day.

TABLE 15-4 Summary of water and the major minerals—cont'd

RDA or minimum requirement*	Nutrient-dense dietary sources	Toxicity
1 ml per kcal expended†	Water as such and in foods	Probably occurs only in those with mental disorders: headache, blurred vision, convulsions
500 mg	Table salt, processed foods, condiments, sauces, soups, chips	Causes hypertension in susceptible individuals, some increase in calcium loss in the urine
2000 mg	Spinach, squash, bananas, orange juice, other vegetables and fruits, milk, meat, legumes, whole grains	Causes slowing of the heartbeat; seen in kidney failure
700 mg	Table salt, processed foods, some vegetables	Causes hypertension in susceptible people when combined with sodium
800 mg (age >24 years); 1200 mg (age 11-24 years)	Dairy products, canned fish, leafy vegetables, tofu, fortified orange juice and other beverages, fortified bread and cereals	Very high intake may cause kidney stones in susceptible people and reduce mineral absorption in general
800 mg (age >24 years); 1200 mg (age 11-24 years)	Dairy products, processed foods, meats, fish, soft drinks, bakery products	Hampers bone health in people with kidney failure; causes poor bone mineralization if calcium intake is low
Men: 350 mg; women: 280 mg	Wheat bran, green vegetables, nuts, chocolate, legumes	Causes weakness in people with kidney failure
None	Protein foods	None likely

providers. Particularly at risk are women living in the northern United States in the winter, because sunlight-generated vitamin D will be in scarce supply for them. It is recommended that dietary daily intake of vitamin D be kept at 400 IU (10 μg).

Mineral deficiencies

Usually, the intake of minerals, especially in the American diet, tends to be adequate, because the required amounts of minerals are relatively small (Roe, 1987). Malabsorption syndromes and drug reactions are causative factors in mineral deficiencies, which may include the following deficiencies in older adults: phosphate, potassium, magnesium, zinc, and iron.

DRUG-NUTRIENT INTERACTIONS

A number of drugs can cause malnutrition, especially when consumed by older adults, for whom multiple drug regimens are often prescribed. Sometimes more than one prescribed drug may deplete the same nutrient, which can result in a serious deficiency. An example of this is potassium depletion caused by use of both diuretics and laxatives. See Table 15-5 for drugs that may cause nutritional deficiencies.

Selected food-drug interactions can alter absorption, distribution, metabolism, and excretion of drugs. More drugs are prescribed for older adults than for any other age group in the United States. The practice of taking medications with very little fluid is not uncommon among older adults. In the presence of such a practice, the absorption of medications may be delayed. Fluids play an important role in drug absorption. Paradoxically, ice water, which is available to patients in the hospital or to residents in nursing homes, delays the dissolution of capsules.

Both food and food components may interact with drugs, and this can affect the drug's bioavailability. Food also may act as a mechanical barrier to medication, preventing the drug's access to the mucosal surface of the gastrointestinal tract. The

potential interaction of the following drugs with food should be considered. Acetaminophen is absorbed 5 times faster in fasting people than in people who have consumed a high-carbohydrate meal. Carbohydrates, particularly *pectin*

TABLE 15-5 Common drugs causing nutritional deficiencies in older adults

Drug group and drug	Deficiency
1. Cardiac glycosides 　　Digitalis	Anorexia→protein 　　energy malnutrition Zinc and magnesium 　　deficiency
2. Diuretics 　　Thiazides→ 　　Furosemide 　　Ethacrynic acid 　　Triamterene→	 Potassium, zinc, and 　　magnesium depletion Folacin deficiency
3. Anti-inflammatory 　　drugs 　　Aspirin 　　Indomethacin→ 　　Colchicine→	 Gastrointestinal blood 　　loss→iron deficiency Malabsorption of fat- 　　and water-soluble 　　vitamins
4. Antacids (antacid 　　abuse)	Phosphate depletion; 　　osteomalacia
5. Laxatives (laxative 　　abuse) 　　Mineral oil→ 　　Phenolphthalein 	 Deficiency of vitamins 　　A, D, and K (potassium 　　deficiency) Multiple nutrient 　　deficiencies due to 　　malabsorption Folacin and vitamin D 　　deficiency

From Roe, D. (1992). *Geriatric nutrition* (3rd ed., pp. 148-150, 167). Englewood Cliffs, NJ: Prentice-Hall. Reprinted with permission.

(an indigestible fiber), delay the absorption of acetaminophen (an analgesic), whereas proteins and lipids do not. Fasting causes a sevenfold increase in absorption of tetracycline (an antibiotic), and food intake reduces the absorption of tetracycline, ampicillin (an antibiotic), and hydrocortisone (a steroid hormone) (Barcheiya & Welling, 1982).

The age-related decrease in hydrochloric acid secretion that occurs in older adults can impair the absorption of calcium and iron and can delay the absorption of some drugs, such as amitriptyline (Elavil), diazepam (Valium), and some analgesics such as pentazocine (Talwin).

Emotional stress can delay gastric emptying. A decrease in gastric emptying in itself may create problems with the metabolism of medications such as penicillin, levodopa, and digoxin, making them less available for absorption in the small intestine (Evans et al., 1981). Alterations in circulation and body composition may have an effect on drug distribution. Total body weight may decrease in the very old, but the ratio of fat to lean tissue is usually greater than in younger years. Adipose tissue increases by about 18% to 30% in men and 35% to 48% in women (Rosenberg, 1994), which may cause an increase in the volume of lipid-soluble drugs such as diazepam and a decrease in the volume of water-soluble drugs such as acetaminophen. In addition, the plasma concentration may be decreased, and this may result in an elevated concentration of drugs such as warfarin (an anticoagulant).

In protein calorie malnutrition the albumin levels may fall. A decrease in the serum level of albumin will also decrease the duration of the action of medications that are bound to protein.

The oxidative capacity of the body also declines with age, and this decline is even greater among older adults who smoke cigarettes. This may affect the function of hepatic enzymes in detoxifying drugs.

High-protein diets can produce an acid urine (pH 5.9), whereas low-protein diets can produce alkaline urine (pH 7.5). If the urine is acidic, weakly alkaline drugs such as amitriptyline are excreted because they form water-soluble salts. Conversely, if the urine is alkaline, the drugs will be reabsorbed (Lamy, 1990a). Thus continued use of such drugs could lead to toxicity if older adults are regularly consuming low-protein diets. The dosage of drugs should be prescribed carefully, individually adjusted for older patients, and strictly monitored.

Drug-nutrient interactions are important to consider when caring for older adults, and identification of any over-the-counter vitamin, mineral, and amino acid supplements that an older adult may have purchased should always be included in a dietary assessment. Many health care professionals are unaware of the potential problems that can be averted by careful consideration of the older adult's dietary and medication habits.

■ Chronic Conditions Influenced by Nutrition

OBESITY

Obesity is a frequent nutritional problem among U.S. citizens and is very often found in the over-65 age group. *Obesity* is defined as being 20% or more over the ideal weight. The importance of body fat composition has also been a focus of recent research, because people with a greater muscle mass–to–fat ratio are not considered overweight, even if they are 20% over ideal body weight.

Problems arise in the understanding of what is the ideal weight and other individual variables because normal values in healthy people vary over a wide range. Two tables have been developed, one to demonstrate the range of normal weights and the other to highlight the difficulties in promoting one normal weight for individuals based only on height. The first table was developed in 1983 by the Metropolitan Life Insurance Company and the second was developed by the Gerontology Research Center. A comparison of these tables is seen in Table 15-6. Recent studies have shed new light on the interesting contro-

lowered ability of the kidneys to concentrate urine, and a decrease in the effectiveness of the antidiuretic hormone (ADH) that helps the body to conserve water. Although these changes by themselves do not cause dehydration, they do contribute to an increased vulnerability in aged individuals and add to the risk of fluid balance problems. A number of acute and chronic diseases prevalent in the older population can inhibit renal function and increase the potential for dehydration. Conditions such as hypertension, congestive heart failure, renal disease, infections, fever, diarrhea, and central nervous system disorders that diminish the thirst sensation are among the many disorders that can affect fluid balance in older people.

Sometimes, diagnostic tests requiring fluid restriction or the use of hypertonic dyes can overtax the older adult's system and can lead to dehydration. A variety of drugs, including diuretics and laxatives, also can alter fluid and electrolyte balance (Todd, 1989). In addition to diseases that directly affect the renal system and fluid balance, other conditions (physical, mental, and psychosocial) may indirectly contribute to water depletion. For example, people with mobility problems might have difficulty obtaining adequate fluids if liquids are not readily accessible. People who are confused and have diminished cognitive ability may not be aware of the need to drink or of the sensation of thirst. Some older people, particularly women who have problems with incontinence, may deliberately restrict their fluid intake to avoid events of incontinence. Unfortunately, this practice adds to their difficulties by facilitating the development of infections and may actually increase the number of episodes of incontinence.

Symptoms associated with fluid and electrolyte imbalance may be attributed to other conditions or to old age if a careful assessment is not done. A fluid balance history is an important component of assessment. Dehydration may be manifested by the following (Kositzke, 1990):

Skin—dry, warm skin; dry oral mucosa; altered tongue turgor

Neurologic symptoms—confusion, disorientation, pathologic reflexes (seizures), change in affect

Cardiopulmonary symptoms—weak rapid pulse, altered respirations, orthostatic hypotension

Genitourinary symptoms—scanty or concentrated urine, with marked ammonia odor

Laboratory values—elevations in sodium, hematocrit, and blood urea nitrogen

Treatment is directed toward reestablishing a normal fluid balance as quickly and safely as possible, before serious complications, such as renal damage, occur. The oral route for fluids is preferred whenever possible. Water is the fluid that is best for patients, although a choice of fluids is important also, especially fruit juices. Tea, coffee, cola, and sweetened beverages are diuretic in nature and should be avoided if possible. For very ill patients, parenteral fluids may be necessary until their condition stabilizes. Careful monitoring assessment of the patient's physical and mental condition and careful monitoring of intake and output are important parts of the treatment regimen. The best treatment for dehydration is prevention. The watchful vigilance of nurses caring for vulnerable older patients may avert this all-too-common disorder, or at least may provide early detection and avoidance of complications (Reedy, 1988).

■ Nursing Process

ASSESSMENT

Nutritional assessment includes the following components:

1. Clinical assessment
2. Dietary assessment
3. Anthropometric assessment
4. Hematologic assessment
5. Biochemical assessment
6. Immunologic assessment
7. Diagnostic assessment

Clinical assessment

Clinical assessment employs the health history, the psychosocial history, and the physical examination to identify signs of nutritional deficiency.

Health history The health history records the patient's or significant other's description of the problems related to nutritional status, such as weight loss or gain, loss of appetite, nausea or vomiting, food intolerance, difficulty in swallowing, drugs being taken, digestive disturbances (e.g., heartburn, bowel problems), sore mouth or tongue, anemia, bleeding problems, and any disabilities that might prevent adequate nutrition.

It is of critical importance to get an accurate history concerning the older person's usual 24-hour intake of food and fluids. A 24-hour dietary diary is an excellent assessment tool if the older person or a caregiver is able and willing to provide the necessary information.

Other pertinent questions to ask about nutritional status are the following:

1. Have you noticed any weight gain?
2. Have you noticed any weight loss?
3. Have you been trying to gain or lose weight?
4. Have you noticed a change in your appetite?
5. Have you had any nausea or vomiting?
6. Have you had any difficulty in swallowing solids or liquids?
7. Have you had any heartburn?
8. Have you had any change in your pattern of bowel movements?
9. Have you noticed any sores in your mouth?
10. Have you had any unexplained bruising?
11. What medications do you take regularly, both prescription and over-the-counter?
12. Are you having any difficulties with nutrition that you would like to tell me about?

Psychosocial history The psychosocial history is concerned with age, sex, lifestyle, activities of daily living, and characteristics that relate to the ability to obtain and prepare food and to live independently, as well as food habits and fads, motivation, job skills, family support, and social skills.

Suggested lifestyle questions concerning nutritional status are the following:

1. How do you obtain your groceries?
2. Do you have anyone to assist you in obtaining groceries?
3. Do you have anyone assisting you in preparing your meals?
4. How many meals do you eat each day?
5. Do you eat alone?
6. How much of your meal do you usually eat?
7. Are you using Meals on Wheels?
8. Do you eat any meals outside of your home?
9. Do you have adequate finances to cover the cost of your food?
10. Is there anything about your food habits that you would like to tell me or that you think I should know?

Physical examination The physical examination includes the measurement of height and weight and the inspection and palpation of the skin and mucous membranes, primarily for signs of dryness, ecchymosis (bruising), and edema. Extremities are examined for weakness or tremor. Mental status is checked for signs of confusion, disorientation, memory loss, or mood disturbances.

The clinical assessment of an older adult can be especially challenging because of the multifactorial etiologies involved and also because the signs and symptoms are more vague and general in older adults and less specific to particular organs and functions. For instance, easy bruising can be the result of vitamin K deficiency, anticoagulant therapy, or simply the increased fragility of aging skin which results in spontaneous bruising. Another possible problem in performing clinical assessment of older adults is the tendency of health care professionals to minimize symptoms or to explain them away as signs of aging.

Dietary assessment

Dietary assessment is done for a number of reasons: to obtain data on food consumption patterns of individuals and groups over a period of time; to obtain actual food energy and nutrient intake information for each individual; to investigate episodes of food poisoning; and to assess the feeding practices of institutions where older adults are housed.

There are a number of methods of obtaining a dietary history, depending on the purpose for which the information is being obtained. In a history interview of an older patient, a record of food intake can be obtained by using a short questionnaire about food items, frequency of intake, methods of preparation, and amounts eaten.

Records of food purchases may also be obtained to determine the adequacy of diet indirectly. If a limited selection is being purchased repeatedly, this could reflect potential deficiencies. Another method of obtaining information from alert people without memory deficits is the 24-hour dietary recall. A food diary may be used with patients who have received complete instructions and understand what they are to record. This has the advantage of reducing dependence on unassisted recall.

The nurse's direct observation at mealtime can also help to assess food intake. This method can be used readily in hospitals and nursing homes.

Anthropometric assessment

Anthropometric assessment includes measurement of height, weight, midarm circumference, and skin folds; these measurements should be as accurate as possible. Special problems with these measurements in older adults are related to change in height caused by aging and the increased compressibility of the fat folds on the older adult's arm (Roe, 1987). In spite of these difficulties, anthropometric measurements can be useful in the initial assessment of nutritional status and in determining therapeutic progress. Combined with other types of assessment, such as gathering dietary and biochemical information, these measurements can be helpful as screening tools.

Hematologic assessment

Hematologic assessment serves as a screen for malnutrition. Determination of a complete blood count (CBC) with differential is needed to diagnose nutritional anemia, as well as to provide supporting evidence for the biochemical status and clinical assessment of the patient. Characteristic changes occur in the structure of the red and white cells, in the hemoglobin level, in the computed red cell indices, and in the packed red cell mass in nutritional anemias (Roe, 1987).

Biochemical assessment

Biochemical assessment can identify recent intake of nutrients, estimate nutrient stores in the body, and yield measures of nutritional adequacy and risk. Levels of albumin, transferrin, and a number of vitamins and minerals can be measured to assess clinical signs of deficiency. Serum albumin levels below 3.5 gm/100 ml may indicate protein malnutrition, although there is evidence of a decline in albumin levels related to age (Rosenberg, 1994). Biochemical measures should always be used in combination with other assessment tools because there are some limitations to these data taken alone (Roe, 1987). These factors, coupled with logistic difficulties in collecting samples and with the inadequate laboratory facilities in some long-term care institutions, should promote conservative interpretations of biochemical findings in older adults.

Immunologic assessment

This assessment involves the use of skin tests to identify delayed reactions to microbial and fungal antigens. Other indications of immune function are lymphocyte and differential white cell counts and albumin levels. Negative reactions on skin tests suggest serious protein energy malnutrition. Positive reactions can be interpreted as positive response to nutritional intervention, but negative findings do not necessarily solely indicate malnutrition. Age-related changes and cancer can also result in a diminished response to antigens.

Diagnostic studies

Diagnostic studies are often made by administration of the suspected deficient nutrient (or nutrients). It is important to consider safety in this type of diagnostic intervention and to avoid obscuring an accurate assessment. For example, administration of folic acid could mask the presence of pernicious anemia, with resultant neurologic damage. Other factors, such as response to treatment, could be the reason for positive outcomes, as well as the administration of a particular nutrient (Roe, 1987).

NURSING DIAGNOSES

Several nursing diagnoses have been identified by the North American Nursing Diagnosis Association (NANDA) for nutrition problems; those with particular relevance for older adults are listed here:

1. Altered nutrition: less than body requirements
2. Altered nutrition: more than body requirements
3. Altered nutrition: potential for more than body requirements

The nursing diagnosis most frequently encountered in older adults, and one of great concern to nurses caring for them, is altered nutrition: less than body requirements. In this state, an individual experiences an intake of nutrients insufficient to meet metabolic needs.

Defining characteristics

Weight loss to a weight 20% or more under ideal weight
Reported food intake less than RDA
Evidence of lack of food intake
Lack of interest in food
Aversion to eating
Reported altered taste sensation
Satiety immediately after ingesting food

Related factors

Advanced age
Depression
Stress in response to living alone
Societal influences

PLANNING AND GOAL IDENTIFICATION

A long-term goal would be that the patient will regain lost weight up to within 10% of ideal weight. A short-term goal would be to have the patient increase intake of nutrients, especially carbohydrates and proteins. Another goal, relating to socioeconomic factors, would be to have the patient gain knowledge about and use resources available in the community.

IMPLEMENTATION
In the acute care setting

There is a high prevalence of malnutrition in hospitalized older patients (Lipkin, 1990). Studies have shown that many older adults have severe protein calorie malnutrition at the time of admission to the hospital (Katz et al., 1986). The method of nutrient administration for the hospitalized older patient depends on the patient's nutritional status, the expected length of illness, the ability to swallow, the available gastrointestinal tract, and the metabolic response to illness (Goodwin & Wilmore, 1988). Nutritional requirements can change over the course of a hospitalization. As the patient recovers from a serious condition, metabolic needs decrease and the role of diet may change from that of restoring health to that of maintaining health.

Normal, oral self-feeding is the desired method for the older adult's obtaining nutritional requirements. Hogstel and Robinson (1989) emphasize the special importance of safety in feeding the hospitalized older adult, as well as the need for meeting essential nutrient requirements. They identify selection and consistency of foods, timing of meals, and the portions of food as considerations in providing safe nutrition for older patients. If the patient has impaired swallowing ability, the nurse assesses for gag and cough reflexes before the patient eats or drinks; these reflexes protect the person from aspiration (Thompson et al., 1989). It is also important for the nurse to ensure that the

cine and gerontology (3rd ed., pp. 1259-1268). New York: McGraw-Hill.

Chandra, R.K. (1992). Effect of vitamin and trace-element supplementation on immune responses and infection in elderly subjects. *Lancet, 340*(2), 1124.

Ciocon, J., et al. (1992). Comparison of intermittent vs. continuous tube feeding among elderly. *Journal of Parenteral Enteral Nutrition, 16*(6), 525-528.

Dawson, J. (1984). Effect of ranitidine on gastric ulcer healing and recurrence. *Scandinavian Journal of Gastroenterology, 19,* 665.

Dykes, M.H.M., & Meier, P. (1975). Ascorbic acid and the common cold: Evaluation of its efficacy and toxicity. *Journal of the American Medical Association, 231,* 1073-1079.

Evans, M.A., et al. (1981). Gastric emptying in the elderly: Implications for drug therapy. *Journal of the American Geriatrics Society, 29,* 201.

Galindo-Ciocon, D. (1993). Tube feeding: Complications among the elderly. *Journal of Gerontological Nursing, 14,* 17-21.

Garry, P.J., et al. (1983). Iron status and anemia in the elderly. *Journal of the American Geriatrics Society, 31,* 389.

Gilinsky, N.H. (1990). Peptic ulcer disease in the elderly. *Gastroenterology Clinics of North America, 19,* 255.

Gilliam, J. (1994). Hepatobiliary disorders. In W.R. Hazzard, et al. (Eds.), *Principles of geriatric medicine and gerontology* (3rd ed., pp. 683-692). New York: McGraw-Hill.

Goodwin, C., & Wilmore, D. (1988). Enteral and parenteral nutrition. In D. Page (Ed.), *Clinical nutrition* (pp. 476-503). St. Louis: Mosby.

Hatchett-Cohen, L. (1988). Nasogastric tube feeding. *Geriatric Nursing, 9*(4), 88-91.

Hogstel, M., & Robinson, N. (1989). Feeding the frail elderly. *Journal of Gerontological Nursing, 15*(3), 16-20.

Katz, P., Dube, D., & Calkins, E. (1986). Special issues in malnutritional therapy. In E. Calkins, P. Davis, & A. Ford (Eds.), *The practice of geriatrics* (pp. 145-148). Philadelphia: W.B. Saunders.

Kerr, R. (1994). Disorders of the stomach and duodenum. In W.R. Hazzard, et al. (Eds.), *Principles of geriatric medicine and gerontology* (3rd ed., pp. 693-705). New York: McGraw-Hill.

Kositzke, J.A. (1990). A question of balance: Dehydration in the elderly. *Journal of Gerontological Nursing, 16*(5), 4-11.

Lamy, P. (1990). Adverse drug effects. *Clinics in Geriatric Medicine, 6*(2), 293-308.

Lamy, P. (1980b). *Prescribing for the elderly.* Littleton, MA: John Wright PSG.

Levine, M. (1986). New concepts in the biology and biochemistry of ascorbic acid. *New England Journal of Medicine, 314,* 892-902.

Lew, E., & Garfinkel, L. (1979). Variations in mortality by weight among 750,000 men and women. *Journal of Chronic Disease, 32,* 563.

Lindenbaum, J., et al. (1988). Neuropsychiatric disorders caused by cobalmin deficiencies in the absence of anemias or macrocytosis. *New England Journal of Nursing, 318,* 1728.

Lipkin, E.W. (1990). Enteral/parenteral alimentation. In W.R. Hazzard, et al. (Eds.), *Principles of geriatric medicine and gerontology* (2nd ed., pp. 269-303). New York: McGraw-Hill.

Lipschitz, D.A. (1994). Anemia in the elderly. In W.R. Hazzard, et al. (Eds.), *Principles of geriatric medicine and gerontology* (3rd ed.). New York: McGraw-Hill.

Logan, R.P., et al. (1991). One week eradication regimen for helicobacter. *Lancet, 338,* 1249.

Lowenstein, F.W. (1986). Nutritional requirements of the elderly. In E.A. Young (Ed.), *Nutrition, aging and health* (pp. 61-89). New York: Liss.

Miller, A.J., et al. (1987). *The national survey of oral health in the United States adults: 1985-1986* (U.S. Department of Health and Human Services, Public Health Service, National Institutes of Health, NIH Pub. No. 87-2868). Washington, DC: U.S. Government Printing Office.

National Research Council. (1989). *Recommended dietary allowances* (10th ed. rev.). Washington, DC: National Academy of Science.

Osato, E., et al. (1993). Clinical manifestations: Failure to thrive. *Journal of Gerontological Nursing, 19*(8), 29-34.

Osborn, C., & Marshall, M. (1993). Self-feeding: In nursing home residents. *Journal of Gerontological Nursing, 19*(3), 7-14.

Porth, C.M. (1990). *Pathophysiology: Concepts of altered health states* (3rd ed.). Philadelphia: J.B. Lippincott.

Reedy, D.F. (1988). How can you prevent dehydration? *Geriatric Nursing, 9*(2), 224-226.

Reif, T.R. (1987). Water and aging. *Clinics in Geriatric Medicine, 3*(2), 403-411.

Roe, D. (1987). *Geriatric nutrition* (2nd ed.). Englewood Cliffs, NJ: Prentice Hall.

Rosenberg, I. (1994). Nutrition and aging. In W.R. Hazzard, et al. (Eds.), *Principles of geriatric medicine and gerontology* (3rd ed.). New York: McGraw-Hill.

Rosenberg, I., & Miller, J. (1992). Nutritional factors in physical and cognitive function in the elderly. *American Journal of Clinical Nutrition, 55,* 1237S.

Shuster, M., & Mancino, M. (1994). Ensuring successful home tube feeding in the geriatric population. *Geriatric Nursing.*

Singer, H. (1991). *A study of the effect of touch during feeding on the food intake of dementia residents.* Unpublished master's study, Georgetown University, School of Nursing, Washington, DC.

Sodeman, W.A. (1989). Bowel habits. In W.A. Sodeman, T.A. Saladin, & W.P. Boyd (Eds.), *Geriatric gastroenterology* (pp. 85-108). Philadelphia: W.B. Saunders.

Sutnick, M.R. (1988). Dietary guidance for the elderly. *Clinics in Geriatric Medicine, 4*(1), 193-202.

Thompson, J.M., et al. (1989). *Mosby's manual of clinical nursing* (2nd ed.). St. Louis: Mosby.

Todd, B. (1989). Diuretics' dangers. *Geriatric Nursing, 10*(4), 212-214.

U.S. Department of Health and Human Services. (1992).

VanderJagt, D.J., Garry, P.J., & Bhagauan, H.N. (1987). Ascorbic acid intake and plasma levels in healthy elderly people. *American Journal of Clinical Nutrition, 46,* 290-294.

Viteri, F. (1988). Vitamin deficiencies. In Paige et al. (Eds.), *Clinical nutrition* (pp. 547-578). St. Louis: Mosby.

Weiffenbach, J., et al. (1990). Oral sensory changes in aging. *Journal of Gerontology, 48,* 45-121.

Williams, S.R. (1989). *Nutrition and diet therapy.* St. Louis: Times Mirror/Mosby.

Wu, W. (1994). Disorders of the esophagus. In W.R. Hazzard, et al. (Eds.), *Principles of geriatric medicine and gerontology* (3rd ed., pp. 683-692). New York: McGraw-Hill.

Yearick, E.S., Wang, M.S.L., & Pesias, S.J. (1980). Nutritional status of the elderly: Dietary and biochemical findings. *Journal of Gerontology, 35*(5), 663-671.

certain hazards associated with its use. One compound that continues to be recommended is tryptophan. This is an amino acid (a protein constituent) that is normally converted to the neurotransmitter serotonin. In 1989 the Food and Drug Administration (FDA) imposed a ban on the sale of isolated tryptophan after an impurity in one batch caused a rare blood disease that killed several people. Although the compound itself is probably harmless, it has no noticeable sedative properties (Harvard Mental Health Letter, 1994a; Tryptophan, 1990).

HYPERSOMNIA

Hypersomnia is classified as a member of the DOES grouping. People with this complaint are concerned that they sleep excessively. The person or a member of the family may report this, or it may be observed by a staff member. The condition may be caused by lack of sleep at night or by boredom, depression, physical confinement, or a number of other causes. If there is a continual feeling of tiredness, lack of energy, and irresistible sleepiness, the person could be suffering from narcolepsy, a chronic, little-known sleep disorder. *Narcolepsy* is a severe form of excessive sleepiness affecting 1 out of every 100 Americans. Over 50% of these cases remain undiagnosed. This condition may be called "sleep attacks," because the individual may find it impossible to remain awake and may fall asleep during almost any activity, even eating, walking, driving, or carrying on a conversation. Narcolepsy tends to be a condition of the early years, however.

Nonetheless, hypersomnia in general is not uncommon in older adults, although what appears to be hypersomnia may actually be a disturbance of the sleep-wake cycle brought on by some of the factors previously mentioned that have disturbed circadian rhythms. With older individuals, hospitalization or admission to a nursing home may cause this disturbance in sleep patterns. Most people will have some disruption in sleep, at least temporarily, if they are moved from their usual sleeping environment. For older individuals, this disruption tends to be more of a problem because of the decreased sleep efficiency, which may already be present, caused by age changes. *Sleep efficiency* is the proportion of time spent actually sleeping, in relation to the overall time spent in bed; this proportion is frequently reduced in older people.

NOCTURNAL MYOCLONUS

Nocturnal myoclonus, also called sleep-related myoclonus or periodic leg movement syndrome (PLMS), is characterized by repetitive leg contractions that occur in clusters during sleep; this is another dysfunction commonly associated with sleep in older adults. The clusters can last from 5 to 60 minutes, and the leg jerks occur at a rate of one every 30 seconds (Buchholtz, 1987). PLMS is sometimes called "restless legs syndrome" and may manifest itself as insomnia with sleep fragmentation.

Nocturnal myoclonus has multiple etiologies. Deficiency diseases such as calcium and potassium deficiencies and iron deficiency anemia can cause sleep-related myoclonus. Diabetes, uremia, withdrawal from some sedative or hypnotic medications, and abuse of caffeine or alcohol may also result in this condition. There are many cases in which there is no known cause, but there are also cases in which the condition occurs in patients with other sleep disorders. Polysomnography, a diagnostic test utilizing an EEG, an electromyogram (EMG), and an electrooculogram (EOG), is required for definitive diagnosis. There should be careful evaluation and search for any associated problems. Treatment involves correcting the underlying cause, if possible, followed by judicious use of medication to suppress the leg jerks. Most medications tend to suppress arousal rather than the contractions and should be used with caution because of the potential for increased drowsiness. Short-acting benzodiazepines are generally used when there is substantial nighttime sleep disruption (Bonnet & Arand, 1990; Snow et al., 1988). In some cases, light exercise before bedtime and quinine at bedtime might be helpful as well (Buchholtz, 1987).

SLEEP APNEA

Sleep apnea is a condition in which there are episodes of cessation of breathing during the night, sometimes as many as 300 times. Sleep apnea is a relatively recent discovery, which fits under the fourth classification of sleep disorder, as a dysfunction associated with sleep or sleep stages. It tends to affect mostly middle-aged, overweight men but may affect either sex at any age (Harvard Health Letter, 1995).

There are two types of sleep apnea: central and obstructive. In *central apnea,* the diaphragm contracts ineffectively or not at all, and thoracic breathing ceases. Respiration resumes as a result of arousal. In *obstructive apnea,* the oropharyngeal airway collapses or the pathway is obstructed by soft relaxed tissue, pressure builds up, and eventually the airway is cleared with a loud snorting sound (Figure 16-2). This condition is becoming more widely recognized in older adults (Ancoli-Israel, 1989; Bliwise et al., 1990; Harvard Health Letter, 1995), and it is potentially life threatening. Sleep apnea is characterized by daytime sleepiness because of interrupted sleep

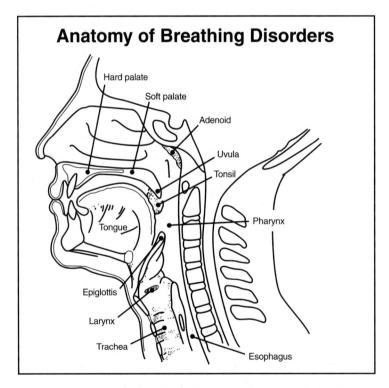

Anatomy of Breathing Disorders

Hard palate
Soft palate
Adenoid
Uvula
Tonsil
Pharynx
Tongue
Epiglottis
Larynx
Trachea
Esophagus

FIGURE 16-2 Snorting occurs when dangling or loose tissue such as that of the *uvula, tonsils, adenoids,* or *tongue* vibrates during breathing. These tissues can also block the airway, causing obstructive sleep apnea. Poor muscle tone or excess weight around the neck can also lead to snorting and apnea by reducing the width of the trachea. (From Harvard Health Letter. [1995, January]. *A special report: Sleep disturbance.* Boston: Harvard Medical School Health Publications Group.)

Buchholtz, D. (1987). Sleep disorders. In T.M. Bayless, M.C. Brain, & R.M. Cherniak (Eds.), *Current therapy in internal medicine,* (pp. 1235-1239). Philadelphia: B.C. Decker.

Carskadon, M. et al. (1986). Guidelines for the multiple sleep latency test (MSLT): A standard measure of sleepiness. *Sleep, 9, 519-524.*

Colling, J. (1983). Sleep disturbances in aging: Theoretic and empiric analysis. *Advances in Nursing Science, 6* (1), 36-44.

Davis-Sharts, J. (1989). The elder and critical care: Sleep and mobility issues. *Nursing Clinics of North America, 24*(3), 755-767.

*Dinner, S.S., Erman, M.K., & Roth, T. (1992). Help for geriatric sleep problems. *Patient Care,* pp. 166-192.

Dowling, G. (1995). Sleep problems in older adults. In *The American Nurse,* (Continuing Education Program: Vol. 27, No. 3, Pt. 5). Washington, DC: American Nurses' Association.

Evans, L. (1987). Sundown syndrome in institutionalized elderly. *Journal of the American Geriatrics Society, 35*(2), 101-108.

Floyd, J.A. (1995, May-June). Another look at napping in older adults. *Geriatric Nursing, 16*(3), 136-138.

Gillin, J.C. (1990, May). Sleeping pills. *Harvard Medical School Health Letter, 15,* 5-8.

Haponik, E.F. (1990). Sleep problems. In W.R. Hazzard et al. (Eds.), *Principles of geriatric medicine and gerontology* (2nd ed., pp. 1213-1228). New York: McGraw-Hill.

Harvard Health Letter. (1995). *Sleep disturbance.* (Available from Harvard Medical School, Boston, MA 02117).

Harvard Mental Health Letter. (1994a, August). *Sleep disorders* (Vol. 11, No. 2, Pt. 1). (Available from Harvard Medical School, Boston, MA 02115).

Harvard Mental Health Letter. (1994b, September). *Sleep disorders* (Vol. 11, No. 3, Pt. 2). (Available from Harvard Medical School, Boston, MA 02115).

Hauri, P., & Linde, S. (1990). *No more sleepless nights.* New York: John Wiley and Sons.

Hoch, C.C. et al. (1992). Sleep disorders and aging. In J. Birren, R. Sloane, & G. Cohen (Eds.), *Handbook of mental health and aging* (2nd ed., pp. 557-581). San Diego: Academic Press.

Kartman, J. (1993). Sleep-rest. In J. Thompson et al. (Eds.), *Mosby's manual of clinical nursing* (3rd ed., pp. 1535-1537). St. Louis: Mosby.

Kartman, J., & McFarlane, E. (1993). Sleep pattern disturbance. In G. McFarland & E. McFarlane (Eds.), *Nursing diagnosis and intervention: Planning for patient care* (2nd ed., pp. 419-425). St. Louis: Mosby.

Kryger, M.Y., Roth, T., & Dement, W.C. (Eds.). (1994). *Principles and practices of sleep medicine* (2nd ed.). Philadelphia: W.B. Saunders.

McCance, K.L., & Heuther, S.E. (1990). *Pathophysiology: The biological basis for disease in adults and children.* St. Louis: Mosby.

McFarland, G.K., & McFarlane, E.A. (1993). *Nursing diagnosis and intervention: Planning for patient care* (2nd ed.). St. Louis: Mosby.

Miller, C.A. (1990). *Nursing care of older adults: Theory and practice.* Glenview, IL: Scott, Foresman.

Monk, T. (1989). Circadian rhythm. *Clinics in Geriatric Medicine, 5*(2), 331-346.

Monk, T.H. (Ed.). (1991). *Sleep, sleepiness and performance.* New York: John Wiley and Sons.

*Morgan, K. (1992). Sleep in normal and pathological aging. In J.X. Brodklehurst, R.C. Tollis, & H.M. Fillit (Eds.), *Textbook of geriatric medicine and gerontology* (4th ed., pp. 122-129). London: Churchill Livingstone.

National Institute on Aging. (1990). *Age page: A good night's sleep.* Bethesda, MD: U.S. Department of Health and Human Services, National Institutes of Health.

Reynolds, C., Hoch, C., & Monk, T. (1986). Sleep and chronobiologic disturbances in late life. In E.W. Busse & D.G. Blazer (Eds.), *Geriatric psychiatry* (pp. 475-488). Washington, DC: American Psychological Association.

*Reynolds III, C.F., & Kupfer, D.J. (1994). Sleep disorders. In J. Oldham & M.B. Riba (Eds.), *Review of Psychiatry* (Vol. 13). Washington, DC: American Psychiatric Press.

Richardson, G.S. (1990). Circadian rhythms and aging. In E.L. Schneider & J.W. Rowe (Eds.), *Handbook of the biology of aging* (3rd. ed., pp. 275-305). San Diego: Academic Press.

Roehrs, T.A., & Roth, T. (1989). Drugs, sleep disorders and aging. *Clinics in Geriatric Medicine, 5*(2), 395-404.

Shaver, J.L.F., & Landis, C.A. (1994). Understanding the behavior of sleep. In *The American Nurse* (Continuing Education Program: Vol. 26, No. 9, Pt. 1). Washington, DC: American Nurses' Association.

Sleep apnea: A new solution. (1989, July). *Harvard Medical School Health Letter, 14*(9), p. 4.

Sleep Disorders Classification Committee. (1979). Association of sleep disorders centers: Diagnostic classification of sleep and arousal disorders. *Sleep, 2,* 1-137.

Snow, T.L. et al. (1988). *Handbook of geriatric practice essentials.* Rockville, MD: Aspen Publishing.

Thelan, L.A. et al. (1990). *Textbook of critical care nursing: Diagnosis and management.* St. Louis: Mosby.

Thelan, L.A. et al. (1994). *Critical care nursing: Diagnosis and management* (2nd ed.). St. Louis: Mosby.

Tryptophan: Natural disaster. (1990, February). *Harvard Medical School Health Letter,* pp. 1-2.

U.S. Pharmacopeia. (1990). *United States Pharmacopeia: Drug information for the consumer.* Rockville, MD: U.S. Pharmacopeial Convention.

Vestal, R.E. (1990). Clinical pharmacology. In W. Hazzard, et al. (Eds.), *Principles of geriatric medicine and gerontology* (2nd ed., pp. 201-211). New York: McGraw-Hill.

Vitiello, M., & Prinz, P. (1989). Alzheimer's disease: Sleep and sleep/wake patterns. *Clinics in Geriatric Medicine, 5*(2), 289-299.

Webb, W. (1989). Age-related changes in sleep. *Clinics in Geriatric Medicine, 5*(2), 275-287.

Wolfe, S. et al. (1988). *Worst pills, best pills: The older adult's guide to avoiding drug induced death or illness.* Washington, DC: Public Citizen Health Research Group.

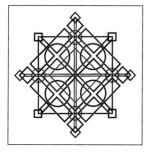

C H A P T E R   17

Where there is despair let me bring hope
Where there is darkness let me bring light
Where there is sadness let me bring joy

Saint Francis of Assisi

Cognition and Mood

■ Learning Objectives

On completion of this chapter, the reader will be able to do the following:

1. Discuss three mental disorders that are frequently experienced by older adults and the relationship between increasing age and the prevalence of these disorders.
2. Differentiate between two cognitive disorders, dementia and delirium, and specify their distinguishing features.
3. Differentiate between cognitive disorders and depression, a mood disorder.
4. Describe the effects of cognitive disorders and depression on the older individual.
5. Discuss the role of the caregiver of the cognitively impaired and/or depressed older person.
6. Discuss the assessment process as it applies to cognitive impairment and the use of instruments to assist in diagnosing the nursing needs of the cognitively impaired or depressed person.
7. Implement nursing interventions that meet the special needs of cognitively impaired older adults.

Just as the anatomic and physiologic changes of the aging process lead to increasing incidence of physical disorders such as arthritis and diabetes, and to sensory impairment from declining visual acuity and hearing loss, so, too, are the brain and other structures of the central nervous system subject to the normal degenerative changes of aging and to pathologic processes. The recognition of cognitive disorders in older adults, the institution of treatment where possible, and the provision of appropriate care and support for the individual, the family, and other caregivers is a major area of concern for all nursing professionals.

A person's state of health, genetic code, past experiences, educational background, cultural influences and beliefs, and current living conditions all influence the level of cognitive ability. Physical changes in the brain caused by the normal process of aging and selected pathologic conditions may affect the cognitive abilities of some older individuals. When cognitive abilities fall to a level that precludes people's ability to care for themselves, health problems are apt to occur.

Cognitive abilities vary among people and across the life span, with a wide range of differences. Language, attention, memory, orientation, visuospatial ability, conceptualization, and general intelligence are all manifestations of cognitive abilities (Albert, 1994).

The nursing care of an older person who has experienced a loss of cognitive ability is a significant challenge. The full knowledge, skills, and interpersonal strengths of the nurse are called upon when the nurse is caring for cognitively impaired people and their families. Society is not tolerant of those older adults who have lost vital cognitive abilities, nor is there a significant role for them within the larger society or even within family units. The fear of cognitive impairment is a recurrent theme in the conversations of the well older adult. Actually, many people of all ages are frightened by those who have suffered cognitive loss, and contact with them is avoided. Nonetheless, each cognitively impaired older person is a unique individual who has the same rights and privileges as any other person.

This chapter presents an overview of the normal structure and function of the neurologic system; age-related changes in the brain; the cognitive disorders of dementia and delirium; and the mood disorder of depression, which may be a symptom associated with cognitive loss or a separate and treatable condition. It also discusses the role of caregivers of cognitively impaired and depressed older adults followed by a description of the nursing process as it applies to the care of these older adults. It is hoped that this presentation may assist the reader in recognizing the complexity of providing nursing care to cognitively impaired or depressed older people.

■ Normal Structure and Function

The neurologic system is divided into two distinct systems, the central nervous system and the peripheral nervous system. The brain and the spinal cord make up the *central nervous system.* The *peripheral nervous system* is composed of the 12 cranial nerves, 31 paired spinal nerves, and the autonomic nervous system, which is subdivided into the sympathetic and parasympathetic divisions. The complex functions of the nervous system encompass analysis of sensory information, response to the internal and external environment, control and coordination of motor function, emotional and intellectual functions, and regulation and communication among body systems.

BRAIN

The cerebrum, the cerebellum, and the brainstem are the three regions that make up the brain. The *cerebrum* consists of four lobes: frontal, parietal, temporal, and occipital; it is the largest part of the brain and controls the higher levels of intellectual functioning. The *cerebellum* functions as the control center for balance and coordination. The *brainstem* and the *spinal cord* form a continuous entity, with the 12 paired cranial nerves emerging from the brainstem. The brainstem comprises the pons, medulla oblongata, midbrain, and diencephalon. The brainstem functions as a connector of the different sections of the brain and as the transmitter of impulses between the spinal cord and the brain. The spinal cord is an important center for the 31 spinal nerves and for reflex action, and serves as the conduction pathway to the brain for sensory and motor impulses.

NEURONS AND NEUROTRANSMITTERS

Neurons are the specialized cells of the nervous system that receive and/or send neural data throughout the human system. *Neurotransmitters* function as a means of communication between neurons. The process of the transmission of information between two neurons involves the synthesis, storage, and release of one or more neurotransmitters (Poirer & Finch, 1994). Catecholamine neurotransmitters, such as dopamine, norepinephrine, and epinephrine, are thought to be involved in the control and modulation of emotion and attention. These neurotransmitters are involved in the control and modulation of visceral function and the cognitive function of attention. The neurotransmitter acetylcholine is thought to play a significant role in mental functions such as learning and memory (Nakamura, 1990). Serotonin, another neurotransmitter, is known to play a role in sleep and memory (Poirer & Finch, 1994). There are at least 30 known neurotransmitters. Science has not yet provided a complete understanding of the mechanism or the dynamics of neurotransmitters.

■ Age-Related Changes

CHANGES IN THE NEUROLOGIC SYSTEM

The neurologic system undergoes changes that are related to the aging process, but scientists disagree about what universal changes occur in the human brain and how these changes relate to cognitive function. The plasticity of the aging brain is without doubt a remarkable feature of the compensatory mechanism related to human aging. The brain undergoes an early period of growth, reaches a plateau of development and stability by adulthood, and then slowly enters a period of decline during senescence (Poirer & Finch, 1994). It has generally been thought that the brain atrophies as a result of the aging process. The most recent studies have challenged that general statement and have proposed that selected and restricted areas of the brain experience atrophy, rather than the entire brain (Poirer & Finch, 1994).

The extent of age-related neuron loss and the effect on function is not clear. Cotman (1990) states, "Neuron loss is not an inevitable consequence of aging, although it occurs." It appears that the age-related change most affecting neurons is shrinkage of large neurons (Terry et al., 1987). The result is a loss of large neurons, with an increase in smaller neurons. The loss is often restricted to specific areas of the brain and is often associated with the compensatory mechanism of dendrite formation (Poirer & Finch, 1994). There is scientific controversy regarding the extent, location, and significance of neuron loss in the aging brain.

There is agreement that the following changes do occur in association with aging: some loss in brain volume and brain weight, enlargement of the ventricles, decrease in enzymes, loss of protein, loss of lipids, and alterations in the amount of and the receptors for some neurotransmitters. The importance of these age-related changes is unknown, as is the extent of their effect on each aging person's cognitive abilities.

Clinical changes exhibited by the older person that are revealed during the examination of the neurologic system and are attributed to the aging process include the following: (1) decreased sensation of vibrations, particularly in the legs, (2) less brisk deep tendon reflexes, with the ankle reflex often absent entirely; and (3) a decreased ability for upward gaze.

There is no doubt that aging brings change. Two examples of functional loss exhibited by most older people and attributed to neurologic age-related change are the slowing of response to tasks and the increase in time needed to recover from physical exertion (Cristofalo, 1990). Nonetheless, the ability of the human body to adjust to age-related alterations and the ability of the human spirit to be resilient in the face of physical loss must not be overlooked or devalued. Clinicians are concerned with the functional everyday abilities of the older adult. The nurse helps older people to adapt to change and to function in a manner that protects their health, promotes their well-being, and ensures their dignity.

CHANGES IN COGNITIVE
AND AFFECTIVE FUNCTIONING

Cognitive functioning is the means by which individuals perceive and react to the world around them, based on the knowledge and skills they have learned and developed since birth, and that most people continue to acquire throughout their lives.

Even though it is normal for individuals to continue to learn from new and changing

Aging Alert
Nursing's challenge— care of the cognitively impaired older person

- Advocate thorough medical evaluation
- Protect existing level of health
- Promote well-being
- Preserve the dignity of the person

experiences, some changes in cognitive functioning do occur over time, as part of the aging process. These changes or declines do not develop uniformly, either across all areas of cognitive functioning, or at the same rate in all individuals. Some cognitive abilities are stable for many decades and decline late in life, whereas other abilities show change in middle age and then remain stable or show less decline with advancing age.

Memory is the first area of cognition to be affected, as the capacity of the brain to process, store, and retrieve information becomes less efficient. Cross-sectional studies have shown that by the age of 50 years, there is a significant decline in ability to recall relatively large amounts of information over long periods. By late in the sixth decade, proficiency declines at tasks that involve series completion. Scores on naming tests and intelligence tests begin to decline by age 70. Perceptual ability, such as the ability to copy complex three-dimensional designs, declines by the mid-60s, as do scores on tests requiring the individual to divide attention among different stimuli (Albert, 1994).

It should be emphasized that although these changes in cognitive functioning are a normal manifestation of aging, there is wide variation among individuals. Some individuals show little decline in cognition, even into their 80s, whereas others show some impairment by age 60.

In regard to affective functioning or change of mood, it is not a normal part of the aging process to develop symptoms of depression. Although older people tend to adhere more to routine, and their lives may become more restricted by physical limitations, most older people continue to have interests and to derive pleasure from life, even within a more limited sphere of activities and social contacts.

■ Common Health Deviations: Mental Disorders

The three most prevalent mental disorders of older adults are the following:

1. Dementia
2. Delirium
3. Depression

These three disorders may exhibit similar signs and symptoms, and the three may coexist within the same patient. The behaviors associated with them are often accepted as a normal part of the aging process, particularly in the older adult. Sometimes the symptoms result from, or are exacerbated by, treatments prescribed for medical conditions. Even though it might be possible to identify some underlying process, which could be treated to ameliorate the condition, this is often left undone. Mental disorders in older adults therefore present a major challenge in terms of accurate diagnosis and management.

Disorders that are the direct result of neurochemical, circulatory, and anatomic changes occurring in the brain are categorized as *organic* disorders and are the predominant form of cognitive illness affecting older adults. In this category are the various *dementias,* with symptoms progressing along a continuum from forgetfulness to a total lack of capacity for self-care, incontinence, and failure to recognize even close family members. These symptoms demonstrate a decline in *cognitive functioning,* or a diminished capacity to discern the common reality. Although symptoms of dementia may occur as the result of some underlying treatable condition, most dementias are progressive and largely unresponsive to treatment.

Delirium is an acute organic disorder, with impairment in cognitive functioning and change in level of consciousness. It is closely related to the dementias and results from either the physiologic effects of other conditions or the treatment administered for these conditions.

The major category of mental disorders, other than those directly attributable to organic processes, is the category described as *functional* disorders. These are diagnosed by identifying the behavioral and emotional symptoms exhibited by the patient, not because the symptoms occur independently of processes taking place in the brain, but because the etiology is unknown (American Psychiatric Association, 1994). The most common functional disorders in older adults are types of *depression,* characterized by loss of interest or pleasure in usual activities or pastimes. Depression can occur at any age, and older people may have a lifetime history of depressive episodes. Older adults are often subject to intense emotional stress from physical pain, disability, loss of independence, bereavement, and other life events associated with advancing age. Furthermore, there is evidence that direct changes in the biochemistry of the brain and the decline in hormone levels that occurs with aging may make older adults less able to cope with stress. Thus emotional stress, combined with the physiologic changes of aging, may put older individuals at risk for developing clinical depression for the first time in their lives.

In contrast with the dementias, depression may, in many cases, be successfully treated. Unfortunately, depression in older adults often manifests itself through signs and symptoms similar to those of dementia, such as memory impairment and self-neglect. In some individuals, both dementia and depression coexist and may be interrelated, with depression developing as a reaction to the stress of progressive loss of cognition caused by dementia.

Both cognitive and affective disorders in older adults can be devastating to the individual, causing loss of dignity, total dependence on others, and changes in behavior that are distressing and unacceptable to family, friends, and caregivers. These disorders are a major cause of institutionalization. They involve implications for the legal status of the individual and major concerns regarding access to and financing of long-term care, whether in nursing homes or in private or family homes. Therefore it is essential that people affected by these disorders receive an accurate diagnosis, so that appropriate treatment may be initiated, and care and support can be provided for the individuals and their families.

DEMENTIA

Dementia is a condition of deteriorating mentality, resulting in a loss of cognitive functioning. Cognitive impairment leading to a diagnosis of dementia should be differentiated from impairment resulting from other causes. *Dementia* is defined as being characterized by the following:

- A *deterioration* from a preexisting level of functioning. By comparison, mental retardation is a lifelong condition.
- A *global* deterioration of functioning, not just impairment of memory or speech, which may be caused by other neurologic conditions affecting specific areas of the brain.
- A state of *full consciousness* (i.e., the person is not comatose and is fully conscious when awake).

Generally, dementia is *not reversible,* although in some less common types of dementia, improvement may result when a precipitating cause, such as malnutrition, is identified and treated.

Prevalence

How common is dementia among older adults? The *prevalence rate,* or the number of cases of a disease found in a defined population at any point in time, is the product of two measures:

1. *Incidence rate*—the number of new cases occurring each year, per unit of the population

2. *Duration*—the length of time that individuals live with the disease

The incidence rate is usually estimated from the number of new cases diagnosed in a particular population. For every case in which a diagnosis of dementia is made, however, there may be an equal or greater number of comparably impaired people living in the community.

Longitudinal studies, in which the same individuals are assessed over a period of years, have established that the incidence of dementia increases with age. The prevalence rate more than doubles between the sixth and eighth decades of life. Projection rates anticipate significant increases, especially in the developed countries. By the year 2000 France is projecting a 9% increase in dementia victims, the United States a 42% increase, and Japan a 76% increase (Rocca et al., 1986). Similarly, studies of prevalence rates at a specific time, in different, older populations, consistently show higher rates of dementia in each successive decade of life. Table 17-1 summarizes the results of surveys carried out in three different settings.

The rates for those living at home and in the retirement community were derived from screening surveys for symptoms of cognitive impairment, carried out within the specific communities (Evans et al., 1989; Pfeffer et al., 1987). The rates determined in the National Nursing Home Survey of nursing homes throughout the United States use a physician's diagnosis of dementia (National Center for Health Statistics [NCHS], 1989). In other studies of the residents of specific nursing homes, up to 65% of residents of nursing homes meet the mental status criteria for dementia (Katzman, 1986).

Recent studies indicate that the prevalence of dementia has been increasing. This has occurred for two reasons:

1. Mortality rates in the older population have declined consistently over the past 30 years, leading to a major increase in the number of individuals age 75 and over, particularly those age 85 and older.
2. Those who develop the disease are likely to live longer because care is available to treat infections and other life-threatening conditions to which older adults are susceptible.

Study results have shown no consistent differences in rates of dementia between men and women or among races. There are, however, significantly more women than men with dementia because a higher proportion of women live to advanced old age. Dementia increases with age and is a major reason for loss of independence and for institutionalization. Risk factors that have consistently emerged from studies are the following: (1) family history of dementia, particularly in a sibling, (2) Down's syndrome, and (3) thyroid disease (Mayeux & Schofield, 1994). In a study of

TABLE 17-1 Reported incidence of dementia in different settings, by age

Type of residence	65 to 74 years	75 to 84 years	85 and over
Home*	3/100	19/100	47/100
Retirement community†	5/100	24/100	57/100
Nursing Homes‡	34/100	45/100	53/100

*Evans et al. (1989). Prevalence of Alzheimer's disease in a community population of older persons: Higher than previously reported. *Journal of the American Medical Association, 262*(18), 2551-2556.
†Pfeffer, R.I., Afifi, A.A., & Chance, J.M. (1987). Prevalence of Alzheimer's disease in a retirement community. *American Journal of Epidemiology, 125*, 420-436.
‡National Center for Health Statistics (1989). *The National Nursing Home Survey.* Washington, DC: U.S. Government Printing Office.

5055 subjects, higher education was found to be a buffering factor in respect to the development of dementia (Zhang et al., 1990). It is postulated that the attainment of higher education acts as a positive factor in delaying the clinical manifestations of the disease.

Symptoms and behaviors

Mental status decline, leading to a diagnosis of dementia, progresses along a continuum of deterioration in cognition, with associated changes in social, physical, and affective behaviors. Dementia is diagnosed when there are multiple cognitive deficits severe enough to cause impairment in occupational or social functioning and when the deficits represent a decline from a previously higher level of functioning. Also, according to recently published criteria, any cognitive deficits must be distinguished from the normal decline in cognitive functioning that occurs with aging in order to establish a diagnosis of dementia (American Psychiatric Association, 1994).

Progression of the disease and the dimensions of any one symptom vary from person to person, but the characteristic symptoms of dementia include the following:

1. Short- and long-term memory impairment (an individual is unable to learn new information, or to remember things that were well known in the past, such as birthdates or addresses)
2. Aphasia, or difficulty with the use of language (this may involve forgetting simple words or substituting one word for another with a similar sound)
3. Apraxia, or difficulty in performing motor activities, despite intact physical capacity for functioning
4. Agnosia, or failure to recognize or identify objects, despite intact sensory function
5. Disturbance in "executive functioning," that is, the ability to plan, organize, or think in abstract terms (this may be manifested as difficulty in defining words or in detecting similarities, as in comparing a dog and a lion)

Symptoms, behaviors, and progress of the disease vary from person to person, but *memory impairment* is the dominant symptom, particularly in the early stages of dementia. As the disease progresses, new information is rapidly forgotten, particularly when attention is distracted, and even long-term memory is retained only selectively. In advanced stages, memory impairment is so severe that individuals may forget the names of close relatives, their own home address, and their date of birth or age.

Aphasia, deficits in spoken and written language skills, frequently occurs. Language may become vague and imprecise, with use of long, rambling sentences to cover loss of words or inability to maintain attention on the topic. Repetitive questions or phrases may come to dominate speech. In the final stages, language and the ability to speak may be entirely lost.

Apraxia, difficulty with motor skills necessary to carry out everyday activities such as bathing, dressing, or eating, is a common symptom as the disease progresses. The person's appearance may become increasingly dirty and unkempt, a distressing symptom when a person was previously meticulous in grooming and behavior.

Agnosia, failure to recognize or identify objects even when sight, hearing, and other sensory systems are intact, means that the individual has increasing difficulty coping with the unfamiliar. Later, there is difficulty with formerly familiar activities, surroundings, and people. The individual may wander, become lost, and finally fail to recognize home and family members.

Disturbance in executive functioning or *impairment in abstract thinking* means that the individual cannot plan or undertake new tasks, and financial and other business affairs may fall into disarray. Judgment often fails as memory loss progresses, and the individual may be at increased risk for accidents. Water may be left running, pots may be left to burn on the stove, and traffic accidents are likely to occur if the individual continues to drive. The mortality rate from motor vehicle accidents for the population age 75 years and over is second only to the rate for those age 24 years and under, even though the number of miles driven by older adults is very low. The very highest mortality rates for motor vehicle accidents are for men age 85 years and over and men age 24 years and under (NCHS, 1990).

It is often reported that personality change occurs, with accentuation of earlier traits, the individual becoming more obsessive, impulsive, or paranoid. Alternatively, an active, energetic person may become apathetic and withdrawn. Along with personality change, social behavior and impulse control may also be affected, as exemplified by such things as inappropriate sexual advances and aggressive behavior.

Depression, anxiety, and other emotional disturbances often accompany the onset of dementia. As individuals become aware of cognitive decline, they may react with fear and withdrawal from social contacts and activities, especially as they recognize the potential for loss of control and as they lose self-esteem. Depressive symptoms associated with dementia further compound cognitive decline because memory impairment is a frequent symptom of depressive disorders in older adults.

In the final stages of a dementing disease, there is usually a total lack of capacity for self-care, with diminished psychomotor activity, visible generalized slowing of movement, incontinence of urine and feces, and almost total lack of communication and interaction with others.

Placement in a nursing home or other institution usually occurs when the person can no longer maintain hygiene or nutrition alone, or a spouse or other family member can no longer cope with the behavioral or personal care demands of the cognitively impaired person. If an accident, such as hip fracture, or other crisis occurs and the person is admitted to the acute care hospital, further physical and cognitive deterioration is likely to result. This may precipitate permanent institutional placement.

Etiology

Dementia is a complex of symptoms for which as many as 60 different causes have been identified (Katzman, 1986). The multiplicity of causes leads to the consideration of dementia as a number of different disease entities. It develops as the result of two different types of processes, giving rise to the use of the categories of primary and secondary dementias.

1. *Primary dementias*—These are the result of primary pathologic changes taking place within the cerebral cortex or the subcortical structures of the brain. Examples of dementing diseases resulting from these processes are Alzheimer's disease, multi-infarct dementia, and Parkinson's dementia. Less commonly, primary dementias may result from tumors of the central nervous system or from circulatory failure suffered during resuscitation from cardiac arrest.
2. *Secondary dementias*—These result from factors external to the brain, such as prescribed medications acting singly or in combination, metabolic disorders such as thyroid disease, or nutritional disorders that may be identified independently or in association with other conditions such as alcoholism.

A subcategory of the secondary dementias is delirium. *Delirium* is characterized by sudden onset of cognitive impairment, with change in level of consciousness, associated with the same etiologic factors as those associated with the secondary dementias.

Primary dementias

Alzheimer's disease Alzheimer's disease is the most common cause of dementia and is the most frequent postmortem diagnosis for hospitalized dementia patients (Mayeux & Schofield, 1994).

In 1907, a German physician (Alzheimer) published the autopsy findings from the brain of a woman suffering from progressive dementia

Alzheimer's disease, versus other causes of dementia, is largely one of exclusion. Investigations are likely to include the following:

1. A careful history is taken from the patient or relative, to determine whether the onset of symptoms was insidious or sudden, and whether these symptoms are more obvious to the patient or to others. It is also necessary to document other physical or cognitive disorders. For instance, a history of high blood pressure or strokes would indicate that multi-infarct dementia should be considered.
2. The possibility of brain tumors or other space-occupying lesions in the brain is excluded, using radiologic and electroencephalography examinations.
3. Neurologic investigation is used to reveal whether the impairment is secondary to other central nervous system disorders, such as Parkinson's disease.
4. A laboratory workup is undertaken, checking renal, hepatic, and other body systems, to determine the overall health and nutritional status of the patient, and to consider whether dementia is secondary to other diseases, to vitamin deficiencies, to alcoholism, or to adverse reactions to medications.

The fact that an individual's loss of cognitive functioning is determined to have been caused by Alzheimer's disease does not preclude further impairment from other causes such as multi-infarct disease or adverse drug reactions. It has been shown that mixed Alzheimer's and multi-infarct dementia occurs in up to 20% of cases. The possibility of further impairment from nutritional or pharmacologic effects should not be overlooked, because the potential effects of cognitive loss from medications, malnutrition, or other causes will be greater where underlying impairment already exists.

A further issue in establishing a diagnosis is the determination of whether the impairment is delirium or dementia, or whether the two disorders coexist in the patient. It is only possible to determine this retrospectively, after any medications or conditions that might be responsible for inducing delirium have been eliminated or treated.

Management of patients with dementia, once reversible causes have been excluded, consists largely of symptomatic treatment and social support for the patient and family.

1. Since the neurotransmitter theory of dementia was advanced in the 1970s, a vast amount of neuropharmacologic research has been undertaken by academic researchers and the pharmaceutical industry with a view to developing drugs to retard or reverse the dementing process. In 1994 (Cognex), tacrine based on the cholinesterase inhibitor tetrahydroaminoacridine (THA), became the first drug treatment available for Alzheimer's disease. A clinical trial indicated that the drug had an effect, although very small, in reducing the rate of cognitive decline (Davis et al., 1992). However, many patients receive no benefit from the drug and there are significant adverse effects, particularly with regard to liver dysfunction.
2. Other medications may be useful in the symptomatic treatment of sleep disorders, agitation, and aggressive behaviors in more advanced stages of the disease. Antidepressants are also sometimes prescribed, particularly for depression associated with multi-infarct dementia. All drug use must be carefully regulated and the patient monitored for adverse effects.
3. Support for patients and families through individual counseling, group therapy, and self-help support groups may assist in maintaining the patient in the private or family home for as long as possible.

Thus far no truly effective drugs for reversing cognitive loss have been developed. However, if the ongoing research is successful, there will be radical changes in the clinical management of patients with dementia, and in particular those with Alzheimer's disease.

DELIRIUM

Delirium has been variously described as *acute brain syndrome, acute brain failure,* and *acute confusional states.* It is characterized by diffuse cognitive dysfunction, with changes in level of consciousness; it is caused by one or more organic etiologic factors; and it is frequently associated with hallucinations and delusions.

Delirium is an organic brain syndrome characterized by global cognitive impairment of abrupt onset, with disturbances of attention, reduced level of consciousness, increased or reduced psychomotor activity, and a disorganized sleep-wake cycle. Duration can be of a matter of a few hours or days, and seldom exceeds 1 month (Lipowski, 1994). Delirium differs from dementia, which is also a state of global cognitive impairment, in the following ways:

1. The onset of delirium is acute or subacute, whereas in dementia, the onset is insidious and the symptoms develop over months or years.
2. In delirium there is alteration in *level of consciousness,* usually shown by difficulty in staying awake, although hypervigilance can also occur. In contrast, dementia is characterized by a state of normal consciousness.
3. There are frequently changes and fluctuations in the symptoms of delirium, with lucid intervals, in which cognition and behavior appear normal, alternating with episodes of confusion, often during a 24-hour period. In dementia, there are no such major alterations in the level of cognitive functioning.
4. If the etiologic factors responsible for the onset of delirium can be identified and treated or withdrawn, improvement occurs in the general physical status of the patient and the state of delirium clears. In dementia, the changes are permanent and progressive.

The etiologic factors that have been implicated in the onset of delirium encompass virtually all diseases or therapeutic interventions with systemic effects, including cancer, chronic lung disease, and diabetes. Surgical interventions, particularly open heart surgery and surgery for hip fracture, are strongly associated with the development of delirium. Many classes of drugs, acting singly or in combination, and particularly exposure to alcohol and other mind-altering substances, are etiologic factors in the occurrence of delirium in certain older adults. Pre-existence of dementia or other organic brain disease has also been found to predispose patients to the development of delirium, and delirium and dementia may well coexist in an older patient. This makes accurate diagnosis difficult, and the relationship between loss of cognition caused by delirium and that caused by dementia can only be determined retrospectively (Foreman, 1986; Lipowski, 1987).

Delirium may occur after surgery or the initiation of treatment, or it may herald the onset of an acute medical emergency. Onset of delirium may be acute or *subacute* (with a slow increase in the number and severity of symptoms). Although it can and does occur at any age, the incidence is higher in older adults, as are mortality rates for those who develop delirium. The symptoms and behaviors associated with delirium can present major problems in the management of patients, who are at high risk for causing injury to themselves and others (Lipowski, 1994).

Prevalence

Although incidence rates for delirium vary, most reports indicate that its occurrence increases with advancing age. It is estimated that between 30% and 50% of older patients experience an episode of delirium during hospitalization. Delirium has been identified in 15% of older patients admitted to general medical wards (Francis & Kapoor, 1990), and up to 10% of nondelirious older patients go on to develop delirium during their hospitalization (Francis et al., 1990). Twenty-five percent of delirious patients have been found to be suffering from dementia, demonstrating that hospitalizations exacerbate the symptoms of mild dementia (Lipowski, 1994).

personal and social ordering of space has significance for the person and is recognized by society (Altman et al., 1984). For most people, sleeping occurs in the bedroom and cooking is done in the kitchen. Families may congregate around the kitchen table to share tales of the day's events, or they may sit on a front porch and watch the world go by. However, whatever the ordering and structuring of space, and whatever the significance and meaning attached, space is important to the cognitively impaired older adult. Wherever older adults live, whether in a private home or in a single room in an institution, their space has meaning for them, and it must be respected. Bernier and Small (1988) found that the behavior that nursing home residents considered most disruptive was the taking away of privacy and control over space in their rooms.

The attaching of significance to environmental objects is an individualized process and changes over time. A special table, a porcelain figurine, a special coffee cup, or a picture may have subjective meaning that is part of how the older adult defines a sense of self. There may be background or history related to an object that communicates the richness of the older person's journey through life. Often, questions or expressions of appreciation by nurses about objects in older adults' living areas may begin the process of sharing that can lead to greater understanding of the meaning attached to the object. Nurses should be open to opportunities to listen and to learn from older adults' expressions of the significance of the space and of the objects that make up their living environment.

The understanding of meaning attached to the environment and its relationship to the well-being of the cognitively impaired older adult is an essential and challenging facet of a wholistic assessment. Observation of behavior, listening to speech despite incoherence, and talking to relatives about the past relationship of the patient to the home environment may assist in understanding the personal significance that the environment has for the cognitively impaired patient.

NURSING DIAGNOSES

Nursing diagnoses are a result of the clinical judgment of the nurse, based on a deliberate process of data collection and analysis. Therefore the diagnosis guides nursing interventions, and the etiologies included in the diagnostic statement, along with the documentation of clinical data that substantiate the diagnosis.

Most of the time, the clinical data to support a diagnosis are observable and measurable. An example is the reporting of a physical change, such as "2-cm reddened area on left great toe." This type of physical data can be observed by another nurse in another environment at another location. Physical data are well understood and respected across the different health professions. Data regarding the patient's mental and emotional status are more difficult to define and are more difficult to communicate to others.

The communication of nursing diagnoses concerning the cognitive function of older patients is made difficult by (1) the diversity of the population, (2) the complexity of both the patient needs and the existing pathologies, and (3) the lack of specificity and conceptual clarity in these kinds of nursing diagnoses. Nonetheless, nurses must diagnose cognitive impairments in order to provide appropriate nursing care for the cognitively impaired older patients and their caregivers.

The following primary nursing diagnoses are applicable to many patients who are afflicted with cognitive impairment:

1. Confusion—acute confusional state or chronic confusional state
2. Altered thought processes
3. Alterations in sensory perception (visual, auditory, kinesthetic, gustatory, tactile, olfactory)

Diagnoses in the previous list are from the approved North American Nursing Diagnosis Association (NANDA) nursing diagnoses list, as are the following significant secondary nursing diagnoses:

1. Altered family processes
2. Ineffective denial
3. Caregiver role strain
4. Risk for caregiver role strain
5. Ineffective family coping
6. Dysfunctional grieving
7. Decisional conflict
8. Personal identity disturbance

These diagnoses are applicable in situations of early recognition of cognitive loss and throughout the period when the nurse is involved in the management of the nursing care for older cognitively impaired patients and their caregivers. Because of the increasing disability many of the cognitively impaired older persons experience, it is impossible to list all the secondary diagnoses that can result from the altered state of cognitive impairment. The alert nurse continually assesses and reassesses the physical, psychosocial, and environmental needs of the adult and the caregivers.

PLANNING AND GOAL IDENTIFICATION
Acute confusional state

Long-term goals include the following:

1. Patient will be free of any signs of confusion.
2. Patient will be aware of etiology of acute episode of confusion and will take appropriate measures to prevent further episodes.

Short-term goals include the following:

1. Patient will not harm self or others.
2. Patient will receive immediate and thorough interdisciplinary assessment to ascertain etiology of confusion.

Chronic confusional state

Long-term goals include the following:

1. Patient will receive environmental stimulation to maximize remaining cognitive abilities.
2. Patient will enjoy daily life.
3. Patient will be treated with dignity and compassion by all staff members.

Short-term goals include the following:

1. Patient will not harm self or others.
2. Patient will be treated with dignity and compassion by all staff members.
3. Patient will attend enjoyable activities.
4. Existing cognitive skills will be reinforced.

Altered thought processes

Long-term goals include having the patient be free of any signs of altered thought processes. Short-term goals include the following:

1. Patient will not harm self or others.
2. Patient will receive immediate and thorough interdisciplinary assessment to ascertain etiology of altered thought processes.
3. Patient will be treated with dignity and compassion by all staff members.

Alteration in visual sensory perception

Long-term goals include having the patient be free of any signs of altered visual perception. Short-term goals include the following:

1. Patient will not harm self or others.
2. Patient will receive immediate and thorough interdisciplinary assessment to ascertain etiology of altered visual perception.
3. Patient will be treated with dignity and compassion by all staff members.

IMPLEMENTATION
In the acute care setting

Acute confusional states are a common occurrence in hospitalized older patients. The patient experiencing an acute confusional state will probably have a medical diagnosis of delirium. Anticipatory mechanisms to identify patients at risk for developing acute confusional states are incorporated into admission assessments. These include identification of the patient's current mental status, prior reactions to hospitalization, and prior postoperative recovery patterns, as well as a detailed history of the use of alcohol and other mind-altering drugs by the older adult.

Early recognition of the fact that the patient is experiencing acute confusion is the next aspect of care. The older patient experiencing an acute confusional state may drift from periods of appropriate cognitive functioning to a state of perceptual disturbance and then to a full state of acute confusion. There is no standard, predictable pattern of behavior (Foreman, 1986).

After diagnosing an acute confusional state, the nurse initiates immediate consultation with the physician for the purpose of ascertaining whether there is a preventable cause of the confusion. It is necessary to review drugs, as well as to review the patient's physical status and physical parameters, such as blood gases, hydration levels, and signs of infection. Sleep-wake disturbances, levels of anxiety, nutritional status, levels of sensory stimulation, and many other factors may contribute to and may exacerbate the confusion.

Constant monitoring of the acutely confused patient ensures the safety of the patient. The environment should be structured so as to alleviate fears and to increase the patient's ability to recognize reality. Often the bedside environment of a modern acute care setting includes a frightening array of highly technologic beeping, flashing monitors, with little personal contact between the patient and the caring health professionals. Actually, because the business of caring for older patients in intensive care units is so demanding, hospitals limit the visitors who care most about the older patient to entering at prescribed and limited times.

Because there may be virtue in a continued orientation of older people during serious illness and subsequent hospitalization, it seems imprudent to exclude capable and mature family members from involvement in the care of their relative. Nurses can advocate use of creative methods of providing care to confused hospitalized older adults, which can involve concerned family members.

Protecting patients from pulling out their intravenous lines and ventilation tubes is important, but it is equally important to find an inter-vention that is less threatening and less injurious than restraining the already confused patient. The first thought should be, Is this line or tube necessary now? Is it part of current medical or nursing care? Consultation between nurses and physicians facilitates collaborative care of the confused patient. It may be appropriate for a family member to be in the room, to sit and hold the patient's hand, and to talk in a soothing and familiar voice. This constant orientation may be beneficial, and hearing a familiar voice may alleviate some of the patient's fear and anxiety. Restraints, if used, must be the last resort to protect the patient from harm. Many patients injure themselves trying to get out of bed when they are restrained, so constant monitoring is the only way to ensure the safety of the restrained older patient. The question to ask before applying restraints is, Would constant monitoring alleviate the need to restrain this patient?

The older patient who is experiencing an acute confusional state is usually hospitalized for an equally acute physical problem—perhaps for a surgical intervention such as a hip replacement. Problems are inherent in care provided by multiple specialists who may each have limited understanding of the comprehensive needs of the older patient. The growing potential for this type of problem increases the need for the one discipline (nursing) that understands the complexity of providing care to the unique and growing population of hospitalized older adults.

In the nursing home

Many of the residents of the nation's nursing homes are afflicted with chronic confusion. There are important areas of challenge for nurses who provide care to cognitively impaired nursing home residents. The ultimate challenge for the nurse is to improve the quality of life for residents who are chronically confused.

Detecting acute physical problems Changes in the pattern of behavior of a nursing home resident who is suffering from dementia may go unnoticed and unrecognized as the sign of an acute problem. Physical causes such as infections, pneumonia, heart attacks, and abdominal pain may be the etiology for an increase in the resident's confused state or a change in behavior. These types of problems, although very amenable to treatment, go unrecognized because of a lack of sensitivity on the part of the nursing staff to considering changes in behavior as a significant sign of a possible physical problem. Communication is difficult for older residents who have lost their cognitive abilities. They are unable to understand pain or discomfort and cannot communicate effectively with staff to call attention to their plight. The nurse must be alert and sensitive to the relationship between pathologic conditions and behavioral changes in cognitively impaired residents. Physical problems must always be considered and investigated when a significant behavior change occurs.

Management of behavior patterns Loss of independence, loss of contact with reality, loss of ability to care for oneself, and loss of a sense of self are the internal stresses that the confused nursing home resident faces on a daily basis. Externally, they face the stresses of an institutional environment: they usually must share their bedroom with another person; all the common living space, no matter how confining, is shared with others; and they confront changing members of nursing, housekeeping, and dietary staff who act as caregivers—some happily and lovingly, and others impersonally at best.

Behavior patterns exhibited by nursing home residents with chronic confusion can be divided into three categories: acting out behaviors, aberrant behaviors, and excess disabilities (Burgio et al., 1988). Specific situations that call for special management therapies include impaired abilities in communication, wandering, and catastrophic reactions (Harvis, 1990).

Impaired abilities in communication Confused residents vary in their abilities to communicate, and the pattern of communication usually contains aberrations. Difficulty in finding the correct word, saying the wrong word, not

being able to respond to a question, and being unable to express an emotion are all frequent experiences of the confused resident. This makes it difficult for meaningful communication to occur between the confused resident and the staff members. The nurse uses therapeutic techniques in communicating with the confused resident and acts as a role model for other staff. Valuing the personhood of the older nursing home resident who is confused is essential to the nurse's ability to teach others to communicate effectively.

Listening for the confused resident's meaning more than the words may help to clarify the true intent of the communication. Often, confused residents will call out a certain person's name or call for a long-lost parent. The nurse should avoid making an immediate response to the words of the resident, and should assess the mood and the intent of the communication. Is the resident seeking attention? Is there an unmet physical need (hunger, thirst, or an urge to use the bathroom)? Is the resident frightened by something unusual in the environment (the unexpected presence of a worker, a change in housekeeping staff, or newly assigned students in the unit)? If the answer to these assessments is negative, then the verbal communication (such as calling for a parent) may be the confused person's expression of profound loss. It is inappropriate to immediately reorient the confused person to the fact that they are in a nursing home and their parent is long since dead. This serves no purpose. The goal of nursing is to promote health, not to cause misery.

The calling out may be loud, annoying to others, and accompanied by pacing or other types of physical behavior. Walking with the resident and then slowing the pace may be the first step in the approach to understanding what the resident is trying to communicate. The ability to enter into the world of the confused person may be facilitated by taking on movements similar to those of the resident, such as walking or swaying with the person. This is a

BOX 17-4 CONDITIONS THAT MAY MANIFEST THEMSELVES WITH DEPRESSIVE SYMPTOMS

Collagen-vascular conditions
  Giant cell arthritis
  Gout
  Periarteritis nodosum
  Rheumatoid arthritis
  Systemic lupus erythematosus
Endocrine conditions
  Acromegaly
  Diabetes mellitus
  Hyperadrenalism
  Hyperparathyroidism
  Hyperthyroidism
  Hypoadrenalism
  Hypoglycemia
  Hypoparathyroidism
  Hypopituitarism
  Hypothyroidism
Gastrointestinal conditions
  Cirrhosis
  Inflammatory bowel disease
  Pancreatitis
  Whipple's disease

Hypovitaminosis
  Ascorbic acid
  Folate
  Iron
  Niacin
  Pernicious anemia
  Pyridoxine
  Thiamin
Infectious conditions
  Brucellosis
  Encephalitis
  Hepatitis
  Influenza
  Malaria
  Pneumonia
  Syphilis
  Tuberculosis
Metabolic conditions
  Decreased bicarbonate
  Hyperkalemia
  Hypocalcemia

Hypokalemia
Hypomagnesemia
Hyponatremia
Increased bicarbonate
Uremia
Neoplastic conditions
  Intracranial
  Leukemia
  Lymphoma
  Oat cell carcinoma
  Pancreatic
Neurologic conditions
  Chronic subdural hematoma
  Huntington's disease
  Multiple sclerosis
  Organic brain syndrome
Miscellaneous
  Amyloidosis
  Psoriasis
  Sarcoidosis
  Wilson's disease

physical health, loss of loved ones through death, loss of social support, and the awareness of time constraints. Erikson's eighth stage—"ego integrity versus despair"—points to the importance of the concept of time. Older adults who are able to integrate and accept aging are viewed as coming to an acceptance of their life's course. On the other hand, older adults who are unable to accept their life course are faced with the reality of a limited amount of time to significantly alter their life. Such a person, in Erikson's view, experiences despair. Whatever the causes of depression, it is paramount that the nurse be able to assess affected older patients and refer them for treatment. Depression is a treatable condition, not an inherent result of old age.

Often the treatment for noninstitutionalized, older, depressed patients consists of antidepressant medications. The most common cardiovascular side effect of the tricyclic antidepressants is orthostatic hypotension. Of all the tricyclic antidepressants, nortriptyline (Pamelor, Aventyl) causes the least hypotension (Chutka, 1990). Other side effects of medications used in the treatment of late-life depression are shown in Table 17-2.

Drugs with anticholinergic effects may have a detrimental effect on the already vulnerable cognitive abilities of the older adult. These drugs can cause delirium in highly sensitive patients. Other anticholinergic side effects that occur over a longer period and therefore are not easily

BOX 17-5 DRUGS THAT MAY CAUSE DEPRESSION AS A SIDE EFFECT

Analgesics and anti-inflammatory
agents
  Ibuprofen
  Indomethacin
  Baclofen
  Opiates
  Pentazocine
  Phenacetin
  Phenylbutazone
Anticonvulsants
Antihistamines
Antihypertensive agents
  Clonidine
  Guanethidine
  Hydralazine
  Methyldopa*
  Propranolol
  Reserpine*

Antimicrobials
  Ampicillin
  Cycloserine
  Dapsone
  Griseofulvin
  Isoniazine
  Methronidazole
  Nalidixic acid
  Nitrofurantoin
  Procaine penicillin
  Streptomycin
  Sulfonamides
  Tetracycline
Antiparkinsonian agents
Cytotoxic agents
Hormones
  Adrenocorticotropic
    hormone (ACTH)*
  Corticosteroids*
  Estrogen

Immunosuppressive agents
Tranquilizers
  Barbiturates*
  Major tranquilizers
  Minor tranquilizers*
Miscellaneous
  Alcohol*
  Amphetamine withdrawal*
  Caffeine
  Cimetidine
  Digitalis
  Disulfiram
  Fenfluramine
  Halothane
  Inderal*
  Methysergide
  Methrizamide
  Phenylephrine

High incidence.

TABLE 17-2 Drugs used to treat late-life depression

| Drug | Dose (mg) | Side effects | |
		Sedative	Anticholinergic
1. Doxepin (Sinequan, Adapin)	50-75	+ + +	+ + +
2. Nortriptyline (Pamelor, Aventyl)	25-50	+ +	+ +
3. Desipramine (Norpramin)	25-50	+	+
4. Trazodone (Desyrel)	100-150	+ + +	0
5. Fluoxetine (Prozac)	20	0	+ +

Adapted from Blazer (1990). Depression. In *Gerontology*. New York: McGraw-Hill.

identified as adverse effects of the drug are dysarthria, decreased gut motility, decreased bladder emptying, decreased visual accommodation, and increased cardiac rate (Maletta, 1988).

Other aspects of treatment for the depressed older adult may be derived from cognitive-behavioral treatment techniques that help the older adult to deal with the here-and-now issues of life. Daily activities and daily diaries engage the older adult in life and begin to reestablish social skills lost through disuse. Assisting older adults in regaining the ability to solve problems through their own actions may help them to feel a sense of self-worth.

Life review therapy is another treatment modality that may help certain older people to master the task of enjoying a mentally healthy old age. *Life review* therapy is considered to be a psychoanalytical intervention and should be instituted by a qualified specialist in mental health. This therapy may include reminiscence as a portion of the process of life review (Butler, 1963).

The single modality of reminiscence is considered a psychosocial intervention and may be used with both alert and cognitively impaired older adults (Burnside, 1988). The focus may be on a variety of subjects that the patient may find beneficial. Subjects can range from the meaning of life to a discussion of trips, or the focus can be directed by a leader of a reminiscence group to topics such as current events or art objects. Demonstrating the ability to listen and to respect the older person's reminiscence is the first step in the nurse's intervention that leads to a significant one-to-one relationship. The goals of reminiscence are to increase self-regard, to improve problem-solving abilities, and to enhance self-understanding. These goals are congruent with needs of most depressed older adults, and therefore, if the patient is a willing participant, reminiscence is an appropriate nursing intervention that is within the scope of nursing practice.

NEEDS OF THE CAREGIVER

The stresses involved in the caregiver role are complex and not easily understood. The nurse should assess five major factors relating to caregiver stress: (1) personal history within the family context of the caregiver-patient relationship, (2) the caregiver's subjective appraisal of stress, (3) change in the caregiver's lifestyle, (4) mastery of the caregiver role, and (5) available social support. These areas of concern are important for the nurse to consider when assessing the strengths of the family caregiver and his or her abilities to provide care and/or support. Several

assessment tools are available for assessing caregiver stress. Three assessment tools are included in the appendix to this chapter to allow the reader to review what has been used in the recent past to assess the caregiver role (Kosberg & Cairl, 1986; Lawton et al., 1989; Zarit et al., 1980). These three scales were developed with a practice orientation for the purpose of assessing the hidden stress experienced by caregivers of older adults. The nurse must be aware of the importance of a systematic assessment of caregivers and the need to be available to the caregiver as an educator and supportive helper.

Legal concerns may present problems for many caregivers. The nurse can suggest that the caregiver discuss with the older adult the option of securing a durable power of attorney for health issues. This allows the caregiver to say how the older adult would have requested to be treated if the person were able to speak for himself or herself. The caregiver should be advised to seek legal advice for interpretations of the laws of a particular state and for legal alternatives that can be used for the benefit of the older adult and the caregiver (Weiler & Buckwalter, 1988).

The twofold goal of nursing interventions involving caregivers of a cognitively impaired older adult is, first, to ensure safe physical, psychologic, and environmental care for the older adult, and second, to safeguard the ability of caregivers to maintain their own health and happiness.

EVALUATION

Evaluation is governed by the stated goals developed during the planning phase. If correctly stated, the goals are observable, measurable, and patient centered. The nursing process is continuous and is centered on the goals of nursing, to provide comfort and to promote, maintain, and restore health. The confused older adult is in need of nursing care on a continuing basis, and the profession of nursing has an obligation to ensure the quality of that care, no matter what the patient's residential setting.

REFERENCES

Albert, M.S. (1994). Cognition and aging. In W.R. Hazzard, R. Andres, E.L. Bierman, J.P. Blass, W. Ettinger, & J. Halter (Eds.), *Principles of geriatric medicine and gerontology* (3rd ed., pp. 1013-1020). New York: McGraw-Hill.

Altman, Lawton, & Wohlwill. (1984). *Elderly people and the environment.* New York: Plenum Press.

American Psychiatric Association. (1994). *Diagnostic and statistical manual of mental disorders DSM-IV* (4th ed.). Washington, DC: Author.

Avorn, J., & Gurwitz, J.M. (1995). Drug use in the nursing home. *Annals of Internal Medicine, 123*(3), 195-205.

Baldwin, B. (1990, July). Family caregiving: Trends and forecasts. *Geriatric Nursing,* 172-174.

Baldwin, B., & Stevens, G. (1990). Family caregiving: Education and support. In C. Eliopoulos (Ed.), *Caring for the elderly in diverse care settings.* Philadelphia: J.B. Lippincott.

Barnes, R., et al. (1982). Efficacy of antipsychotic medications in behaviorally disturbed and dementia patients. *Psychiatry, 139,* 1170-1174.

Baumgarten, M., Hanley, J., Infante-Rivard, C., Battista, R., Becker, R., & Gautier, S. (1994). Health of family members caring for elderly persons with dementia: A longitudinal study. *Annals of Internal Medicine, 120*(2), 126-132.

Bernier, S., & Small, N. (1988). Disruptive behaviors. *Journal of Gerontological Nursing, 14*(2), 8-13.

Biegel, D., Sales, E., & Schulz, R. (1991). *Family caregivers in chronic illness.* Newbury Park, CA: Sage Publications.

Bienenfeld, D. (1987). Alcoholism in the elderly. *American Family Physician, 6*(2), 163-169.

Billig, N. (1995). *Growing older and wiser: Coping with expectations, challenges and change in the later years.* New York: Lexington Books.

Blazer, D.G. (1982). *Depression in late life.* Toronto: Mosby.

Blazer, D.G. (1994). Depression. In W.R. Hazzard, R. Andres, E.L. Bierman, J.P. Blass, W. Ettinger, & J. Halter (Eds.), *Principles of geriatric medicine and gerontology* (3rd ed., pp. 1063-1070). New York: McGraw-Hill.

Blazer, D.G., Federspiel, C.F., Ray, W.A., et al. (1983). The risk of anticholinergic toxicity in the elderly: A study of prescribed practices in two populations. *Journal of Gerontology, 38*(1), 31-35.

Blessed, G., Tomlinson, B.E., & Roth, M. (1968). The association between quantitative measures of dementia and of senile change in the cerebral grey matter of elderly subjects. *British Journal of Psychiatry, 114,* 797-811.

Brody, E. (1985). Parent care as a normative family stress. *Gerontologist, 25*(1), 19-29.

Brower, B. (1987). Intergenerational caregiving: Adult caregivers and their aging parents. *Advances in Nursing Science, 9,* 20-31.

Burgio, L., Jones, L., Butler, F., & Engel, B. (1988). Behavior problems in an urban nursing home. *Journal of Gerontological Nursing, 14,* 31-34.

Burke, M. (1994). Nurse Practitioner: *Journal of Primary Health Care, 19*(2), 9-16.

Burks, T.F. (1979). Autonomic agents: Neuropsychiatric side effects of drugs in the elderly. *Aging, 9,* 69-78.

Burnside, I. (1988). *Nursing and the aged: A self-care approach* (3rd ed.). St. Louis: Mosby.

Butler, R. (1963). The life review, an interpretation of reminiscence in the aging. *Psychiatry, 26,* 25-28.

Chutka, D. (1990). Cardiovascular effects of the antidepressants: Recognition and control. *Geriatrics, 45*(1), 55-67.

Cohen, G.D. (1985). Toward an interface of mental and physical health phenomena in geriatrics: Clinical findings and questions. In C.M. Gaitz & Samorajski (Eds.), *Aging 2000: Our health care destiny: Vol. 1. Biomedical issues.* New York: Springer-Verlag.

Collins, P., Stemmel, Wang, & Givern. (1994). Caregiving transitions: Changes in depression among family caregivers of relatives with dementia. *Nursing Research, 43*(4), 220-225.

Cotman, C. (1990). The brain: New plasticity/new possibility. In R. Butler, M. Oberlink, & M. Schechter (Eds.), *The promise of productive aging: From biology to social policy* (pp. 70-85). New York: Springer.

Cristofalo, V. (1990). Biological mechanisms of aging: An overview. In W. Hazzard, R. Andres, E. Bierman, & J. Blass (Eds.), *Principles of geriatric medicine and gerontology.* New York: McGraw-Hill.

Davis, K.L., Thal, L.J., Gamzu, E.R., et al. (1992). A double-blind, placebo-controlled multicenter study of tacrine for Alzheimer's disease. *New England Journal of Medicine, 327*(18), 1253-1259.

Dreyfus, J. (1988). Depression: Assessment and interventions in the medically ill frail elderly. *Journal of Gerontological Nursing, 14*(9), 27-36.

Dura, J.R., et al. (1991). Anxiety and depressive disorders in adult children caring for demented parents. *Psychology Aging, 6,* 467.

Evans, D.A., Funkenstein, H.H., Albert, M.S., et al. (1989). Prevalence of Alzheimer's disease in a community population of older persons: Higher than previously reported. *Journal of the American Medical Association, 262*(18), 2551-2556.

Folstein, M.F., Folstein, S.E., & McHugh, P.R. (1975). "Mini–mental state": A practical method for grading the cognitive state of patients for the clinician. *Journal of Psychiatric Research, 12,* 189-198.

Foreman, M.D. (1986). Acute confusional states in hospitalized elderly: A research dilemma. *Nursing Research, 35*(1), 34-38.

Francis, J., & Kapoor, W. (1990). Delirium in hospitalized elderly. *Journal of General Internal Medicine, 5,* 65.

Francis, J., et al. (1990). A prospective study of delirium in hospitalized elderly. *Journal of the American Medical Association, 263,* 1097.

Gandy, S. (1994). The degenerative disorders of the nervous system. In W.R. Hazzard, R. Andres, E.L. Bierman, J.P. Blass, W. Ettinger, & J. Halter (Eds.), *Principles of geriatric medicine and gerontology* (3rd ed., pp. 1063-1070). New York: McGraw-Hill.

Garrad, J., Chin, V., & Dowd, B. (1995). The impact of the 1987 federal regulation on the use of psychotropic drugs in Minnesota nursing homes. *American Journal of Public Health, 85*(6), 771-776.

George, L., & Gwyther, L. (1986). Caregiver well-being: A multidimensional examination of family caregivers of demented adults. *Gerontologist, 6,* 253-259.

Gold, D., Reis, M., Markiswiez, D., & Andres, D. (1995). When home caregiving ends: A longitudinal study of outcomes for caregivers of relatives with dementia. *Journal of the American Geriatrics Society, 43,* 1.

Hachinski, V.C., Iliff, L.D., Zilkha, E., et al. (1975). Cerebral blood flow in dementia. *Archives of Neurology, 32,* 632-637.

Hamilton, M. (1967). Development of a rating scale for primary depressive illness. *British Journal of Social and Clinical Psychology,* 278-296.

Harvis, K. (1990). Care plan approach to dementia. *Geriatric Nursing, 11*(2), 76-79.

Hollister, L.E. (1979). Psychotherapeutic drugs: Neuropsychiatric side effects of drugs in the elderly. *Aging, 9,* 79-88.

Horowitz, A. (1985). Family caregiving in the frail elderly. In C. Eisdorfer (Ed.), *An annual review of gerontology and geriatrics* (Vol. 5). New York: Springer.

Intrieri, R.C., & Rapp, S.R. (1994). Self-control skillfulness and caregiver burden among help-seeking elders. *Journal of Gerontology, 49*(1), 19-23.

Jacobs, J.W., Bernhard, B.A., Delgado, A., & Strain, J.J. (1977). Screening for organic mental syndromes in the medically ill. *Annals of Internal Medicine, 86,* 40-46.

Katzman, R. (1986). Alzheimer's disease. *New England Journal of Medicine, 314*(15), 964-973.

Kosberg, J., & Cairl, R. (1986). The cost-of-care index: A case management tool for screening informal care providers. *Gerontologist, 26*(3), 273-278.

Lawton, P., Klebian, M., Moss, M., Rovine, M., & Glicksman, A. (1989). Measuring caregiving appraisal. *Journal of Gerontology, 44*(3), 61-71.

Levkoff, S.E., et al. (1992). Delirium: The occurrence and persistence of symptoms among elderly hospitalized patients. *Archives of Internal Medicine, 152,* 334.

Lipowski, Z.J. (1987). Delirium (acute confusional states). *Journal of the American Medical Association, 258*(13), 1789-1792.

Lipowski, Z.J. (1994). Delirium. In W. Hazzard, A. Andres, E. Bierman, J. Blass, W. Ettinger, & J. Halter (Eds.), *Principles of geriatric medicine and gerontology* (3rd ed., pp. 1021-1026). New York: McGraw-Hill.

Maletta, G. (1988). Management of behavior problems in elderly patients with Alzheimer's disease and other dementias. *Clinics in Geriatric Medicine, 4*(4), 719-747.

Mayeux, R., & Schofield, P. (1994). Alzheimer's disease. In W. Hazzard, A. Andres, E. Bierman, J. Blass, W. Ettinger, & J. Halter (Eds.), *Principles of geriatric medicine and gerontology* (3rd ed., pp. 1035-1050). New York: McGraw-Hill.

McDowell, F.H. (1994). Parkinson's disease and related disorders. In W. Hazzard, A. Andres, E. Bierman, J. Blass, W. Ettinger, & J. Halter (Eds.), *Principles of geriatric medicine and gerontology* (3rd ed., pp. 1051-1062). New York: McGraw-Hill.

Mentes, J., & Ferrario, J. (1989). Calming aggressive reactions: A preventive program. *Journal of Gerontological Nursing, 15*(2), 22-27.

Moore, J.T., Bobula, J.A., Short, T.B., et al. (1983). A functional dementia scale. *Journal of Family Practice, 16,* 499-503.

Nakamura, S. (1990). The brain: Neurochemical aspects. In R. Butler, M. Oberlink, & M. Schechter (Eds.), *The promise of productive aging: From biology to social policy* (pp. 85-101). New York: Springer.

National Center for Health Statistics. (1990). *Health, United States, 1989.* Hyattsville, MD: U.S. Public Health Service.

National Center for Health Statistics. (1989). In Hing, E., Sekscenski, E., & Strahan, G. (Eds.), *The National Nursing Home Survey, 1985: Summary for the United States. Vital and health statistics* (Series 13, No. 97, DHHS Pub. No. [PHS] 89-1758). Washington, DC: U.S. Government Printing Office.

Pallet, P. (1990). A conceptual framework for studying family caregiver burden in Alzheimer's-type dementia. *Image, 22*(1), 51-58.

Palmateer, L., & McCartney, J. (1985). Do nurses know when patients have cognitive deficits? *Journal of Gerontological Nursing, 11*(2), 10-12.

Pearlin, L., Mullan, J., Semple, S., & Skaff, M. (1990). Caregiving and the stress process: An overview of concepts and their measures. *Gerontologist, 30*(5), 583-591.

Perry, E.K., Tomlinson, B.E., & Blessed, G. (1978). Correlation of cholinergic abnormalities with senile plaques and mental test scores. *British Medical Journal, 2,* 1457-1459.

Petrie, et al. (1982). Loxapine in psychogeriatrics. A placebo and standard controlled clinical investigation. *Journal of Clinical Psychopharmacology, 2,* 122-126.

Pfeffer, R.I., Afifi, A.A., & Chance, J.M. (1987). Prevalence of Alzheimer's disease in a retirement community. *American Journal of Epidemiology, 125,* 420-436.

Pfeiffer, E. (1975). A short portable mental status questionnaire for the assessment of organic brain deficit in elderly patients. *Journal of the American Geriatrics Society, 23,* 433-441.

Phillips, L. (1989). Elder-family caregiving relationships: Determining appropriate nursing interventions. *Nursing Clinics of North America, 24*(3), 795-807.

Phillipson, M., Morganville, J., Jeste, D., & Harris, M. (1990). Antipsychotics. *Clinics in Geriatric Medicine, 6*(2), 411-422.

Piest, S. (1995). Rewards, costs and coping of African American caregivers. *Nursing Research, 44*(3), 147-152.

Poirer, J., & Finch, C. (1994). Neurochemistry of the aging brain. In W. Hazzard, A. Andres, E. Bierman, J. Blass, W. Ettinger, & J. Halter (Eds.), *Principles of geriatric medicine and gerontology* (3rd ed., pp. 1005-1012). New York: McGraw-Hill.

Rader, J., Doan, J., & Schwab, M. (1985). How to decrease wandering: A form of agenda behavior. *Geriatric Nursing, 6*(4), 196-199.

Ray, Taylor, Meador, Lichtenstein, Griffin, Fought, Adams, & Blazer. (1993). Reducing antipsychotic drug use in nursing homes: A controlled trial of provider education. *Archives of Internal Medicine, 153*(6), 713-721.

Reisberg, B., Schneck, M.K., Ferris, S.H., et al. (1983). The brief cognitive rating scale: Findings in primary degenerative dementia. *Psychopharmacology Bulletin, 19,* 47-50.

Rocca, W., et al. (1986). Epidemiology of clinically diagnosed Alzheimer's disease. *Annals of Neurology, 19,* 415.

Rovner, S.W., Edelman, B.A., Cox, M.P., & Shmuely, Y. (1992). The impact of antipsychotic drug regulations on prescribing practices in nursing homes. *American Journal of Psychiatry, 149*(10), 1390-1392.

Schor, J.D., et al. (1992). Risk factors for delirium in hospitalized elderly. *Journal of the American Medical Association, 267,* 827.

Shanas, E. (1979). Social myth as hypothesis: The case of the family relations of old people. *Gerontologist, 19,* 3-9.

Soldo, B., & Manton, K. (1985). Health status and service needs of the oldest old: Current patterns and future trends. *Milbank Memorial/Fund Quarterly/Health and Society, 63,* 286-319.

Stone, R., Cafferata, G., & Sangl, J. (1987). Caregivers of the frail elderly: A national profile. *Gerontologist, 27*(5), 616-626.

Stone, R., & Kemper, P. (1990). Spouses and children of disabled elders: How large a constituency for long-term reform? *The Milbank Memorial/Fund Quarterly/Health and Society, 67*(34), 485-506.

Suiter, J., & Pillemer, K. (1993). Support and interpersonal stress in the social network of married daughters caring for parents with dementia. *Journal of Gerontology, 18*(1), 81-89.

Terry, R., DeTeresa, R., & Hansen, L. (1987). Neocortical cell counts in normal human adult aging. *Annals Neurology, 21,* 530-539.

Weiler, K., & Buckwalter, K. (1988). Care of the demented client. *Journal of Gerontological Nursing, 14*(7), 26-31.

Williams, J.M. (1987). *Cognitive behavior rating scales.* FL: Psychological Assessment Resources.

Yesavage, J.A., Brink, T.L., Rose, T.L., et al. (1983). Development and validation of a geriatric depression screening scale: A preliminary report. *Journal of Psychiatric Research, 17,* 37-49.

Zarit, S., Reever, K., & Back-Peterson, J. (1980). Relatives of the impaired elderly: Correlates of feelings of burden. *Gerontologist, 20,* 649-655.

Zarit, S., Todd, P., & Zarit, J. (1986). Subjective burden of husbands and wives as caregivers: A longitudinal study. *Gerontologist, 26*(3), 273-278.

Zhang, M., et al. (1990). The prevalence of dementia and Alzheimer's disease in Shanghai: Impact of age, gender, and education. *Annals of Neurology, 27,* 428.

Zung, W.W.K. (1965). A self-rating depression scale. *Archives of General Psychiatry, 12,* 63-70.

BIBLIOGRAPHY

Abraham, I., & Neundorfer, M. (1990). Alzheimer's: A decade of progress, a future of nursing challenges. *Geriatric Nursing, 11*(3), 116-119.

Colman, P.D., & Flood, D.G. (1987). Neuron numbers and dendrite extent in normal aging and Alzheimer's disease. *Neurobiological Aging, 8* , 521.

Folstein, M., Anthony, J.C., Parhad, I., et al. (1985). The meaning of cognitive impairment in the elderly. *Journal of the American Geriatrics Society, 33,* 228-235.

Ford, C.V., & Folks, D.G. (1985). Psychiatric disorders in geriatric medical/surgical patients: Part II. *Southern Medical Journal, 78*(4), 397-402.

Fox, P. (1989). From senility to Alzheimer's disease: The rise of the Alzheimer's disease movement. *Milbank Quarterly, 67*(1), 58-102.

Gallagher, D., Rose, J., Rivera, P., Lovett, S., & Thompson, L. (1989). Prevalence of depression in family caregivers. *Gerontologist, 4,* 438-448.

Hirst, S., & Metcalf, B. (1989). Whys and whats of wandering. *Geriatric Nursing, 10*(5), 237-238.

Kolcaba, K., & Miller, C. (1989). Geropharmacology treatment: Behavioral problems extend nursing responsibility. *Journal of Gerontological Nursing, 15*(5), 29-35.

Nagley, S., & Dever, A. (1989). What we know about treating confusion. *Applied Nursing Research, 1,* 80.

Smith, L.W., & Dimsdale, J.E. (1989). Postcardiotomy delirium: Conclusions after 25 years? *American Journal of Psychiatry, 146,* 452-458.

Wolanin, M., & Phillips, L. (1981). *Confusion: Prevention and care.* St. Louis: Mosby.

■ Appendix: Screenings

SCREENING FOR DEMENTIA AND DELIRIUM

Over the years, numerous tools have been devised to test individuals of all ages in the various dimensions of cognitive functioning, including memory, conceptualization, verbal fluency, and motor performance. The administration of many of these tests requires specialized neuropsychologic training and equipment. In recent years, however, several questionnaires have been developed specifically for preliminary assessment of cognitive functioning in older adults. They were designed to test for signs of the existence of organic brain disease, resulting in either dementia or delirium.

Among the most commonly used test questionnaires are the following:

1. The Short Portable Mental Status Questionnaire (SPMSQ) (Pfeiffer, 1975) (shown in this appendix)
2. The Mini–Mental State Examination (MMSE) (Folstein et al., 1975)
3. The Cognitive Capacity Screening Examination (CCSE) (Jacobs et al., 1977)

All of these questionnaires are easily administered at the bedside and can provide nurses and other health care professionals with some information on the patient's level of cognitive functioning. It should be stressed, however, that low scores on these test instruments provide only an indicator of the existence of organic brain syndromes. Lack of education, language difficulties, and poor hearing also may lead to low scores in individuals without significant impairment. Similarly, there is evidence of lack of sensitivity in these instruments for detecting impairment in individuals with higher levels of education, even though behaviors would indicate that impairment exists.

Follow-up neurologic or psychiatric assessment is therefore always required when individuals obtain low scores, to establish that there is real impairment. Similarly, when there are symptoms and behaviors associated with dementia or delirium, without obvious loss of cognitive functioning as evidenced by preliminary screening, further investigation should be undertaken.

The SPMSQ is shown herein. It has an advantage over the MMSE in that it does not require the patient to write and can therefore be more easily administered to patients with physical impairments or restricted mobility. It also has an advantage over the CCSE, in that it is shorter and less demanding on the patient.

It should be noted that the SPMSQ does have adjustment scores for level of education, as well as for race.

Caregiver-relative questionnaires

Loss of cognitive functioning resulting from dementia is important to the extent that it affects the physical and social functioning of the individual and the person's relationships with other people. Observations by family members and other caregivers are therefore important in determining the level of functional impairment shown by an older adult, particularly where the individual is resistant to testing, or where loss of cognition is suspected but not detected by preliminary screening tests.

Several instruments have been developed for assessment of the severity of symptoms of dementia by family members or other caregivers. These include the following:

1. The Functional Dementia Scale (Moore et al., 1983)
2. The Cognitive Behavior Rating Scale (Williams, 1987)
3. The Brief Cognitive Rating Scale (Reisberg et al., 1983)

The Brief Cognitive Rating Scale assesses impairment in concentration, recent and remote memory, orientation, social functioning, and self-care. It is, however, administered by a trained observer during a structured clinical interview. An alternative is the Cognitive Behavior Rating Scale, which asks a family member to rate the severity of symptoms, covering orientation, memory, aggression, need for routine, and other symptoms and behaviors. The length of this instrument, which has more than 100 items, may be unacceptable to many caretakers.

The Functional Dementia Scale (shown in this appendix) has advantages over the other two. It has only 20 items to be rated by the caregiver, covering activities of daily living, orientation, and emotional factors. It is therefore easily completed and can provide useful supplementary information in determining the level of impairment in the person being assessed.

SCREENING FOR DEPRESSION

Older adults seldom complain of feeling depressed. They often go to primary care physicians with somatic complaints of insomnia, constipation, or lack of energy. Some may be seen by social workers when they seek assistance for perceived financial or other problems that are precipitated by depression. The depressed patient in the hospital or nursing home may appear to the nursing staff as apathetic and uncooperative. Depression screening instruments or tests are therefore valuable in detecting symptoms of depression in older adults.

There are two types of depression scales—those that are self-rated and those that are rated by an interviewer or observer. Among the screening tests that have been devised are the following:

1. The Geriatric Depression Scale (Yesavage et al., 1983)
2. The Zung Self-Rating Depression Scale (Zung, 1965)
3. The Hamilton Rating Scale for Depression (Hamilton, 1967)

The Hamilton scale has the disadvantage that it must be administered by a trained observer, and the Zung self-rating scale may be somewhat confusing to many older people because each symptom must be ranked on a 4-point scale. Furthermore, neither was specifically designed for detection of depression in older adults.

In contrast, the Geriatric Depression Scale was designed to include items that are characteristic of depressive symptoms and behaviors in older people and was tested for reliability against the Hamilton and Zung scales. It requires only simple yes-or-no answers and can be self-administered. If an older adult has poor vision or reading skills, another person, without specialized training, may ask the questions.

Of the 30 questions on the Geriatric Depression Scale, 20 indicate depression when answered yes, and 10 indicate depression when answered no. A depression score of 0 to 10 is considered to be in the normal range. A score of 11 or more is indicative of clinical depression and merits further evaluation of the patient to determine whether a clinical depression does exist and treatment should be initiated.

SCREENING FOR CAREGIVER STRESS

Three assessment tools are included herein to assist the nurse in providing an opportunity for caregivers to express their needs and concerns. The degree of stress or burden can only be inferred through these tools. The tools may be helpful in providing the caregiver with a sense that others are experiencing similar stresses and that their negative feelings, if any, are not abnormal.

The tools are as follows:

1. The Burden Interview (Zarit et al., 1980)
2. The Cost-of-Care Index (Kosberg & Cairl, 1986)
3. The Caregiver Appraisal Scale (Lawton et al., 1989)

SHORT PORTABLE MENTAL STATUS QUESTIONNAIRE (SPMSQ)
ERIC PFEIFFER, M.D.

Instructions: Ask questions 1-10 in this list and record all answers. Ask question 4A only if patient does not have a telephone. Record total number of errors based on ten questions.

+	−

1. What is the date today? _____
                                       Month   Day   Year

2. What day of the week is it? _____

3. What is the name of this place? _____

4. What is your telephone number? _____

4A. What is your street address? _____
   (Ask only if patient does not have a telephone)

5. How old are you? _____

6. When were you born? _____

7. Who is the president of the United States now? _____

8. Who was president just before him? _____

9. What was your mother's maiden name? _____

10. Subtract 3 from 20 and keep subtracting 3 from each new number, all the way down.

_____ Total Number of Errors

To Be Completed by Interviewer

Patient's Name: _____ Date: _____

Sex: 1. Male   Race: 1. White
              2. Female   2. Black
                                        3. Other

Years of Education: _____ 1. Grade School
                                         2. High School
                                         3. Beyond High School

Interviewer's Name: _____

From Pfeiffer, E. (1975). SPMSQ for the assessment of organic brain deficit in elderly patients. *Journal of the American Geriatrics Society, 23,* 433-441.

INSTRUCTIONS FOR COMPLETION OF THE SHORT PORTABLE MENTAL STATUS QUESTIONNAIRE (SPMSQ)

Ask the subject questions 1 through 10 in this list and record all answers. All responses to be scored correct must be given by subject without reference to calendar, newspaper, birth certificate, or other aid to memory.

Question 1 is to be scored correctly only when the exact month, exact date, and the exact year are given correctly.

Question 2 is self-explanatory.

Question 3 should be scored correctly if any correct description of the location is given. "My home," correct name of the town or city of residence, or the name of hospital or institution if subject is institutionalized, are all acceptable.

Question 4 should be scored correctly when the correct telephone number can be verified, or when the subject can repeat the same number at another point in the questioning.

Question 5 is scored correct when stated age corresponds to date of birth.

Question 6 is to be scored correct only when the month, exact date, and year are all given.

Question 7 requires only the last name of the president.

Question 8 requires only the last name of the previous president.

Question 9 does not need to be verified. It is scored correct if a female first name plus a last name other than subject's last name is given.

Question 10 requires that the entire series must be performed correctly in order to be scored as correct. Any error in the series or unwillingness to attempt the series is scored as incorrect.

From Pfeiffer, E. (1975). SPMSQ for the assessment of organic brain deficit in elderly patients. *Journal of the American Geriatrics Society, 23,* 433-441.

MEASURING CAREGIVER APPRAISAL—cont'd

Caregiving satisfaction
   You really enjoy being with [IP]?
   [IP] shows real appreciation of what you do for [her]?
   [IP's] pleasure over some little thing gives you pleasure?
   Helping [IP] has made you feel closer to [her]?
   It makes you happy to know that [IP] is being cared for by [her] family?
   You take care of [IP] more because you want to than out of a sense of duty?
   [IP's] old self is showing through in spite of [her] current condition?
   The knowledge you are doing your best gets you through the rough times with [IP]?
   I do pretty much what I have to do, not what I want to do, in relation to [IP].
Cognitive reappraisal (traditional caregiving ideology)
   A strong reason for taking care of [IP] is to be true to family traditions?
   Taking care of [IP] is a way for you to live up to religious principles?
   A strong reason to care for [IP] is to provide a good model for your own children to follow?
   You think of the help you give [IP] as an opportunity to repay [her]?

From Lawton, P., Klebian, M., Moss, M., Rovine, M., & Glicksman, A. (1989). Measuring caregiving appraisal. *Journal of Gerontology, 44*(3), 61-71.
*Identified patient.

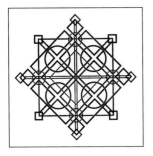

C H A P T E R 18

More humane, we assert, than to take care of the hurt,
Is the plan of removing the danger.

AUTHOR UNKNOWN, *Parable of the dangerous cliff*

Safety

■ Learning Objectives

On completion of this chapter, the reader will be able to do the following:

1. Discuss the concept of safety as it applies to the older adult.
2. Discuss the incidence of injury in the older population.
3. Recognize the older adult who is at risk for falling.
4. Discuss interventions to diminish the risk of falling for older adults.
5. Identify the susceptibility of the older adult to sustaining an injury as a result of a traffic accident and/or burns.
6. Recognize signs and symptoms of elder abuse.
7. Discuss the use of restraints with older patients.

Safety generally connotes protection from hazards to health and well-being. More specifically it can mean protection from unintentional injury or harm to one's physical or psychologic well-being. Safety, despite various definitions, is a recognized universal human need. Maslow (1954) listed safety, as a human need, right after the most basic physiologic needs such as food, air, and water. In this context, higher social needs of love and belonging can be realized only after physiologic and safety needs have been met. Safety provides a sense of stability and manageability to one's world—in other words, security.

The risk of actual injury or harm is variable at any given time for any given individual. In turn, a person's susceptibility to harm or injury will be affected by that individual's own personal characteristics, as well as the offending agent and the environment of the agent and susceptible person (host). Epidemiologically derived models that consider the interrelationship of hazardous agent, host (person), and environment are helpful in providing a wholistic framework for examining hazards to safety. Box 18-1 provides an example of an epidemiologic model of factors involved in safety. Activities to promote safety will employ methods to control the hazardous

BOX 18-1 FACTORS INVOLVED IN SAFETY

AGENT

Kinetic force
Thermal energy
Electrical energy
Gravitational energy
Radiation
Chemicals
Microbes

PERSON

Consciousness
Cognitive and emotional status
Developmental stage
Knowledge
Physiologic status
Health status
Nutritional status
Biologic defense mechanisms
Attitude

ENVIRONMENT

Space
Ventilation
Cleanliness
Sanitation
Lighting
Temperature
Weather
Shelter
Furnishings
Pets
Other people

ter will focus on those that have particular relevance to older people: unintentional injuries, particularly falls; automobile accidents; and abuse. The use of physical restraints as they relate to safety in older adults also will be discussed.

■ Ethical Considerations

As people age, they experience age-related changes that alter what constitutes a threat or risk to their safety. The family home environment can be dangerous for an older adult, not because the aspects of the home have changed, but because of the change in the physical abilities of the older adult. Older adults with intact cognitive abilities may choose to take the risk of staying in their familiar home environments, with full knowledge of increased risk. The dilemma for others, especially family members and health care providers, is the definition of what constitutes the acceptable level of risk for older adults.

Balancing the rights of individuals and the need to provide for their safety is not an easy task and may pose ethical dilemmas for older adults, their families, and health care providers. An ethical dilemma exists when one must choose between two equally desirable or undesirable alternatives. Resolving such a dilemma requires consideration of a number of ethical principles. Autonomy, beneficence, and nonmaleficence are ethical principles that are considered in making decisions about the older adult's safety.

Autonomy refers to an individual's right to determine his or her own course of existence, as long as that right does not infringe on the autonomy of another (Beauchamp & Childress, 1994). Most Western ethicists view autonomy as the supreme and overriding principle in ethical decision making. Exercise of the right of autonomy requires rational decision making. For some older adults the capacity for rational decision making may be compromised or diminished. In these cases the decision making may have to be assumed by another.

agent, decrease the susceptibility of the host, and/or modify environmental factors.

Because numerous factors pose hazards or threats to one's health and well-being, this chap-

In the older adult with diminished decision-making capability, not all areas of self-determination are necessarily compromised to the same degree. Those assuming decision making for the older adult must use care to ensure that the individual maintains the right to self-determination whenever and wherever possible. Overriding an individual's right to self-determination and exercise of autonomy is rarely, if ever, justified.

Beneficence and its corollary principle of nonmaleficence require one to do good for others and to do no harm (Beauchamp & Childress, 1994). In the case of those with diminished decision-making capabilities, those assuming the decision making must weigh the risk of doing harm against the benefits of any given action. Most ethicists concede that the duty to prevent harm is stronger than the duty to do good (Hogstel & Gaul, 1991).

This chapter is written within the framework of acceptance of the older adult's individual right to make choices. When there is a question of the extent of risk inherent in the decision or in the older adult's behavior, family members and care providers must employ ethical principles to guide their actions. The right to be treated with dignity is a basic human right, and it must rarely be breached in the name of safety and beneficence by violating principles of autonomy or nonmaleficence.

Chapter 22 provides a more detailed discussion of ethical principles related to the care of older adults.

■ Injury

Accidents are usually viewed as random events in which individuals have little or no control either to prevent them or to influence their outcome. On the other hand, injury can be thought of as having three phases of development: preevent, event, and postevent. Injury prevention is possible in the preevent phase and may decrease the number of serious injuries. Whether the term *unintentional injury* or *accident* is the label

Health Promotion

Increase vigilance for potential injury when these psychosocial factors are present
- Cognitive impairment
- Depression
- Grief
- Anniversary date of significant loss
- Psychologic stress
- Anger
- Loss of social roles, or social isolation
- Loss of independence
- Hazardous behavior

used to describe these random events, the prevention of their occurrence is a significant challenge for nursing and is the main focus of this chapter.

Unintentional injuries (accidents) are the seventh leading cause of death in people over 65 years of age, and their incidence increases dramatically with advancing age. The rate for those age 65 and older is twice that of middle-aged people (U.S. Census Bureau, 1994). In the over-85 age group, it is the fifth leading cause of death. Close to two thirds of all injury-related deaths and more than 80% of hospitalizations resulting from injury involve unintentional injuries (U.S. Department of Health and Human Services [USDHHS], 1991). Motor vehicle accidents account for half of the deaths resulting from unintentional injuries, and falls are the second most frequent cause of injury-related death. Unintentional injuries cost the United States close to $400 billion each year, with one third attributable to falls and 28% to motor vehicle accidents (U.S. Census Bureau, 1994).

FALLS

Falls and fall-related injuries account for a considerable amount of morbidity and death in older adults. Longer recovery periods and greater severity of injuries related to falls in older people pose particularly serious threats to the older person's health and functional abilities. Although most falls do not result in serious physical injury or death (Nevitt et al., 1991), they very often lead to decreased physical and social activity and loss of confidence in functional independence.

Falls in older adults are a major risk factor for hip fracture. Four physical factors have been found to be related to increased risk of fracture: inability to rise from a chair without using arms, a faster resting pulse, poor depth perception, and poor low-frequency contrast sensitivity (Cummings et al., 1995). The number of hip fractures (200,000) yearly in the United States is substantial, costly, and serious. Hip fractures lead to death in 12% to 20% of cases, and the mortality rate increases with age. Those over 80 years of age have a mortality rate from falls 8 times greater than those 60 years of age or under (Urton, 1991). Only about a fourth of older adults who sustain a hip fracture will fully recover (Ross, 1991). Box 18-2 lists some of the more serious physiologic, psychosocial, and functional consequences of falls.

Most falls occur in the home. Stairs account for a large proportion of falls, and most serious falls on stairs occur during descent. Many falls occur because the older individual misses the last step. The risk of falling is generally recognized to be significantly greater for hospitalized older adults than for other hospitalized age groups. In the nursing home population, more than one half of the ambulatory nursing home residents fall during a 1-year period (Tinetti, 1990).

A myriad of environmental and personal factors contribute to fall susceptibility. Poorly or inappropriately soled footwear; unstable furniture; elevated bed positions; side rails; highly polished floors; loose floor coverings (e.g., scat-

BOX 18-2 CONSEQUENCES OF FALLS

PHYSIOLOGIC

Fractures, especially of the hip, wrist, vertebrae, and ribs
Soft-tissue injury: hematomas, lacerations
Concussion, subdural or epidural hematoma
Exacerbation of arthritis or cardiovascular or pulmonary problems
Death

PSYCHOSOCIAL

Loss of confidence
Depression
Fear of falling
Social withdrawal
Dependency
Compromised autonomy
Institutionalization

FUNCTIONAL

Immobility, which may lead to the following:
  Thrombosis
  Dehydration
  Contracture
  Pressure ulcers
  Urinary and bowel incontinence or retention
  Infection
Deconditioning
Decreased righting reflex

Adapted from Hough, J.C. (1992). Falls and falling. In R.J. Ham & P.D. Sloane (Eds.), *Primary care geriatrics: A case based approach* (2nd ed., pp. 362-379). St. Louis: Mosby.

ter rugs and broken tiles); dimly lighted bathrooms, halls, and stairways; clutter, ice, water, or grease in walking areas; use of ambulatory assistive devices; and even pets are environmental factors that have been generally cited as contributing

Aging Alert

Factors to address when older adults have complaints of instability and/or falls

Assessment and treatment of physical injury

Treatment of underlying conditions

Provision of physical therapy and education

  Gait retraining

  Muscle strengthening

  Aids to ambulation

  Properly fitted shoes

  Adaptive behaviors

Alteration of the environment

  Safe and proper-sized furniture

  Elimination of obstacles

  Proper lighting

  Rails (stairs, bathroom) (Figure 18-1)

Provision of increased assistance and monitoring

to falls (Brady et al., 1993; Keene-Payne, 1994; Ross, 1991). Being 75 years of age or older, having a history of falls, and having gait problems are personal factors that have been identified repeatedly in the literature as increasing the risk of falls (Brady et al., 1993). Sensory impairments, diminished position and postural control, decreased muscle strength and coordination, increased bone fragility, and alterations in gait are age-related physiologic factors that may increase fall susceptibility. Many medications have also been identified as increasing the risk of falling. Examples include diuretics, antihypertensives, hypoglycemics, sedatives, and psychotropic drugs. The older person's risk of falling may be compounded further by cognitive deficits; urinary or bladder dysfunction; cancer; or cardiovascular, cerebrovascular, or neurologic diseases.

TRAFFIC INJURIES AND BURNS

The same physiologic changes that increase older people's risk of falls, such as decreased response time, sensory impairments, and alterations in the musculoskeletal, nervous, and cardiovascular systems, increase their risk of traffic accidents and burns. Approximately 25% of accidental deaths in those over the age of 65 are attributed to motor vehicle accidents, whereas burns account for about 8%. Injuries incurred from motor vehicle accidents and burns affect multiple organ systems and can quickly overwhelm the older person's physiologic reserves. Increased metabolic, cardiopulmonary, renal, and immunologic requirements of injury have more severe consequences and result in higher case mortality rates for older people, as compared to younger people with similar injuries.

The older person's driving an automobile is often a vital link in maintaining independence and a necessity for socializing and obtaining goods and services (Carr, 1993). However, deficits in visual-spatial skills, psychomotor coordination, cognition, and attention increase the risk of traffic accidents. Intersections are particularly hazardous to older adults, whether as pedestrian or as vehicle passenger or driver (Figure 18-2). Curb height, increased complexity of visual and auditory stimuli at intersections, and increased time needed for crossing on foot are factors that increase the risks to older adults. There are some indications that older drivers tend to ignore red lights and more often disregard the right-before-left priority at intersections than do younger drivers (Schlag, 1993). Identifying conditions that increase the likelihood of vehicle accidents and modifying driving practices or seeking alternative transportation should be included in any attempt to ensure the safety of older people.

Burns are another category of injury that poses a significant safety threat to older adults. Decreased sensory perception (hearing, vision, touch, and smell), decreased reaction time, and decreased mobility and agility make older adults

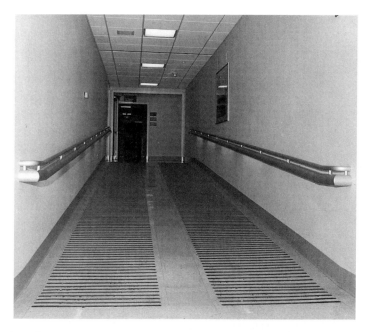

FIGURE 18-1 Handrails and non-skid surfaces in hallways help the older adult to avoid accidents. *Courtesy Loy Ledbetter, St Louis.*

particularly prone to burn injuries (Potter, 1993). The most common burn injuries are scalds (from hot baths, showers, fluids on the stove) and flame burns (from ignition of clothing, flammable liquids, house fires) (Reynolds, 1994). Smoking, cooking, heating, and use of electrical equipment account for a large percentage of older adult burn casualties. Because of the poor prognosis associated with burns in older adults, a greater effort needs to be directed toward prevention (Reynolds, 1994).

■ Abuse and Neglect

Two million older Americans are abused or neglected each year (Gilman, 1993), and the number of reports has been increasing annually. Furthermore, it is estimated that only between 1 in 8 and 1 in 14 cases are reported (Tatara, 1995). A significant problem in identification of abuse has been the lack of a clear definition. Elder abuse is defined by state laws, yet definitions vary considerably from state to state.

Most broadly, the terms *elder abuse* and *elder neglect* refer to any action that brings harm to people over the age of 65. Elder abuse is further categorized into three broad areas: (1) domestic elder abuse, (2) institutional elder abuse, and (3) self-neglect or self-abuse. Domestic elder abuse occurs in the older person's own home or the home of a caregiver and usually consists of any of five types of maltreatment (Box 18-3) of an older person by someone with a special relationship to the person (e.g., a spouse, a sibling, a child, a friend, or a caregiver) (Tatara, 1995). *Institutional abuse* generally refers to any of the five types of maltreatment when they occur in residential facilities (nursing homes, foster homes, group homes, and assisted living facilities) for older people. The perpetrators of institutional abuse are usually paid caregivers or others with a legal or contractual obligation to provide care and protection to the older person. *Self-neglect* or *self-abuse,* on the other hand, refers to older people's conduct that threatens

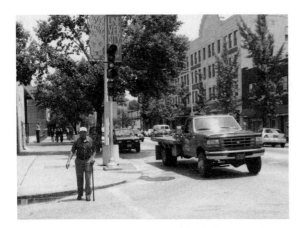

FIGURE 18-2 Crossing a busy intersection can be hazardous to the older adult. *Courtesy Loy Ledbetter, St. Louis.*

Health Promotion
Measures to prevent fire and burns

- Do not smoke in bed or when sleepy.
- When cooking, do not wear loose-fitting clothing (robes, nightgowns, pajamas).
- Set hot water thermostat at 120° Fahrenheit.
- Install a portable hand fire extinguisher in the kitchen.
- Keep access to outside doors unobstructed.
- Identify emergency exits in public buildings.
- If considering moving to a boarding home or foster home, check to see that it has smoke detectors, a sprinkler system, and fire extinguishers.
- Wear clothing that is nonflammable or treated with a flame-retardant finish. Wear less flammable materials of animal hair, wool, or silk.
- Avoid the use of electrical extension cords and do not overload electrical outlets.
- Install and maintain smoke detectors.
- Do not store flammable materials in the home.
- Call in an alarm before attempting to extinguish a fire, regardless of its size.

their own health or safety and is often the result of physical or mental impairment. Examples include the refusal to eat or to seek and receive appropriate medical and personal care.

The majority of confirmed cases of elder abuse are self-abuse, whereas approximately 16% are physical abuse (Tatara, 1995). Elder abuse or neglect occurs in all racial, religious, and socioeconomic groups. Those at highest risk appear to be female, living with the caregiver, and dependent on the caregiver for personal care, health care, and financial decision making. More than two thirds of elder abusers are family members, and over one third are the adult children of the abused older person. The median age of the victims was 76.4 years and those over the age of 80 accounted for more than one third of the victims in 1994 (Tatara, 1995).

A complex variety of factors contributes to the occurrence of elder abuse, and no single theory best explains its occurrence. However, abuse is generally attributed to a combination of personal, psychosocial, and economic factors that affect interpersonal and intrafamilial relationships. Caregiver stress, in combination with other factors such as unresolved conflicts with the older person, inadequate coping skills, emotional problems, financial burden or concerns, and lack of family and community support, may lead to frustration and abuse or neglect. Stress and frustration may be heightened by the increasing mental and/or physical disabilities of the older person and thus lead to abuse. Other theories propose that the abuse is part of a learned behavior of violence toward others and is the expression of a normative behavior pattern in some families. Among abusers, a high incidence of mental and emotional problems that have led to their dependence on the older person for finances and housing has been observed

(All, 1994). In these cases it may be that the abuse is an inappropriate response of the adult children to their own inadequacies. The abuse may be the result of the abuser's poor self-control or ineffective coping mechanisms. Regardless of the etiology, abuse and neglect can pose significant risks to the safety of the older adult and should be considered in any effort to meet the safety needs of the older adult.

Elder abuse laws exist in all 50 states, and more than 85% of the states include provisions for mandatory reporting of abuse or suspected abuse. Health care personnel are designated as mandated reporters of suspected elder abuse in most states with a mandatory reporting law. Most statutes require confidentiality for people who report suspected abuse and protect reporters from civil or criminal liability (Tatara, 1995).

■ Restraints

Physical devices, euphemistically labeled *protective devices,* have been used for years to restrain and protect people. Vests, belts, wrist ties, mitts, straitjackets, side rails, nets, and locked geriatric chairs are just some of the devices used to control wandering, prevent falls, facilitate treatment, and control disruptive and agitated behavior. Yet the use of such devices may, more often than not, be a form of physical and psychologic abuse that violates the dignity and autonomy of the restrained person (Strumpf & Evans, 1991). Rather than promoting safety, in many instances such devices cause depersonalization, unintentional injury, diminished quality of life, and even death (Brower, 1991; Miles & Irvine, 1992; Strumpf & Evans, 1992; Weick, 1992). Between 100 and 200 deaths a year are associated with the use of physical restraints (Weick, 1992). In fact, "restraints are an under recognized, under reported, avoidable, and proximate cause of death in at least 1 in 1,000 nursing home deaths" (Miles & Irvine, 1992, p. 762).

Growing research findings indicate that the hazards of restraint use outweigh perceived benefits. Those who exhibit confusion, poor judgment, or behavioral problems and have concurrent physical impairments are those most likely to be restrained (Mion & Strumpf, 1994; Tinetti et al., 1992). Those who exhibit behavioral problems of verbal and physical aggression are not only the most likely to be restrained, but also the least likely to be released from restraints or appropriately monitored and attended to while restrained—in other words, neglected by staff (Schnelle et al., 1992). Furthermore, restraint use has been linked to impeded mobility; loss of muscle strength, balance, and gait; new-onset bowel and bladder incontinence; pressure ulcers;

nerve injuries; contractures; and nosocomial infections (Janelli et al., 1994; Mion & Strumpf, 1994; Tinetti, 1990; Tinetti et al., 1992). Restraints do not appear to decrease injuries from falls or wandering and actually increase the seriousness of injuries in those who do fall (Mion & Strumpf, 1994; Tinetti et al., 1992). Significant psychologic distress, confusion, depression, anger, fear, loss of self-esteem, and increased agitation may also be related to restraint use. Despite an increased awareness of the physical, psychologic, and ethical problems of restraint use, the practice continues, and conflicts between the decision to restrain and the preservation of patient dignity and autonomy persist (Scherer et al., 1991).

Use of restraints must be accompanied by more rigid and explicit criteria for their use, proper application by trained personnel, and more staff monitoring of the restrained person. Otherwise, their use may be abusive, unnecessary, and punitive and actually constitute a greater risk to safety than any problem they are meant to control. The Omnibus Budget Reconciliation Act (OBRA) of 1987, the Health Care Financing Administration (HCFA), the Commission on Accreditation of Rehabilitation Facilities (CARF), and, more recently, the Joint Commission on Accreditation of Healthcare Organizations (JCAHO) and the Food and Drug Administration (FDA) have set forth standards and guidelines regarding restraint use (Stolley, 1995; Weick, 1992). In addition to recommendations for thorough evaluation of the need for restraints, appropriate application, and documentation related to their use, these standards and guidelines require development and implementation of suitable alternatives to the use of restraints (CARF, 1992; HCFA, 1992; U.S. FDA, 1992). See Box 18-4 for a practice protocol developed to address these standards and guidelines.

The movement of many health care facilities to becoming virtually "restraint-free environments" is increasing. Since passage of the Nursing Home Reform Law of OBRA in 1987, the prevalence of restraint use in nursing homes has declined 47% to 54% ("Nursing Homes Report," 1992; Strumpf & Evans, 1992). That still means that nearly a quarter million U.S. older adults are being restrained to their beds or chairs. Nurses can continue the movement to safer, more humane protection of older people only with diligent assessment of older people's behavior and awareness and implementation of alternative interventions.

Companionship, supervision, the elimination of bothersome treatments, environmental manipulation, psychosocial interventions, diversion, and physical activities must be considered and tried before physical restraint. See Box 18-5 for more specific examples of restraint alternatives.

Consistent with Maslow's ideas, safety and security are needs for all humans, but they are important to older people in a unique way. Activities that are often taken for granted by younger people can become major challenges as people age. All age groups are concerned about controlling hazardous agents, decreasing the susceptibility of the host, and/or modifying the environment. Approaches to each and all of these factors take on a different degree of emphasis for the older adult.

Injuries, accidents, falls, burns, and abuse are threats to the comfort and well-being of older adults. It behooves the health care provider to be aware of the hazards that precipitate any one or more of these events. Preventing these incidents enables greater comfort for the older person, as well as fewer challenges in the provision of health care.

There is increased awareness of the problems that can and do result in the use of restraints in the care of older adults. The creative health care provider is willing to accept the challenge of coping with the health care of the older adult through means other than the use of restraints.

Care of the person who may be prone to any or several of these threats to safety and security requires a systematic, orderly pursuit of care,

BOX 18-4 NURSING STANDARD OF PRACTICE PROTOCOL: USE OF MECHANICAL RESTRAINTS WITH OLDER ADULTS

I. Background
  A. Physical restraint is the use of any manual method or physical or mechanical device that the older person cannot remove, that restricts the older person's physical activity or normal access to his or her body, and that
    1. Is not a usual or customary part of medical, diagnostic, or treatment procedure indicated by the older person's medical condition or symptoms
    2. Does not serve to promote the older person's independent functioning
  B. The standard of care for institutionalized older people is nonuse of mechanical restraints, except under exceptional circumstances, after all reasonable alternatives have been tried.
  C. Risk factors involved in use of mechanical restraints in the institutional setting include the following:
    1. Fall risk
    2. Tubes or intravenous (IV) lines that need stability
    3. Severe cognitive or physical impairments
    4. Diagnosis or presence of a psychiatric condition
    5. Surgery
    6. Lack of staff education regarding restraint use
  D. Morbidity and mortality risks associated with mechanical restraint use include the following:
    1. Nerve injury
    2. New-onset pressure ulcers
    3. Pneumonia
    4. Incontinence
    5. Increased confusion
    6. Inappropriate drug use
    7. Strangulation or asphyxiation
  E. Appropriate alternatives exist to the use of mechanical restraints.
II. Assessment parameters
  A. Request information about the use of mechanical restraints from preinstitutional settings.
  B. On admission, identify as "at risk for restraint use" any older person who is agitated, at risk for falling, or disrupting therapy.
  C. Use one-to-one observation or behavior monitoring logs to identify and document specific risks. For example, for fall risk, assess impaired cognition, poor balance, impaired gait, orthostatic hypotension, impaired vision and hearing, and the use of sedative and hypnotic agents.
III. Care strategies
  A. Prevention
    1. Develop a nursing plan tailored to the older person's presenting problem or problems and specific risk factors.
    2. Consider and implement several alternative interventions.
    3. Refer to occupational and physical therapy for self-care deficits or mobility impairments; use adaptive equipment as appropriate.
    4. Document use and effect of alternatives to restraints.

Continued

BOX 18-4 NURSING STANDARD OF PRACTICE PROTOCOL: USE OF MECHANICAL RESTRAINTS WITH OLDER ADULTS—cont'd

B. Treatment
1. Use restraints only after exhausting all reasonable alternatives.
2. Obtain informed consent from the older person or the person's guardian before using restraints.
3. Use restraints only under the supervision of a licensed health care provider and only for a strictly defined period.
4. When using restraints do the following:
   a. Choose the least restrictive devices.
   b. Use the correct size and follow manufacturer's directions.
   c. Reassess the older person's response at least every hour.
   d. Remove restraints at least every 2 hours.
   e. Renew orders every 24 hours.
5. Modify the care plan to compensate for restrictions imposed by restraint use:
   a. Change person's position frequently and provide skin care.
   b. Provide adequate range of motion.
   c. Assist with ADLs, such as eating and use of toilet.
6. Continue to address underlying condition or conditions that prompted restraint use (e.g., gait impairment). Refer to gerontologic nurse specialist, occupational or physical therapist, etc., as appropriate.

IV. Evaluation of expected outcomes
A. Older person: Mechanical restraints will be used only under well-documented, exceptional circumstances, after all reasonable alternatives have been tried.
B. Health care provider: Providers will use a range of interventions other than restraints in the care of older people.
C. Institution
1. Incidence and prevalence of physical restraint use will decrease.
2. Use of chemical restraints will not increase.
3. The number of serious injuries related to falls, agitated behavior, and other problems indicating use of restraints will not increase.
4. Referrals to occupational and physical therapy will increase, as will availability of adaptive equipment.
5. Staff will receive ongoing education on the prevention of restraint use.

V. Follow-up to monitor condition
A. Document incidence of restraint use on an ongoing basis.
B. Educate caregivers to continue assessment and prevention.
C. Identify older people's characteristics and care problems that continue to be refractory, and involve consultants (e.g., gerontologic nurse specialist, recreational therapist) in devising an expanded range of alternative approaches.

Adapted from: Mion & Strumpf, L.C.N. (1994), Use of physical restraints in the hospital setting: Implications for the nurse. *Geriatric Nursing, 15*(3), 127-131.

BOX 18-5 ALTERNATIVES TO RESTRAINT USE

Provide companionship and supervision.

- Have staff, family, friends, or volunteers stay with the patient.
- Assess times that the older person needs more individual attention (typically early evening and at night) and intervene accordingly.
- Answer call bells promptly.

Change or eliminate bothersome treatments.

- Initiate oral (as opposed to IV or nasogastric [NG]) feedings.
- Remove catheters and drains as soon as possible.
- Provide more frequent nasal, oral, and skin care to reduce irrigation.

Modify the environment.

- Modify the amount of light in the room to reduce glare, accommodate visual deficits, and avoid interruption of sleep.
- Position the bedside tables, personal articles, and commode for easy patient access.
- Move the patient nearer the nurses' station, unless the situation triggers agitation or worsens confusion.
- Keep the bed at its lowest height or place the mattress on the floor so that the older person can move about freely in bed without falling.
- Leave the bed rails down if the older person tends to climb over them, or use half rails to prevent the patient's rolling out of bed.
- Reduce environmental stimulation, such as unnecessary noise or use of the wall intercom (many older people have difficulty understanding what is said over an intercom).
- Keep the call button accessible and review its use frequently.
- Use special furniture (low bed, special chairs).

Use reality orientation and psychosocial interventions.

- Involve the patient in conversation and therapeutic communication to elicit feelings, fears, and perceptions.
- Explain procedures to reduce fear and misperceptions.
- Provide reality links when appropriate (TV, radio, calendar, clock, newspaper).
- Use relaxation techniques (therapeutic touch, massage, warm baths).

Offer diversionary and physical activities.

- Use TV, radio, or music appropriate to the older person's preferences and cognitive status.
- Enlist the aid of a recreational therapist.
- Schedule appropriate exercise and ambulation into the daily routine.
- Institute training in ADLs.
- Use physical and occupational therapy to increase strength and endurance and promote a sense of accomplishment.

Continued

BOX 18-5 ALTERNATIVES TO RESTRAINT USE—cont'd

Design creative alternatives.

- Use rocking chairs to provide diversion and expend energy.
- Use music, audiobooks, or videotapes chosen specifically for the patient to reduce agitation or to provide diversion.
- Use a pressure-sensitive bed or chair pads with alarms for alerting staff to an unsteady patient who is standing without help.
- Develop, implement, and periodically evaluate toileting routines to eliminate sense of urgency and reduce falls related to elimination.
- Consult with other disciplines for other suggestions.

Adapted from Evans, L., et al. (1993). Limiting use of physical restraints: A prerequisite for independent functioning. In E. Calkins, et al. (Eds.), *Practice of geriatrics* (2nd ed.). Philadelphia: W.B. Saunders. Stolley, J.M. (1995). Freeing your patients from restraints. *American Journal of Nursing, 95*(2), 27-31. Strumpf, N., et al. (1992). Physical restraint of the elderly. In C. Chenitz, et al. (Eds.), *Clinical gerontological nursing* (pp. 329-344). Philadelphia: W.B. Saunders. Strumpf, N., et al. (1992). *Reducing restraints: Individualized approaches to behavior.* Huntington Valley, PA: Whitman Group.

---

whether in the acute care setting, the long-term care facility, or the person's own home. This care is best achieved by following the nursing process: assessing, diagnosing, identifying goals or outcomes, implementing, and evaluating.

■ Nursing Process

ASSESSMENT

Data for the identification of threats to safety are obtained from individual and environmental assessments. A comprehensive health history is necessary and should include both a medical and social history with information on existing medical conditions and their past and current treatment; over-the-counter and prescription drug use; previous falls (Box 18-6); and any episodes of vertigo or dizziness. The physical assessment should encompass the cardiovascular, neurologic, and musculoskeletal systems. Postural blood pressures, performance-based assessment of posture, and sensory-motor testing are essential (Kane et al., 1994) (Box 18-7).

Environmental assessment (Box 18-8) should identify any item or factor that puts the older person at risk, such as scatter rugs, inadequate lighting, clutter, or wet floors. Environmental assessments are most easily accomplished in institutional settings. For those living at home, some information on the environment may be obtained from the older adult, caregiver, or family member. In some cases an in-home assessment may need to be arranged through a home care agency such as a visiting nurses association.

There is no easy formula for the assessment of abuse and neglect of an older person. One reason is that both the older victim and the abuser tend to deny the mistreatment. Older women who are cognitively impaired and exhibit difficult behaviors such as wandering, belligerence, and insomnia should be considered at greatest risk for abuse or neglect. Unexplained bruises or burns, poor skin care, severe dehydration, malnutrition, poor hygiene, and the patient's fearful response to the caregiver should alert the health care provider to the possibility of abuse or neglect. Other cues are listed in Box 18-9. Caregiver characteristics should also alert the health care provider to the increased risk of abuse or neglect (Box 18-10).

BOX 18-11 SCREENING TOOL FOR ABUSE—cont'd

Additional comments: _____

_____

_____

_____

_____

4. *Social assessment*
   - Narrative statement regarding older person–identified social problems: _____

   _____

   - Family or nursing home perception of problem: _____

   _____

	Very good quality	Good quality	Uncertain	Poor quality	Very poor quality	No basis for judgment
a. Financial situation						
b. Interaction with family						
c. Interaction with friends						
d. Interaction with nursing home personnel						
e. Living arrangement						
f. Observed relationship with care provider						
g. Participation in daily social activities						
h. Support systems						
i. Ability to express needs						

Additional comments (recent changes in life situation): _____

_____

_____

_____

_____

Continued

BOX 18-11 SCREENING TOOL FOR ABUSE—cont'd

5. *Medical assessment*

	Definite evidence	Evidence	Possibility	Probably no evidence	No evidence	No basis/not applicable
a. Duplication of similar medications (e.g., multiple laxatives, sedatives)						
b. Unusual doses of medication						
c. Alcohol or other substance abuse						
d. Greater than 15% dehydration						
e. Bruises and/or fractures beyond what is compatible with alleged trauma						
f. Failure to respond to warning of obvious disease						
g. Repetitive admissions because of probable failure of health care surveillance						

NOTE: ATTACH DESCRIPTION OF ANY ADDITIONAL PHYSICAL FINDINGS.

Additional comments (if either 5a or 5b has been answered in the affirmative, please elaborate and be *as specific as possible*): _____

_____

_____

_____

_____

_____

_____

_____

_____

_____

BOX 18-11 SCREENING TOOL FOR ABUSE—cont'd

	Definite evidence	Evidence	Possibility	Probably no evidence	No evidence	No basis/not applicable

6. *Summary assessments*

    a. Evidence of financial and/or possession abuse

    b. Evidence of physical abuse

    c. Evidence of psychologic abuse

    d. History of recent life crisis

Additional comments: _____

_____

_____

_____

_____

	Yes	No

7. *Disposition*

    a. Referral to elder assessment team

    b. Referral to clinical advisor

8. General comments (nursing home contact person and date): _____

_____

_____

_____

_____

_____

From Fulmer, T., Street, S., & Carr, K. (1984). Abuse of the elderly: Screening and detection. *Journal of Emergency Nursing, 10*(3), 131-140.

high risk for injury, defining characteristics may include any of the following:

- Sensory impairment: visual, auditory, tactile, olfactory
- Cognitive impairment
- Physical impairment: reduced muscle mass, muscle weakness, musculoskeletal system abnormalities or limitations; peripheral neuropathies, irregular heart rhythms; dehydration, electrolyte disorders; malnutrition; anemia, fever
- History of falls, family violence, affective disorder, drug abuse
- Unexplained or repeated trauma
- Recent environmental change
- Declining functional ability
- Lack of safety education
- Family stress: interpersonal, material, financial
- High fall-risk appraisal profile
- Fatalistic attitude

PLANNING AND GOAL IDENTIFICATION

The planning phase of the nursing process involves specifying expected patient goals or outcomes. The goals or outcomes will guide the nurse in selecting appropriate interventions to achieve the desired goals or outcomes.

Identification of goals or outcomes for older people at high risk for injury will facilitate the nurse's ability to develop and evaluate nursing interventions. Individualized goals and outcomes may also be thought of as subcategories of national health goals for older adults, because the health of the nation ultimately depends on the health of individuals. Prevention of injury is one of the major strategies identified for improving the health of the nation (USDHHS, 1991). Objective 9.4a of *Healthy People 2000* is to reduce the number of fall-related deaths and injuries to no more than 14.4 per 100,000 people age 65 to 84 (1987 baseline 18). This would require a 20% decrease from the 1987 figures. A related and equally relevant objective is 9.21: to increase to at least 50% the proportion of primary care

providers who routinely provide age-appropriate counseling on safety precautions to prevent unintentional injury. Counseling is particularly urged for individuals at increased risk for motor vehicle injury, alcohol and other drug users, and patients whose medical conditions diminish motor vehicle safety. Objective 7.12 focuses on increasing the use of protocols for identifying, treating, and referring victims of violent and abusive behavior, including older adults. These broad, long-range objectives should be kept in mind as more specific, individualized goals and outcomes are formulated. Examples of more specific goals and outcomes include but are not limited to the following:

- The older adult will remain injury free.
- The older adult or caregiver will be able to identify factors or people that increase the potential for injury (e.g., falls, motor vehicle accidents, neglect, or abuse).
- The older adult or caregiver will eliminate physical risks from the environment (e.g., loose carpeting, poorly lighted areas, or unnecessary restraints).
- The older adult or caregiver will install and maintain safety devices (e.g., railings, grab bars, elevated toilet seats, or smoke detectors).
- The older adult will engage in appropriate exercises to promote and maintain flexibility and mobility.
- The older adult will demonstrate appropriate use of devices to enhance mobility.
- The older adult will discontinue behaviors that place him or her at risk for injury (e.g., driving at night, on major highways, or during peak traffic hours; climbing on chairs; or wearing inappropriate footwear).
- The older adult will obtain regular periodic evaluation of hearing, vision, and functional ability.
- The older adult or caregiver will utilize appropriate community services or agencies (e.g., Adult Protective Services, Meals on Wheels, transportation services, or home health aides).

IMPLEMENTATION

The four broad areas of the OMAHA system nursing intervention scheme can provide the nurse with guidance for organizing and implementing interventions for the older adult at risk for injury (Martin & Scheet, 1992). Although originally developed for use in community health settings, these categories can be very helpful to nurses in other settings. The four categories of interventions are as follows: (1) health teaching, guidance, and counseling; (2) treatments and procedures; (3) case management; and (4) surveillance.

In the acute care setting

Older patients are at significant risk for sustaining an injury as a result of a fall during the time they are hospitalized. Any decline in the physical condition or mental status of an older patient should be identified as a risk factor. Precipitating factors, especially the interaction of physical and environmental hazards such as a sense of urgency to urinate at night when unfamiliar side rails are in place, can increase the occurrence of falls. Studies have found a relationship between falls and a sense of urgency in older, hospitalized patients (Janken et al., 1986). Most nurses' ability to assess and identify those who might fall are relatively well developed; the difficulty is in developing realistic interventions that will decrease the number of falls.

Labeling the patient's chart to alert staff to the fact that the patient is classified as being at high risk for falling, with subsequent close monitoring, is a standard intervention. Scheduling accompanied trips to the bathroom is another frequently used intervention. Educating patients to be aware of the risk of falling and to take precautions, such as always dangling legs before getting out of bed, is an important intervention that often may be overlooked. The use of restraints has been demonstrated to be counterproductive in preventing falls. Furthermore, the use of side rails contributes to falls rather than being an instrument of protection. The ordinary hospital, with its high-tech and high-speed orientation, may be viewed as a hazardous environment for many older patients. Falls by older patients in acute care settings are difficult problems that require continued education of staff, patients, and families, as well as constant surveillance. Clinical nursing research should investigate interventions that both decrease the number of falls and maintain the dignity and autonomy of the older patient.

In the nursing home

All of the interventions used in the acute care setting can be utilized in the nursing home. The major difference is the transitional nature of the hospital experience. The hospital is an acute, time-limited experience. In contrast, the nursing home may well be the older person's residence for an extended period; it is *home,* which should be a safe haven, not a dangerous harbor.

The second category of the OMAHA interventions—treatments and procedures—would include nursing activities aimed at identifying risk factors for injury and preventing, decreasing, and/or alleviating signs and symptoms of injury. Examples of interventions in this category might include such actions as implementing alternatives to physical restraints; instituting a fall protection protocol; or modifying or making recommendations for the modification of the environment. Surveillance, another OMAHA intervention classification, will also be effective and necessary in a long-term care facility setting.

The resident who is independent is clearly more at risk for falling than the resident who is confined to bed or to a wheelchair. Meeting the safety needs of nursing home residents is a difficult problem for all health care professionals because of the conflicting goals of seeking to protect the resident from sustaining an injury as a result of a fall and seeking to meet the resident's need for a sense of independence. The nursing staff must make the adjustments in the environment that are necessary to diminish the likelihood of falling, while fostering the independence and preserving the dignity of the older resident.

In the private or family home

Case management, the third category of the OMAHA system nursing intervention scheme, includes nursing activities involving advocacy, coordination, and referral. Many times, the case manager will be a nurse making a home visit.

Prevention of falls may not be the primary reason for the home care visit, but the nurse should always be alert to the older person's increased risk of falling. Intervention in the pre-injury phase is an appropriate independent nursing action. Observation of the patient's physical abilities and detection of significant changes are key functions of the home care nurse's visit.

The house in which the family and the patient have been living may be assessed by the nurse as having many hazards. It is good for the nurse to stress that there is a need to reassess the home environment because of the changes in the patient's abilities. This approach may be less threatening to family members who may regard an assessment of their home as an unwarranted intrusion and as a judgment that they have not provided a safe environment for their family member. Working within the family structure and with the community of the homebound older person is crucial to the nurse's effectiveness.

Many older people live alone in an apartment or in a house. The nurse must remember the importance of preserving the patient's dignity and self-esteem, along with assisting the patient to maintain a safe environment. In regard to home hazards, with some support, teaching, follow-up, and appropriate referral, the nurse can make a significant impact in the area of prevention of falls.

Patients need to have information concerning the effects of drugs that they are taking, and they need to consider their risk of orthostatic hypotension. Instruction concerning how to decrease the effects of orthostatic hypotension, such as dangling feet before getting out of bed and rising slowly from a sitting or a reclining position, is important in the prevention of falls.

Nurses are among the few professionals who are welcomed into older adults' homes. Nurses have the opportunity to make a significant difference in older people's efforts to remain in an independent living arrangement. The prevention of injury from falls should always be a segment of every nurse's visit when home care is provided for an older person.

EVALUATION

The last step of the nursing process is evaluation. Goals or outcomes and nursing interventions are planned to reduce the risk of injury. The evaluation of the extent to which these goals or outcomes have been achieved indicates the effectiveness of the interventions. Evaluation of outcome achievement is ongoing and should be used to direct further assessment, outcome revision, and/or changes in interventions. Data for the evaluation of outcomes may come from reassessment of the patient and environment, subjective reports from the older adult and caregiver, chart reviews, and incident reports.

REFERENCES

All, A.C. (1994). A literature review: Assessment and intervention in elder abuse. *Journal of Gerontological Nursing, 20*(7), 25-31.

Beauchamp, T., & Childress, J.E. (1994). *Principles of biomedical ethics* (4th ed.). New York: Oxford University Press.

Brady, R., Chester, F.R., Pierce, L.L., Salter, J.P., Schreck, S., & Radziewicz, R. (1993). Geriatric falls: Prevention strategies for the staff. *Journal of Gerontological Nursing, 19*(9), 26-32.

Brower, H.T. (1991). The alternatives of restraints. *Journal of Gerontological Nursing, 17*(2), 18-22.

Carr, D.B. (1993). Assessing older drivers for physical and cognitive impairment. *Geriatrics, 48*(5), 46-51.

Carroll-Johnson, R.M. (Ed.). (1991). *Classification of nursing diagnoses: Proceedings of the Ninth Conference.* Philadelphia: J.B. Lippincott.

Commission on Accreditation of Rehabilitation Facilities. (1992). *Standards manual for organizations serving people with disabilities.* Tucson: Author.

Cummings, S.R., Nevitt, M.C., Browner, W.S., Stone, K., Fox, K.M., Ensiud, K.E., Cauley, J., Black, D., & Vogt, T.M. (1995). Risk factors for hip fracture in white women. *New England Journal of Medicine, 332*(12), 767-773.

Fulmer, T., Street, S., & Carr, K. (1984). Abuse of the elderly: Screening and detection. *Journal of Emergency Nursing, 10*(3), 131-140.

Gilman, L. (1993). Elder abuse. *American Health, 1*(7), 84.

Health Care Financing Administration. (1992). *State operations manual.* Baltimore: U.S. Department of Health and Human Services.

Hogstel, M.O., & Gaul, A.L. (1991). Safety of autonomy: An ethical issue for clinical gerontological nurses. *Journal of Gerontological Nursing, 17*(3), 6-11.

Janelli, L.M., Kanski, W.G., & Neary, M.A. (1994). Physical restraints: Has OBRA made a difference? *Journal of Gerontological Nursing, 20*(6), 17-21.

Janken, J., Reynolds, B., & Sweich, K. (1986). Patient falls in the acute care setting: Identifying risk factors. *Nursing Research, 35,* 215-219.

Kane, R.L., Ouslander, J.G., & Abrass, I.B. (1994). *Essentials of clinical geriatrics* (3rd ed.). New York: McGraw-Hill.

Keene-Payne, R. (1994). Hospitalized older adults. In M.O. Hogstel (Ed.), *Nursing care of the older adult* (3rd ed., pp. 250-264). Albany, NY: Delmar.

Martin, K., & Scheet, N. (1992). *The OMAHA system: A pocket guide for community health nursing.* Philadelphia: W.B. Saunders.

Maslow, A. (1954). *Motivation and personality.* New York: Harper.

McFarlane, E.A. (1993). Nursing diagnosis: The critical link in the nursing process. In G.K. McFarland & E.A. McFarlane (Eds.), *Nursing diagnosis and intervention* (2nd ed., pp. 10-20). St. Louis: Mosby.

Miles, S.H., & Irvine, P. (1992). Deaths caused by physical restraints. *Gerontologist, 32,* 762-766.

Mion, L.C., & Strumpf, N. (1994). Use of physical restraints in the hospital setting: Implications for the nurse. *Geriatric Nursing, 15*(3), 127-132.

Nevitt, M.C., Cummings, S.R., & Hudes, E.S. (1991). Risk factors for injurious falls: A retrospective study. *Journals of Gerontology, 46,* M164-M1701.

Nursing homes report decreased restraint use. (1992). *American Geriatrics Society Newsletter, 21*(2), 1.

O'Brien, J.G. (1992). Elder abuse. In R.J. Ham & P.D. Sloane (Eds.), *Primary care geriatrics: A case based approach* (2nd ed.). St. Louis: Mosby.

Potter, P., & Perry, A. (1993). *Fundamentals of nursing* (3rd ed.). St. Louis: Mosby.

Reynolds, C.A. (1994). Emergency care. In M.O. Hogstel (Ed.), *Nursing care of the older adult* (3rd ed., pp. 265-287). Albany, NY: Delmar.

Ross, J.E. (1991). Iatrogenesis in the elderly: Contributors to falls. *Journal of Gerontological Nursing, 17*(9), 19-23.

Scherer, Y.K., Janelli, L.M., Kanski, G.W., Neary, M.A., & Morth, N.E. (1991). The nursing dilemma of restraints. *Journal of Gerontological Nursing, 17*(2), 14-17.

Schlag, B. (1993). Elderly drivers in Germany: Fitness and driving behavior. *Accident Analysis and Prevention, 25*(1), 47-55.

Schnelle, J.F., Simmons, S.F., & Ory, M.G. (1992). Risk factors that predict staff failure to release nursing home resident from restraints. *Gerontologist, 32,* 767-770.

Stolley, J.M. (1995). Freeing your patients from restraints. *American Journal of Nursing, 95*(2), 27-31.

Strumpf, N.E., & Evans, L.K. (1991). The ethical problems of prolonged physical restraint. *Journal of Gerontological Nursing, 17*(2), 27-30.

Strumpf, N.E., & Evans, L.K. (1992). Alternatives to physical restraints. *Journal of Gerontological Nursing, 18*(2), 4, 27-30.

Tatara, T. (1995). *Elder abuse: Questions and answers* (5th ed.). Washington, DC: National Center on Elder Abuse.

Tinetti, M.C. (1990). Falls. In W. Hazzard, R. Andres, E. Bierman, & J. Blass (Eds.), *Principles of geriatric medicine and gerontology* (2nd ed., pp. 1192-1199). New York: McGraw-Hill.

Tinetti, M.C., Liu, V., Marottolil, R.A., & Ginter, S.F. (1992). Mechanical restraint use among residents of skilled nursing facilities: Prevalence, patterns, and predictors. *Journal of the American Medical Association, 265,* 468-471.

Urton, M.M. (1991). A community home inspection approach to preventing falls among the elderly. *Public Health Rep, 106*(2), 192.

U.S. Department of Health and Human Services, Public Health Service. (1991). *Healthy people 2000: National health promotion and disease prevention objectives—Full report, with commentary* (DHHS Pub. No. [PHS] 91-50212). Washington, DC: U.S. Government Printing Office.

U.S. Food and Drug Administration. (1992). *FDA safety alert: Potential hazards with restraint devices.* Rockville, MD: U.S. Department of Health and Human Services.

Weick, M.D. (1992). Physical restraints: An FDA update. *American Journal of Nursing, 92*(11), 74-80.

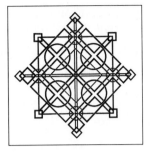

C H A P T E R 19

The soul has no rainbow
If the eyes have no tears.
NATIVE AMERICAN SAYING

Cancer in the Older Adult

■ Learning Objectives

On completion of this chapter, the reader will be able to do the following:

1. Understand the problem of cancer, its myths, and its biases as they relate to the older adult.
2. Discuss biologic aspects of aging as they relate to cancer incidence, morbidity, and mortality.
3. Recognize major issues (e.g., age, gender, extent of disease, and comorbidity) that may influence decisions concerning eligibility for screening, extent of diagnostic workup, treatment, and treatment aggression for the older adult experiencing cancer.
4. Address (1) the major therapeutic modalities employed in cancer treatment; (2) the major cancers affecting the older adult; and (3) the nurse's role in caring for the older adult experiencing cancer.
5. Identify patterns of care for the older adult, family, and community experiencing cancer.
6. Project future goals for approaches to cancer prevention, control, treatment, and research in the older adult.

The burden of cancer is disproportionately carried by the older adult. It is a leading cause of morbidity and death in individuals over 65 years of age. Age is the most important determinant of cancer risk. The overall cancer incidence rate for individuals 65 years of age or older is 2085.3 per 100,000, compared to a rate of 193.9 per 100,000 for individuals younger than 65 years of age (Miller et al., 1994). With projections that one in five individuals will be over 65 by the year 2020, cancer presents a major health problem. Nursing is well positioned to play a role in all aspects of

cancer care, from prevention, through active treatment, to providing care at the end of life. The purposes of this chapter are to frame the problem of cancer within the context of aging, to identify the major issues related to providing care to this population, and to discuss strategies that may be helpful to nurses caring for older adults, families, and communities experiencing cancer.

Older adults faced with a diagnosis of cancer pose a challenge to those responsible for their care. The individual over age 65 generally has

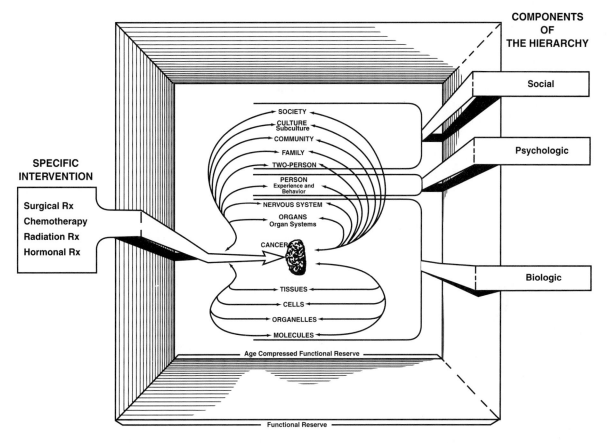

FIGURE 19-2 Comprehensive Geriatric Model. (From Cohen, H.J. [1994b]. Oncology and aging: General principles of cancer in the elderly. In W.R. Hazzard, et al. [Eds.], *Principles of geriatric medicine and gerontology* [3rd ed., p. 85]. New York: McGraw-Hill.)

versies, pay particular attention to changes in the recommendations, and be prepared to educate patients and their families about the current guidelines.

As can be seen in Table 19-1, recommendations for cancer screening frequently begin after age 50 (Fink, 1991). Only recently have upper age limit restrictions been lifted from screening guidelines. It must be recognized that screening for cancer is not an exact science and decisions concerning whether or not to screen rely on a comprehensive evaluation of each individual.

Factors that should be considered when deciding whether or not to screen include the cost of the test, the specificity and sensitivity of the test, the ability to treat the cancer if a diagnosis is made, and the discomfort and potential risk to the individual from the test. Evaluation of these factors contributes to the screening decisions made for all individuals, not just the older adult. In addition to the preceding factors, other factors that influence a screening decision for an older individual include the presence or absence of comorbidity, ability to perform activities of daily

TABLE 19-1 American Cancer Society recommendations

| Examination | Target population | | Interval |
	Gender	Age	
Sigmoidoscopy (preferably flexible)	M and F	50 and older	Every 3 to 5 years (per physician's recommendations)
Fecal occult blood test	M and F	50 and older	Every year
Digital rectal examination	M and F	40 and older	Every year
Pap test	F	18 and older; currently or having been sexually active	Every year (may be performed less frequently, at discretion of provider, after three or more consecutive negative examinations)
Pelvic examination	F	18 to 40	Every 1 to 3 years with Pap test
		40 and older	Every year
Endometrial tissue sample	F	At menopause (high-risk women*)	At menopause
Breast self-examination	F	20 and older	Every month
Clinical breast examination	F	20 to 40	Every 3 years
		40 and older	Every year
Mammography†	F	40 to 49	Every 1 to 2 years
		50 and older	Every year
Health counseling and cancer checkup‡	M and F	20 and older	Every 3 years
	M and F	40 and older	Every year

Adapted from *Guidelines for the cancer related checkup* (ACS, 1992).
*History of infertility, obesity, failure to ovulate, abnormal uterine bleeding, or estrogen therapy.
†Begin screening mammography at age 40.
‡Includes examination for thyroid, testicular, prostate, ovarian, head and neck, skin and lymph node cancers.

living (ADLs), and life expectancy. Although determining life expectancy for a particular individual is ambiguous, some attempt should be made to correlate the life expectancy with the potential for development of a specific cancer in the future. The decision to treat is separate from deciding how aggressive that treatment should be. The prevention of morbidity and enhancement of quality of life as a result of early detection must be weighed carefully against the morbidity caused by screening. For example, there is no reason not to screen for breast cancer regard-less of age in an otherwise healthy individual. It may make more practical sense to screen a healthy 75-year-old, who may have a life expectancy of 7 to 10 years, than to screen a 55-year-old who has severe debilitating cardiovascular disease, suffers from diabetes, and has a limited life expectancy. Breast cancer can be detected relatively inexpensively, with little discomfort or risk. The early detection of a small breast cancer in the older adult can result in effective treatment and minimal impact on quality of life. On the other hand, undetected breast cancer has the potential to cause significant morbidity, requiring more extensive therapy and costing more. Health care professionals must weigh the costs and benefits of screening for a particular individual, with a particular risk profile, within the context of that person's preferences. Recommendations exist for screening for many cancers, and these serve only as a starting place for the practitioner. "Differences in decisions may be entirely appropriate in certain situations but must be based on specific individualized patient information, not on categorical decisions made on the basis of chronological age" (Cohen, 1994b, p. 84).

To serve their purpose effectively, guidelines must be individualized. Three other factors influence decisions regarding screening for cancer. First, the older adult may choose not to participate in routine cancer screening. This decision may be related to lack of complete information about a particular screening test (e.g., a perception that, because of age, screening is not necessary), fears or other myths or biases about cancer or a cancer diagnosis (see Box 19-1), or inability to pay for screening tests. Second, physicians and other health care professionals may also lack correct information concerning eligibility for screening. Third, older individuals tend to be seen for episodic rather than preventive services. Therefore physician and patient alike tend to focus more on attending to presenting symptoms than on whether or not an individual has had a Pap test or mammogram. Educating physicians and the public about the value of early detection of cancer in the older adult is essential.

DECISION TO DIAGNOSE CANCER IN THE OLDER ADULT

Once the decision has been made to screen the older adult for a particular type of cancer, one must next decide which screening tests should be used for the purpose of diagnosis. Again, more than just the older adult's chronologic age should be considered when making this decision. The decision should consider the social, psychologic, and biologic factors portrayed by the comprehensive gerontologic model (see Figure 19-2). In addition, the following factors should be evaluated when making a decision concerning whether to pursue diagnosing a cancer: (1) the efficacy of the screening test, its cost, and its potential for causing morbidity; (2) how extensive the workup should be (or how many tests to include); and (3) the availability of appropriate treatment once a diagnosis is made. The preferences of the older adult individual, in consultation with the appropriate health care provider, are an integral part of this decision-making process.

Consider the following case scenario: A 75-year-old woman comes to the clinic complaining of a breast lump that she says she discovered while doing her monthly breast self-examination. She is in good health with no significant comorbidities, is married, and is fully active. The goal in this situation is to obtain clear-cut evidence as to whether or not a malignancy is present. The primary decision that faces the practitioner in this scenario is whether to order a diagnostic mammogram or to go directly to a biopsy. The practitioner must weigh the risks and benefits of choosing one or both of these diagnostic tests.

The previously discussed paradigm may provide some guidance in evaluating whether one or both of these diagnostic tests should be used. The mammogram has a high specificity and sensitivity, is of relatively low cost, and is generally risk-free. If a diagnosis of breast cancer is made, efficacious treatment is available. There are no significant factors described in this case that would preclude the use of a mammogram for this particular individual. The major factor that needs consideration is whether a mammogram is needed given the fact that a clinically palpable lump is present. If the additional clinical information that might be obtained from the mammogram would possibly alter approaches to therapy, then a decision to perform this diagnostic test seems appropriate. If, however, no additional treatment-relevant information is expected, then not to perform a mammogram may be an appropriate decision. Because the mass is clinically palpable, a biopsy is the only method available that will provide conclusive data as to whether or not it is malignant, what its cytologic characteristics are, and if prognostic parameters are present. Therefore, in this situation, it may be most appropriate to avoid the expense and possible discomfort of a mammogram.

If there is any question about whether the lump might be cystic, either a needle aspiration or a sonogram might be appropriate. However, the addition of the mammogram would only be important to detect occult disease in either the affected breast or the contralateral breast. These factors must be weighed within the context of the social, psychologic, and biologic parameters of the individual. The possible discovery of an occult cancer, which might not be clinically detectable for many years, may not be a sufficient reason to proceed with extensive diagnostic testing. This reasoning may be appropriate even in a healthy 75-year-old individual such as the one discussed in the scenario. Decisions such as this remain controversial.

Additional factors that might influence a decision to have additional diagnostic tests include when the individual had her most recent mammogram, and the existence of financial and insurance constraints. It is beyond the scope of this chapter to discuss all the possible scenarios that might influence decisions concerning what approach or approaches to take to make a diagnosis. It is essential, however, to discuss each possible approach with the patient, discuss the risks and benefits of each approach, and present expected outcomes from each approach. Providing accurate information is essential so that the older adult is equipped with sufficient data with which to make an informed decision.

DECISION TO TREAT THE OLDER ADULT WITH A DIAGNOSIS OF CANCER— AND HOW AGGRESSIVELY

Research suggests that a significant age bias exists in relation to treatment decisions for the older adult (Bergman et al., 1991; Greenfield et al., 1987; Guadagnoli et al., 1990; Mor et al., 1985; Samet et al., 1986; Yancik et al., 1989). This age bias is reflected in decisions physicians make concerning whether or not to treat the older adult with cancer, the type of therapy offered, and the aggressivity of this therapy. Findings from studies suggest that physicians tend to offer older women more conservative therapy and refer them to specialists less frequently than they do comparable younger women. Although older women may refuse chemotherapy and certain types of surgical procedures more frequently than do younger women, these decisions tend, in part, to be related to the type of recommendations made by the physician. Chronologic age should not be the sole factor used in deciding on cancer treatment in the older adult (Ganz, 1993).

Consider the following case scenario: The 75-year-old woman described in the previous scenario received a biopsy with a resultant diagnosis of infiltrating ductal carcinoma of the breast. The interaction of the biologic, social, and psychologic factors should guide decisions concerning appropriate treatment options. In addition, patient factors (e.g., personal preferences and physician recommendations) need to be carefully weighed. Other factors include expected outcomes from each therapy, impact of the chosen therapy on the patient's quality of life, and economic factors.

Assume that the following therapies are equivalent in this situation. The possible approaches to treatment include breast-conserving therapy alone (removal of the mass), breast-conserving therapy with radiation therapy, or modified radical mastectomy. Also, the addition of chemotherapy and/or tamoxifen may be considered. Just as the decisions to screen and to diagnose are made independently, so are treatment decisions. The first decision is to treat the local disease. A decision must be made as to which of the approaches will afford the individual the best local control of her breast cancer, with the least morbidity and maintaining the best quality of life. Second, the decision of whether or not to treat the woman with chemotherapy is dependent on the characteristics of the tumor and the presence or absence of tumor-positive axillary nodes. In most situations tamoxifen is prescribed for postmenopausal women with a diagnosis of breast cancer. Each of these decisions is made within the context of what is in the best interest of the individual woman. The decision concerning the extent of therapy, in particular, whether to treat the older adult with adjuvant radiation or chemotherapy, remains uncertain. Little data exist for the older person concerning the outcome from aggressive treatment for the various cancers. This lack of data is due, in part, to the lack of clinical trials that include a significant sample of older adults in the study (Ganz, 1993). Therefore studies that include a significant sample of older individuals are needed. Data from these studies would assist providers and patients in the difficult treatment decisions with which they are often faced.

The health care team must weigh the interaction of a composite of factors when determining the efficacy of screening, making decisions concerning which tests to use for diagnosis, and deciding whether to and how aggressively to treat the older adult. Throughout this process the preferences of the older adult must be included in the decision-making process.

■ Major Therapeutic Modalities

The major therapeutic modalities used in the treatment of cancer include surgery, radiation therapy, chemotherapy, hormonal therapy, and biologic therapy. The choice of therapy is dependent on such factors as the type of cancer, the extent of disease at diagnosis (i.e., presence or absence of metastasis), tumor aggressivity, and the presence of certain prognostic factors.

SURGERY

Surgery has been and remains one of the mainstays of cancer therapy. Its use can be traced to ancient times. For example, at the beginning of the Christian era, surgery for breast cancer was described by Leonides (De Moulin, cited in Lippman et al., 1989). Although surgery is frequently the first approach to therapy, an enhanced understanding of tumor biology, introduction of new therapeutic techniques, earlier stage of disease at diagnosis, and a greater reliance on interdisciplinary approaches to care have all contributed to changing the overall complexion of cancer therapy (Kalinowski, 1993). Surgery is used to establish a diagnosis of cancer, to determine the extent of disease (stage), to treat the primary cancer with curative intent, and to provide palliation in more advanced stages of disease. Although in some situations surgery is the only therapy, it must be remembered that it is a local therapy. Therefore surgery is frequently followed by additional therapies that are discussed in the following sections. The use of combination therapy in the older adult has not been well studied. Clinical trials that examine the effects of combination therapies on quality of life and morbidity and mortality in the older person are needed.

Two major factors may influence the choice of surgery as a therapeutic modality in the older adult. First, research has demonstrated that surgery in the older adult carries morbidity and mortality similar to those seen in the younger adult when controlled for comorbid conditions and other physiologic parameters (Cohen, 1994). Second, older adults may choose surgery over other modalities, such as radiation therapy. This choice is frequently related to a desire to treat the cancer in the most expeditious manner and "get on with one's life." This choice of surgical treatment over more time-consuming breast-conserving surgery with adjuvant radiation therapy was observed in older women with a diagnosis of breast cancer who described their experiences during participation in focus groups (C.B. Burnett, B. Kraling, & J.H. Rowland, personal communication, 1995).

RADIATION THERAPY

Radiation therapy is a local modality that can be used as primary therapy with curative intent, as

Aging Alert
Warning signs for potential surgical complications

- Existence of comorbid conditions
- Extensive surgery
- Psychologic distress or fear of surgery
- Potential risk of anesthesia
- Potential for infection

Aging Alert
Warning signs of complications from radiation therapy

- Skin: potential dryness, desquamation, infection
- Mucous membranes: sloughing, alterations in taste, decreased saliva
- Alterations in nutrition, weight loss
- Target organ injury (e.g., cardiac or pulmonary)
- Weakness and/or fatigue

adjuvant therapy with surgery and/or chemotherapy, or as palliative therapy. Radiation therapy, particularly in the older adult, may be the initial treatment of choice to help decrease tumor size and reduce the need for extensive surgery that may convey significantly more morbidity. In some situations (e.g., in prostate and breast cancers), radiation therapy and surgery have been shown to provide equivalent outcomes with regard to overall survival. Choices that have emerged in such therapies are particularly beneficial to the older adult for whom biologic, social, and psychologic factors may limit the feasibility of one particular modality. The side effects that accompany radiation therapy must be considered when suggesting this as a therapeutic modality. The effects of radiation therapy on normal tissue are said to be more pronounced in the older adult (Cohen, 1994). It should be remembered that side effects from radiation therapy are generally limited to the site at which the therapy is delivered. However, when radiation therapy is delivered to organs that are experiencing the normal decline that occurs with aging (e.g., salivary glands, mucous membranes, and skin), the effects potentially will be magnified. Fatigue is another type of side effect experienced by most people who receive radiation therapy. In the older adult,

fatigue may result in significant alterations in the quality of life and the ability to carry out ADLs.

CHEMOTHERAPY

Chemotherapy administration poses significant management problems for all individuals, not just older adults. A major reason for the problems relates to the issues of pharmacokinetics and pharmacodynamics. Pharmacokinetics refers to the action taken by the body on the drug, and pharmacodynamics refers to the action of the drug on the body (Egorin, 1993). The pharmacodynamic effects of chemotherapy are both therapeutic and potentially toxic. Drug therapy in general is designed to have a maximum therapeutic effect with little or no side effects. In cancer chemotherapy, this goal is modified somewhat. The aim is still to have a maximum therapeutic effect; however, there is an expectation that there will be side effects. The level or degree of side effects is closely monitored.

No studies have clearly demonstrated a difference in tumor response from chemotherapy in older versus younger adults (Cohen, 1994). However, in the older adult the dosing is complicated by (1) the effects of normal aging on body systems, (2) the presence of comorbid conditions, and (3) polypharmacy. The changes associated with normal aging may affect the processes of absorption, distribution, metabolism, and excretion. Specifically, the changes may include decreases in body tissue mass, decreases in renal and hepatic functioning, changes in gastric absorption and motility, and alteration in bone marrow reserve (Egorin, 1993). Measuring the effects of these changes is less than an exact science and requires the practitioner to carefully evaluate the physiologic age of the individual.

The effects of comorbidity and polypharmacy are frequently linked. For example, the older adult is more likely to have made long-term use of such agents as allopurinol, barbiturates, or acetaminophen that may minimize or exaggerate age-related hepatic changes (Egorin, 1993).

Clearly, providing for the correct dose that produces an appropriate therapeutic level within some acceptable range of toxicity is essential. To achieve this goal, approaches to therapy must be individualized. As stated earlier, chronologic age, in and of itself, is not a sufficient parameter to guide therapeutic management. Physiologic age, to the extent possible, needs to be determined by assessing body system functions. Table 19-2 provides an overview of body systems, alterations related to aging, assessment factors for chemotherapy, and some of the major chemotherapy drugs that affect those systems.

Health care professionals must be willing to accept the underlying principle inherent in cancer chemotherapy that there will be some toxicity. Underdosing as a means to prevent side effects may cause patients more harm in that they are receiving medication designed to kill cancer cells in less than therapeutic doses. Decisions to treat with chemotherapy must be made with the older adult, providing sufficient information so that informed decisions are possible. Nurses must be able to monitor the response to the drug, record and treat its side effects, and educate patient and family concerning their individual responsibilities.

Aging Alert
Warning signs of complications from chemotherapy
- Nausea and vomiting resulting in malnutrition
- Depletion in marrow reserve resulting in infection
- Alopecia resulting in alterations in body image
- Pain as a result of therapy
- Constipation as a result of altered elimination
- Mucositis

■ Future Goals in Cancer Prevention, Control, and Treatment

Projections on the number of older adults by the year 2030 indicate that there will be more than 55 million people 65 years of age or older. This number will account for approximately 20% of the population (Monfardini & Yancik, 1993). Also, an increased number of individuals will be at risk for the development of cancer. Improved treatments for cardiovascular diseases and those of infectious origin result in more individuals surviving and subsequently being at risk for cancer. The significant increase in older adults who will require cancer care clearly makes research on aging a national priority.

A variety of initiatives have evolved in response to these factors. The significance of these factors for nursing lies in the implications for clinical practice and research. Specifically, nurses in general, as well as advanced practice nurses, will need to educate themselves to the needs of the older adult as they relate to aging and the potential development of cancer, and to develop

TABLE 19-2 Chemotherapy and the older adult

System	Alterations related to aging	Assessment factors	Therapeutic measures
Cardiovascular	Decreased compliance and elasticity in both peripheral vessels and heart; decreased maximum heart rate; increased peripheral vascular resistance	Blood pressure; pulse; electrocardiogram volume	Doxorubicin
Pulmonary	Decreased elasticity; decreased ciliary activity; decreased respiratory muscular strength	Tidal volume; vital capacity in total oxygen consumption; sensitivity skin test	Bleomycin
Wound healing	Slower healing due to decreased cell proliferation and collagen production and to decreased skin thickness and loss of subcutaneous tissue; decreased muscle and bone weight and mass	Mobility	Surgery resulting in immobility
Endocrine	Changes most likely to occur during time of stress (increase in basal and stimulated plasma norepinephrine concentrations; impaired release of insulin resulting in impaired use of glucose)	Blood chemistry	Surgery and chemotherapy
Central nervous	Loss of neurons in cerebral cortex, cerebellum, and hippocampus; lipofuscin pigment accumulation; loss of brain weight and cerebral blood flow; confusion; postoperative delirium	Mental status; peripheral neuropathy	Cerebellar toxicity from cytosine, arabinoside; peripheral toxicity from vincristine
Special senses	Visual and hearing changes; changes in taste and smell; decreased pain sensation	Hearing and visual testing before, during, and at completion	Chemotherapy; radiation therapy to head and neck
Hematopoietic	Diminished hematopoiesis during increased demand	Complete blood counts	Chemotherapy; radiation therapy
Gastrointestinal	Decreased nausea	Nutritional status	Cyclophosphamide
Hepatorenal	Decreased drug metabolism	Liver function tests; creatinine clearance	Platinum methotrexate

From Cohen, 1994a.

BOX 19-2 RESEARCH REGARDING PATTERNS OF CARE FOR OLDER ADULT CANCER PATIENTS

National Institute of Medicine priority areas	Subjects of National Cancer Institute and National Institute on Aging funded projects
Basic biomedical research	Altered drug metabolism and enhanced toxicity
	Pharmacokinetics and metabolism of antineoplastic agents
Clinical research	Toxicity of chemotherapy
	Patterns of care and incidence of comorbidity
Behavioral and social research	Analysis of relationships between age, diagnosis, and treatment
	Symptom management
	Social support and relation to outcome
Research on the delivery of health services	Variations in patterns of medical care between older adults and the young
	Effects of age on stage of disease at diagnosis
Research in biomedical ethics	Decision making in older adults and responses to treatment
	Physicians' attitudes toward treatment of older adults and relation to treatment choice
General	Survey in patterns of care in radiation therapy

appropriate intervention strategies designed to meet these needs. Collaboration among nurses and other health care personnel is essential to this process.

In 1984 the National Institutes of Health's National Cancer Institute (NCI) and the National Institute on Aging supported 11 projects designed to identify patterns of care for older adult cancer patients. These projects focused on the natural history of cancer in the older adult; treatment patterns; the interaction of comorbidity, aging, and cancer; and the professional skills necessary to provide optimum cancer care for the older adult (NCI, 1987). Findings from these studies provided some of the first information concerning patterns of care for individuals age 65 years and older. Box 19-2 summarizes these initiatives.

In 1991 the Institute of Medicine of the National Academy of Sciences released a report that delineated 15 high-priority research areas designed to increase knowledge of the aging process and enhance understanding of factors that contribute to quality of life (QOL) in the older adult (Lonergan & Krevans, 1991). Of the 15 areas, the majority of them are relevant to the individual at risk for the development of cancer. These areas focus on biologic aspects of oncogenesis, prevention and control, clinical management, social and psychologic factors, ethical issues concerning allocation of resources and treatment decisions, and access to and costs of care. Box 19-3 summarizes these areas.

In 1991 the U.S. Department of Health and Human Services (USDHHS) published *Healthy*

BOX 19-3 A NATIONAL AGENDA FOR RESEARCH ON AGING: RELEVANCE TO CANCER

High-priority research areas	Specific research areas
Basic biomedical research	Cellular regulation and repair
Clinical research	Prevention, management, and rehabilitation
	Mismanagement of medications: lack of compliance; polypharmacy; underdosing and overdosing
	Interaction of age-dependent physiologic changes and cancer
	Health service delivery systems designed to reduce morbidity and mortality
	Targeted diseases such as cancer, infectious diseases, and diminished immunologic competence
Behavioral and social research	Relations among social, psychologic, and biologic factors in aging
	Effects of changes in the social structure on performance, productivity, health, and well-being
Research on the delivery of health services	Long-term care and continuity of care
	Cost and financing of care
	Availability of drug therapy and its costs
	Prevention of disability and disease and promotion of health
Research in biomedical ethics	Decisions on life-sustaining therapies
	Decision making concerning appropriateness and availability of therapies
	Equity of access to care, clinical trials, and research
General	Adequate resources for delivery of appropriate care
	Sufficient funds for centers of education and research
	Increased support for research infrastructure

Adapted from Lonergan, E.T., & Krevans, J.R. (1991). A national agenda for research on aging. *New England Journal of Medicine 324*(25), 1825-1828. Copyright 1991. Massachusetts Medical Society. All rights reserved.

People 2000: National Health Promotion and Disease Prevention Objectives. A major focus of this initiative was to provide health promotion and disease prevention guidelines for major diseases across the life span and among special populations. The most important aspect of health promotion among older people is to maintain health and functional independence (US-DHHS, 1991). Determining why cancer incidence and death rates differ with advancing age is the only high-priority research need that specifically focuses on older individuals. Five "key

Healthy People 2000 Objectives

General categories		Specific categories
General health status	17.1	Increase years of healthy life to at least 65 years. (Baseline: An estimated 62 years in 1980.)
Risk reduction	21.1f	Increase to at least 40% the proportion of adults aged 65 and older who have received . . . all of the screening . . . appropriate for their age and gender . . .
Key services: general	8.8	Increase to at least 90% the proportion of people aged 65 and older who had the opportunity to participate during the preceding year in at least one organized health promotion program through a senior center, lifecare facility, or other community-based setting that serves older adults.
Key services: breast cancer screening	16.11	Increase to at least . . . 60% those aged 50 and older who have received [a clinical breast examination] within the preceding 1 to 2 years. (Baseline: 25% of women aged 50 and older "within the preceding 2 years" in 1987.)
Key services: cervical cancer screening	16.12b	Increase to at least 95% the proportion of women aged 70 and older with uterine cervix who have ever received a Pap test, and to at least 70% those who received a Pap test within the preceding 1 to 3 years. (Baseline: 76% "ever" and 44% "within the preceding 3 years" in 1987.)
Key services: fecal occult blood testing	16.13	Increase to at least 50% the proportion of people aged 50 and older who have received fecal occult blood testing within the preceding 1 to 2 years, and to at least 40% those who have ever received proctosigmoidoscopy. (Baseline: 27% received fecal occult blood testing during the preceding 2 years in 1987; 25% had ever received proctosigmoidoscopy in 1987.)
Key services: primary care	16.14	Increase to at least 40% the proportion of people aged 50 and older visiting a primary care provider in the preceding year who have received oral, skin, and digital rectal examinations during one such visit. (Baseline: An estimated 27% received a digital rectal exam during a physician visit within the preceding year in 1987.)

From U.S. Department of Health and Human Services. (1990). *Healthy People 2000: National health promotion and disease prevention objectives* (DHHS Pub. No. [PHS] 91-50212). Washington, DC: U.S. Government Printing Office.

Health Promotion
Cancer prevention

- Avoid overexposure to the sun.
- Eliminate smoking.
- Cut down on excessive alcohol use.
- Eat a diet high in fruits, vegetables, and fibers.
- Exercise daily.
- Participate in regular screenings and self-examinations to detect cancers at an early stage. Early detection can lead to a better prognosis.

services and protection objectives" that specifically target older adults are presented in the *Healthy People 2000 Objectives* box.

The Oncology Nursing Society has long been a champion of care issues for special populations. In 1992 the organization published a fact sheet on cancer and the older adult. This fact sheet serves as a resource for nurses, other health care providers, and other disciplines interested in care of the older adult with cancer. The background material summarizes major issues of concern in providing care to this population. Some of these issues include insufficient financial resources that influence compliance with treatment regimens; problems related to more advanced stage of disease at time of diagnosis as a result of delay in seeking health care; lack of accurate and complete information about cancer, its risks, and the need for early detection and treatment; and limited access to care (*Fact Sheet*, 1992). Also in 1992, the society published the *Oncology Nursing Society Position Paper on Cancer and Aging* (Boyle, et al., 1992), which delineated ten position statements that serve to guide the nurse caring for individuals 65 years of age or older throughout their experiences with cancer. Box 19-4 presents these statements.

A number of research initiatives supported by the NCI and the American Cancer Society have subsequently focused on various aspects of older adult cancer care (NCI, 1987, 1993). Most recently the Agency for Health Care Policy and Research funded an initiative designed to examine the care and cost outcomes of older adult women with a diagnosis of early-stage breast cancer (PORT, 1994). The American Cancer Society has convened several conferences that focus on older adults at risk for cancer and on issues surrounding their diagnosis, treatment, and supportive care (Cancer, 1991 & 1994). Relevance of the guidelines and findings from these conferences has been discussed throughout the chapter.

National attention on issues facing the older adult with cancer, partly as a result of lobbying efforts by groups such as the American Association of Retired Persons (AARP), has contributed to changes in approaches to care and to dispelling myths and biases. Research initiatives have been supported by the federal government and professional organizations. Future research efforts must continue to focus on the special needs of the individual facing a diagnosis of cancer. In particular, efforts must be championed toward enhancing the early detection of cancer throughout the individual's life span. Nursing's role in this effort is clear. Primary care and political advocacy are but two areas in which nurses are well positioned to effect change.

■ Cancer Risk Assessment

Because the incidence of cancer increases with age, performing a cancer risk assessment in older adults is as important as it is in younger individuals. Basic elements of a cancer risk assessment include obtaining a detailed personal and family medical history (White & Spitz, 1993). In addition, the nurse should obtain information about the older adults' level of understanding of cancer and their potential risk, physical ability to perform routine screening procedures (e.g., breast self-examination), and desire to participate in cancer screening.

BOX 19-4 POSITION STATEMENTS ON CANCER AND AGING,
ONCOLOGY NURSING SOCIETY (1992)

1. It is imperative that oncology nurses recognize personal biases toward aging and older adults that may interfere with the delivery of quality nursing care.
2. It is imperative that oncology nurses advocate cancer prevention and early detection activities for older adults.
3. It is imperative that oncology nurses acknowledge the dynamic and complex interrelationships between cancer and aging that affect cancer nursing care.
4. It is imperative that oncology nurses intervene to prevent or minimize the unique age-specific sequelae of cancer and its management.
5. It is imperative that oncology nurses integrate comprehensive gerontologic assessment into the nursing care of older adults.
6. It is imperative that oncology nurses assess the availability and capability of the support networks of older patients and their significant others.
7. It is imperative that oncology nurses increase communication with colleagues about older adults with cancer to enhance problem solving in a variety of settings and at different points along the cancer continuum.
8. It is imperative that oncology nurses consider age-related factors that affect learning and performance of self-care activities related to the cancer experience.
9. It is imperative that oncology nurses maximize their advocacy role in ethical decision making relative to quality of life of older people with cancer.
10. It is imperative that oncology nurses recognize the effects of health care policy on the nursing care of older adults who have or who are at risk for cancer.

A goal of cancer risk assessment is to avoid the consequence of missed opportunities. Missed opportunities result if there is a failure to perform cancer risk assessment when an opportunity presents itself. These missed opportunities occur when an individual seeks episodic or chronic care from a provider, sees a provider who assumes that primary health care needs are being given by another provider, relies on misinformation concerning efficacy of screening for the older adult, and/or is fearful of and resistant to having screening examinations performed. Data suggest that compliance with screening guidelines can be increased if these examinations are incorporated into routine health care (Mandelblatt et al., 1993). This section focuses on elements of a cancer risk assessment and describes approaches designed

to incorporate this assessment for older adults into routine care so as to avoid these missed opportunities.

A variety of reminder systems have been reported that are designed to increase the frequency with which an older adult is screened for cancer. Some of these include chart reminder flow sheets, personal contact by telephone and/or mail, and other, more general approaches such as use of clinic posters, mass media, and community agencies. A recent study found that when nurse practitioners (NPs) personally approached underserved older women attending a primary care clinic about participating in breast and cervical cancer screening, the compliance rate was significantly higher for those approached by the NP than for those seeing physicians who were using a standard chart reminder card (Mandelblatt et al., 1993). Findings such as these have significant implications for nursing practice. These findings suggest that nurses are well positioned to perform a cancer risk assessment on patients who are attending a clinic for routine or episodic care; to determine the date of a previous mammogram, Pap test, digital rectal examination, prostate-specific antigen (PSA), stool blood test, and/or sigmoidoscopy; to recommend appropriate screening tests that are consistent with ACS guidelines; to schedule necessary screening tests; and to follow up to ensure that the appropriate tests have been obtained. Refer to Table 19-1 for recommended ACS screening guidelines.

■ Nursing Process

ASSESSMENT

Assessment of cancer risk status is appropriate whether a patient is being seen for the first time in a clinic, is being admitted to an acute care setting, or is a resident of a long-term care facility. It is essential to carefully differentiate between normal symptoms of aging and those that suggest early-stage cancer. Cancer checkups, as recommended by the ACS, should be completed every year for individuals over 40 years of age. This checkup includes collection of standard demographic information (e.g., age, gender, marital status, height, weight, alcohol and/or smoking history, and exposure to environmental risk factors); recording of personal and family history of cancer; a physical assessment for cancers of the breast, ovary, prostate, lymph nodes, oral cavity, skin, testicles, and thyroid according to recommended ACS guidelines (Mettlin & Dodd, 1992); recording of changes in body functions (e.g., weight loss, blood in stools, and changes in appetite); and assessment of general cancer knowledge, myths and biases, cultural factors, previous screening behavior patterns, and changes in cognition and physical ability that might influence ability to perform self-examination. See Table 19-3. For the purpose of

example, many of the responses used in the table are vague and might easily give the impression of merely reporting symptoms associated with normal aging.

NURSING DIAGNOSES

The potential for development of cancer exists for all older adults. A review of the findings from the assessment will enable the nurse to determine a cancer risk profile for the individual patient. The data may reveal a strong family history of cancer (i.e., first-degree relatives with a history of breast, ovarian, and colorectal cancers), significant environmental exposure to known carcinogens, long history of tobacco use, or severe sunburns as a young child or adult. Although many of the familial cancers would be expected to have occurred at an earlier age, a strong family history might be an indication that members of the family other than the patient are at increased risk. It would be important to gather specific information concerning age at onset, type of cancer, and outcome for each affected individual so that appropriate action might be taken.

To accurately determine a person's cancer risk, a variety of factors, including the individual's age, must be considered (Fink, 1991; Frank-Stromberg & Rohan, 1992):

HIGH RISK FOR THE DEVELOPMENT OF BREAST CANCER

- Age
- Family history of breast cancer or genetic predisposition
- Young age at menarche, first full-term pregnancy after 30 years of age, late menopause
- Nulliparity
- History of ovarian or colorectal cancer
- Alcohol use

RISK FOR THE DEVELOPMENT OF OVARIAN CANCER

- Age
- History of breast or colorectal cancer

TABLE 19-3 Cancer risk assessment for the older adult

Assessment factors	Sample questions	Possible responses	Action
Demographic factors date of birth, gender, height and weight (changes), marital status	Has your weight changed in the past 6 months?	Lost 10 lb	Assess changes in eating and bowel habits
Date of last exam Reason for current exam	What was the date of your most recent health exam? What brought you to the clinic today? What do you expect from today's visit?	May 1, 1995 Tired all the time, no appetite To find out what's wrong	Assess changes in emotional, sleep, and physical activity patterns
Smoking history: cigarettes, cigars, pipes, other	Do you currently use any tobacco products? Have you ever used any tobacco products? How many cigarettes do you smoke a day?	Yes	Assess presence or absence of cough, sputum, shortness of breath
Alcohol history: amount, type, frequency	Do you currently drink alcohol? What type? How many drinks per week?	15 to 20 Yes Wine 5 glasses a week	Is this your usual amount?
Nutrition history	How would you describe your eating habits? What types of food do you eat a lot of? What foods do you avoid?	Nibble frequently Chicken Meat No	Assess whether easily satiated, feelings of bloating, stool composition
History of cancer	Have you ever been diagnosed with cancer?		
Family history of cancer	Has anyone in your family been diagnosed with cancer? If yes, obtain details of age at diagnosis and primary site	Yes (father: colon; sister: ovarian)	Assess personal risk factors for these and other familial cancers
Cancer knowledge, cultural biases and myths	Can you describe what you think cancer is? What do you believe causes cancer? Do you think that you are at risk for cancer?	Refer to Box 19-1	Correct misinformation, myths, and biases
Cognitive and physical abilities	Have you noticed any changes in your ability to take care of yourself (either emotional or physical)?	Arthritis limits mobility and sensation	Plan for teaching self-examination methods according to limitations

- Family history of ovarian cancer
- Low parity

RISK FOR THE DEVELOPMENT OF CERVICAL CANCER

- Multiple sexual partners
- Intercourse before age 20
- HPV infection (human papilloma virus)
- Smoking

RISK FOR THE DEVELOPMENT OF COLORECTAL CANCER

- Personal or family history (first-degree relatives) of polyps
- History of polyposis syndromes
- High-fat diet
- Personal history of inflammatory bowel disease

RISK FOR THE DEVELOPMENT OF PROSTATE CANCER

- Age
- Being black North American man

RISK FOR THE DEVELOPMENT OF ORAL CANCER

- Poor dental hygiene
- Tobacco use
- Alcohol use

RISK FOR THE DEVELOPMENT OF LUNG CANCER

- Age
- Smoking
- Asbestos and other environmental or occupational exposures

RISK FOR THE DEVELOPMENT OF MELANOMA AND NONMELANOMA SKIN CANCERS

- Age
- Dysplastic nevi
- Family history
- Being white and fair-skinned
- Severe sunburns, particularly before age 18

The risk for development of cancer and the stage at which it is diagnosed may be influenced by frequency and adequacy of cancer screening. A woman who has not had a Pap test since the birth of her last child, or a man who avoids a digital rectal examination of his prostate, increases the chances that disease, when detected, will be at a more advanced stage. Therefore the nurse compiles the data gathered in the initial assessment and determines appropriate action for screening.

PLANNING AND GOAL IDENTIFICATION

Compliance with cancer screening guidelines is the primary desired outcome or goal. Increased knowledge on the part of the patient about cancer, its causes, and its risks is another desired outcome, which contributes to compliance with screening guidelines.

Providing the older adult with feedback is a key aspect of conducting a cancer risk assessment. This feedback provides older adults with an opportunity to ask questions concerning their understanding of the findings from the assessment and enables the nurse to validate the findings. A plan might include a review of the assessment at the time it is conducted or the scheduling of a future meeting. Studies that have looked at compliance with screening guidelines—in particular, guidelines for mammograms—show that tests that are performed at the time of an initial visit, rather than scheduled in the future, have a higher compliance rate (Mandelblatt et al., 1993). One might suggest from these findings that immediate discussion of the findings from the cancer risk assessment with the older adult would have a greater impact on compliance. Therefore it is suggested that at least a preliminary review of the assessment be conducted on the same day it is completed. If feasible, set aside time for discussion of the results of the cancer risk assessment at the conclusion of the examination, and inform the patient beforehand of this arrangement.

Discuss possible approaches to cancer screening and risk behavior modification with the patient after reviewing the findings from the assessment. Assist the patient in setting achievable goals that consider demographic, personal, social, and fiscal factors.

IMPLEMENTATION

Intervention strategies include education of the older adult about cancer, cancer screening tests, and self-examination. Provide the individual with appropriate educational materials (e.g., copies of ACS cancer screening guidelines or other NCI and ACS publications), resource telephone numbers (1-800-4-CANCER, National Institutes of Health, or local ACS and screening clinics), and information on availability of financial assistance.

Strategies have been developed for increasing compliance with guidelines among economically disadvantaged older adults. These include the elderly educator (EE) method, adaptation for aging changes (AAC) method, and combination method (Weinrich et al., 1992). The elderly educator method was designed to use older adults as educators in an ACS colorectal cancer program (Weinrich et al., 1992). The underlying tenet of this approach is that through the use of role models with whom individuals can identify, common myths and misinformation concerning colorectal screening can be dispelled. The adaptation for aging changes method uses approaches to education that account for changes occurring with aging (i.e., increased time needed for processing information, and changes in sensory abilities, such as visual acuity and tactile sensitivity). The combination method is the EE and AAC methods combined. The findings from the study clearly demonstrate that the combination method produces a higher level of participation in colorectal screening by socioeconomically disadvantaged older adults. Nurses can adapt these methods to develop and implement intervention strategies for the variety of cancers for which approaches to screening and early detection are available.

EVALUATION

Evaluation of intervention strategies provides information necessary both for improving the effectiveness of the educational approach and ultimately for improving older adults' adherence to cancer screening guidelines. Evaluation will uncover factors that influence compliance—for example, lack of comprehension of educational material, altered sensory or motor ability necessary to perform self-examination, cultural factors, lack of desire, or a combination of factors that contribute to misunderstanding the importance of carrying out these screening behaviors.

Knowledge of personal cancer risk and appropriate screening guidelines can be evaluated by a test designed to measure comprehension. Return demonstrations can be used to determine an individual's ability to perform self-examination procedures. Evaluation of compliance with cancer screening guidelines can be accomplished by checking with individual patients (verbal report) during routine primary or episodic care, checking patient records to see if the results of a screening test have been reported, or checking with the relevant department (e.g., x-ray or laboratory) for the test results.

In summary, the nursing process provides an organized approach to performing a cancer risk assessment. A cancer risk assessment should be carried out for any individual over 40 years of age; however, it increases in importance for those over 65. Patients need to be made aware that they are never too old to alter outcomes; for example, stopping smoking can always have beneficial effects. Practitioners need to be educated on the fact that patients are never too old to be screened for cancer. The combination of patient and practitioner education about cancer prevention and control is one approach that will work toward decreasing morbidity and mortality from those cancers for which screening is efficacious.

REFERENCES

Bergman, L., Dekker, G., van Kerkhoff, E.H.M., Peterse, H.L., van Dongen, J.A., & van Leeuwen, F.E. (1991). Influence of age and comorbidity on treatment choice and survival in elderly patients with breast cancer. *Breast Cancer Research and Treatment, 18,* 189-198.

Berkman, B., Rohan, B., & Sampson, S. (1994). Myths and biases related to cancer in the elderly. *Cancer, 74*(Suppl. 7), 2004-2008.

Boyle, D.M., Engelking, C., Blesch, K.S., Dodge, J., Sarna, L., & Weinrich, S. (1992). Oncology Nursing Society position paper on cancer and aging: The mandate for oncology nursing. *Oncology Nursing Forum, 19*(6), 913-933.

Brawley, O.W. (1995). Are mass cancer screenings effective? Con. *ONS News, 10*(1), 7.

Cohen, H.J. (1994a). Biology of aging as related to cancer. *Cancer, 74*(Suppl.), 2092-2100.

Cohen, H.J. (1994b). Oncology and aging: General principles of cancer in the elderly. In W.R. Hazzard, E.L. Bierman, J.P. Blass, W.H. Ettinger, J.B. Halter, & R. Andres (Eds.), *Principles of geriatric medicine and gerontology* (3rd ed., pp. 77-89). New York: McGraw-Hill.

Cutler, R.G. & Semsei, I. (1989). Development, cancer and aging: Possible common mechanism of action and regulation. *Journals of Gerontology, 44*(1), 25-34.

Egorin, M.J. (1993). Cancer pharmacology in the elderly. *Seminars in Oncology, 20*(1), 43-49.

Fact sheet: Cancer and the elderly. (1992, April). Oncology Nursing Society.

Fink, D.J. (1991). Guidelines for the cancer related checkup: Recommendations and rationale. Reprinted from *American Cancer Society textbook of clinical oncology.* (91-50M, No. 3347-PE). Atlanta: American Cancer Society.

Frank-Stromberg, M. & Rohan, K. (1992). Nursing's involvement in the primary and secondary prevention of cancer: Nationally and internationally. *Cancer Nursing, 15*(2), 79-108.

Ganz, P.A. (1993). Age and gender as factors in cancer therapy. *Clinics in Geriatric Medicine, 9*(1), 145-155.

Greenfield, S., Blanco, D.M., Elashoff, R.M., et al. (1987). Patterns of care related to age of breast cancer patients. *Journal of the American Medical Association, 257,* 2766-2770.

Guadagnoli, E., Weitberg, A., Mor, V., Silliman, R.A., Glicksman, A.S., & Cummings, F.J. (1990). The influence of patient age on the diagnosis and treatment of lung and colorectal cancer. *Archives of Internal Medicine, 150,* 1485-1490.

Holmes, F.F., Wilson, J., Blesch, K.S., Kaesberg, P.R., Miller, R., & Sprott, R. (1991). Biology of cancer and aging. *Cancer, 68*(Suppl.) 2525-2526.

Kalinowski, B.H. (1993). Surgical therapy. In S.L. Groenwald, M.H. Frogge, M. Goodman, & C.H. Yarbro (Eds.), *Cancer nursing: Principles and practice* (3rd ed., pp. 222-234). Boston: Jones and Bartlett.

Lippman, M.E., Lichter, A.S., & Danforth, D.N. (1989). *Diagnosis and management of breast cancer* (p. 96). Philadelphia: W.B. Saunders.

Lonergan, E.T., & Krevans, J.R. (1991). A national agenda for research on aging. *New England Journal of Medicine, 324*(25), 1825-1828.

Mandelblatt, J., Traxler, M., Lakin, P., Thomas, L., Chauhan, P., Matseoane, S., Kanetsky, P., & Harlem Study Team. (1993). A nurse practitioner intervention to increase breast and cervical cancer screening for poor, elderly black women. *Journal of General Internal Medicine, 8*(4), 173-178.

Mettlin, C. & Dodd, G.D. (1992). Guidelines for the cancer related checkup: An update. Reprinted from *Ca-A cancer journal for clinicians, 41,* 279-282. (92-10M, No. 3402).

Miller, R.A. (1991). Gerontology as oncology: Research on aging as the key to the understanding of cancer. *Cancer, 68*(Suppl.), 2496-2501.

Miller, R.A. (1994). The biology of aging and longevity. In W.R. Hazzard, E.L. Bierman, J.P. Blass, W.H. Ettinger, J.B. Halter, & R. Andres (Eds.), *Principles of geriatric medicine and gerontology* (3rd ed., pp. 3-18). New York: McGraw-Hill.

Monfardini, S., & Yancik, R. (1993). Cancer in the elderly: Meeting the challenge of an aging population. *Journal of the National Cancer Institute, 85*(7), 532-538.

Mor, V., Masterson-Allen, S., Goldberg, R.J., et al. (1985). Relationship between age at diagnosis and treatments received by cancer patients. *Journal of the American Geriatrics Society, 33,* 585-589.

Padberg, R.M. (1995). Are mass cancer screenings effective? Pro. *ONS News, 10*(1), 7.

PORT. (1994). *Care, costs, and outcomes of localized breast cancer in elderly women.* (Report 1 RO1 HSO8395-0115). Agency for Health Policy and Research.

Samet, J., Hunt, W.C., Key, C., et al. (1986). Choice of cancer therapy varies with age of patient. *Journal of the American Medical Association, 255,* 3385-3390.

Schwab, R., Walters, C.A., & Weksler, M.E. (1989). Host defense mechanisms and aging. *Seminars in Oncology, 16*(1), 20-27.

Weinrich, S.P., Weinrich, M.C., Boyd, M.D., Atwood, J., & Cervenka, B. (1992). Effective approaches for increasing compliance with American Cancer Society recommendations in socioeconomically disadvantaged populations. In *Proceedings of the Second National Conference on Cancer Nursing Research.* Atlanta: American Cancer Society. (92-50M, No. 3320.01-PE).

NAME OF BEREAVED _____ DATE OF BIRTH _____

ADDRESS _____ PHONE _____

NAME OF DECEASED _____ DATE OF BIRTH _____

RELATIONSHIP TO DECEASED _____ DATE OF BIRTH _____

LENGTH OF RELATIONSHIP _____ ANNIVERSARY _____

PRIMARY NURSE _____

LIVING ARRANGEMENTS

OWN HOME _____ APARTMENT _____ OTHER _____

LIVING WITH _____ RELATIONSHIP _____

_____

_____

PHYSICAL STATUS

1. Sleeping pattern _____

2. Appetite _____ Weight-gain _____ loss _____

3. Substances used — alcohol _____ change in intake _____

cigarettes _____ change in intake _____

drugs _____ change in intake _____

4. Appearance — neat _____ unkempt _____

5. Health _____

ACTIVITY LEVEL

Increased _____ Decreased _____ Employed _____

Hobbies _____

PSYCHOLOGICAL EMOTIONAL STATUS

1. Affect: Appropriate _____ Flat _____ Labile _____

2. Expression of grief: Discussion of loss _____

guilt _____

anger _____

suicide _____

SUPPORT SYSTEMS

1. Family _____

2. Clergy _____

3. Quantity of contacts _____

4. Perceived quality of contact _____

ADDITIONAL CONCERNS

1. Other losses _____

2. Financial _____

3. Living arrangements _____

4. Major problems _____

OVERALL IMPRESSION

_____

_____

PLAN/INTERVENTION STRATEGY

_____

_____

_____

SIGNATURE _____

DATE _____

FIGURE 20-2 Bereavement—initial assessment form. (From Amenta. [1986]. *Nursing care of the terminally ill.* [pp. 247-262]. Philadelphia: Lippincott-Raven Publishers.)

NURSING DIAGNOSES

Numerous nursing diagnoses may be associated with bereavement in older adults. Among the possible nursing diagnoses are the following:

- Dysfunctional grieving
- Anxiety
- Denial, ineffective
- Fear
- Health maintenance, altered
- Role performance, altered
- Social interaction, impaired
- Spiritual distress (distress of the human spirit)

For each diagnosis, the nurse records the appropriate cause or related factors according to the patient data gathered during the assessment. The nursing diagnosis that is most directly related to bereavement following a loss is that of dysfunctional grieving. However, the focus of this chapter is on normal bereavement. By changing this from an actual nursing diagnosis to a potential nursing diagnosis (i.e., potential for dysfunctional grieving), it is possible to maintain the emphasis on normal bereavement.

PLANNING AND GOAL IDENTIFICATION

The plan of care depends on the nursing diagnoses identified as a result of the assessment. The nursing goals and strategies described here are meant to facilitate normal grieving and to prevent dysfunctional grieving.

Long-term goals for a diagnosis of potential for dysfunctional bereavement include the following:

1. The person will accommodate to the loss.
2. The person will reinvest in a new life.

Short-term goals include the following:

1. The person will verbalize feelings.
2. The person will cope adequately with the immediate physical and psychologic demands of bereavement.
3. The person will verbally acknowledge the loss.
4. The person will agree to use available social support.

IMPLEMENTATION

Nursing interventions for the bereaved span all settings. The major responsibilities of the nurse are encouragement and support, as this is an attempt to acknowledge loss. This may be accomplished by being physically and psychologically present and available to provide a sense of security. The nurse demonstrates an understanding of the loss and provides freedom to express the loss in an individual and unique way. If the person gives evidence of experiencing spiritual pain, the nurse can acknowledge presence of the pain and encourage the expectation that eventually it will subside.

There may be need for support and assistance in verbalizing feelings about the loss. To enable the verbalization, the nurse gives the person permission to identify, accept, and express all of the various emotions connected with grief. Opportunity can be provided for the person to cry or to talk if need be. It is not unusual to review and re-review the situation without interruption.

Nurses can provide the grieving person with factual information about bereavement. Realistic and practical help with immediate problems resulting from the loss can assist in moving through the grieving process. The person may experience frustration with self or others, and it is important to encourage patience.

Allow grievers to give themselves a respite from their grief, and encourage them to accept help and consolation from others. Maximum utilization of social support networks can often be key in the person's adaptation to loss. When appropriate, the nurse can provide information about bereavement support groups.

Accommodating to loss can be accomplished by helping the griever to develop a perspective on what it will mean to resolve the grief. This may include helping the person to develop a new identity and to learn new life skills. The nurse can help the person (1) to develop a new relationship with the deceased, based on the changed reality; (2) to find and utilize ways to

Family consent laws are different in every state. In some states, family members may make all health care decisions, whereas in others, a family member's authority to make health care decisions for an incapacitated relative is limited to situations in which a physician has certified that the patient is terminally ill. There is also usually a requirement that before a family member is authorized to act, the resident or patient must be certified as lacking capacity to make a health care decision. State law specifies both who can make such a certification and how.

Although physicians labor with a respect for life, which is the impetus for saving many lives, on occasion it appears to the medical provider that further treatment would be useless. The term often used is *medical futility*. And the issue is being debated "in multiple arenas: in courtrooms, in legislative halls, and at the bedside" (Darr, 1995). It is an issue that will call for understanding on the part of caregivers, patients, and patients' families if the difficult circumstances surrounding death are not to be made more extreme by arguments, lay and legal, over the bed of the dying person.

Even more emotionally charged is the issue of physician assistance in dying. The courts and legislatures are already grappling with this issue, in part because of the activities of Jack Kevorkian, M.D., and such groups as the Hemlock Society. The issue is a continuing and complex one, and one that our society is having a difficult time resolving. But it is also one about which a caregiver may be questioned by patients or their families. It is also one in which a caregiver may become personally involved through circumstances. Therefore it would be prudent to have thought through the issues as they apply to the patient involved, and to have formed one's views and reached an opinion calmly, before being asked in a difficult situation for advice, opinion, or assistance.

It may be helpful in trying to form conclusions in this area for the caregiver to reflect on the patient and to attempt to see the patient's view. Although not always agreeing with the patient's conclusions, the caregiver can always seek to enhance patient autonomy and respect any advance directives put in place by the patient for ensuring a death with dignity.

FINANCIAL AND PROPERTY MANAGEMENT PLANNING

Often compounding the problems that challenge older adults with respect to failing health is the situation of failing financial abilities. The costs of necessities such as food, lodging, and medical care often take an ever-increasing share of the older adult's income as prices rise and inflation takes its toll. Preserving savings and minimizing costs are ever-present goals that take careful management. Many older adults recognize this situation and desire to make plans to manage their finances and property.

One of the most common signs that people are thinking of their own death is their interest in making a will. Wills are commonly understood as disposing of the person's estate after death, offering an opportunity for the deceased to influence the disposition of the property, and serving as a last communication of the person's wishes. Although wills may be prepared by individuals on their own behalf, such wills often encounter difficulties in probate because of their failure to meet some arcane requirement of state law. Will law is notorious for its unique development in each state and for its complexities of execution. Older adults should be advised to obtain legal assistance in the preparation of their wills. Preparing a will is an overt step that a person takes toward acknowledging his or her mortality, and it is usually the first step of a planning nature that people take in response to their recognition of the fact that there are things they can do to influence how their affairs will be managed when they are no longer capable of managing them themselves. The peace of mind that comes from having taken a concrete step toward the uncertain future is important and may serve to make the person more inclined to make other types of plans.

The older adult may also take any of the steps that all citizens are entitled to take to manage their affairs. A "trust," a type of surrogate, to manage property, including real estate properties, can be established. A trust is a "person" as seen by the law and so can act as a surrogate for another person. Of course, there is a real person who takes the actions on behalf of the older adult, the "trustee," and the trustee can exercise the trust powers either now or in the future. If a trust is established by a living person, the powers and the resources given the trustee are detailed in a document called an "inter vivos" (living) trust, which is effective when signed. If the trust is established in the will of a person who has died, the powers and the resources given the trustee are detailed in a document called a "testamentary" trust, which is effective upon the death of the person making the will and trust. Trusts are also classified as revocable and nonrevocable, depending on whether the grantor has retained the power to modify or revoke the trust. For example, an older adult can prepare a revocable living trust that allows him or her the flexibility of revoking the trust if not satisfied with the arrangement, but that becomes irrevocable upon the older person's loss of capacity. The different types of trusts can have similar effectiveness in managing the affairs of the older adult, but choosing the type of trust to use has income and estate tax consequences and therefore requires professional assistance.

There are often specific things that the older adult or the surrogate can do to better manage the available resources, or to prepare for the eventual need to qualify for the Medicaid program discussed in a later section. For example, the older adult, or the older adult's surrogate, may be advised to prepare, and perhaps pay for, funeral arrangements in advance. Such a step often has the benefit of allowing older adults to express their desires in an effective way, whereas wills, which may contain instructions, are often not located or read until after the burial. And prepayment eases the burden survivors face in making decisions as to arrangements while under the stresses related to the death of the older person. Prepayment of funeral arrangements also removes countable assets from the Medicaid calculations.

Two types of commercial offerings are widely available to assist the older adult with financial concerns. Long-term care insurance is offered by various health insurance companies in response to the perceived concern on the part of older adults and their families regarding meeting the large, and increasing, costs of long-term care. These are insurance-type contracts designed to provide funds for paying the expenses of care provided in nursing homes or at home. Long-term care contracts are complex contracts with both a potential impact on the older adult's Medicaid eligibility and tax implications. A qualified advisor should be consulted in the selection and purchase of such insurance.

Another type of contract, sometimes confused with the long-term care insurance, is the contract for continuing care. This is a contract for services, such as care and housing, and it is discussed in the section on living arrangements.

Reverse mortgages are, in effect, loans on the equity of the older adult's home. These mortgages are offered by banks and have many of the characteristics of a typical mortgage, such as interest payments and claim on the property by the lender. The unique feature is that the amount borrowed is not paid all at once to purchase the home and repaid with interest over time, but rather, the amount "borrowed" is paid monthly to the borrower in amounts dependent on the interest rate, value of the equity, and term of the loan. Upon the death of the borrower, or sale of the home if earlier, the lender recoups the loan and interest from the value of the home that is then sold. As with the long-term care insurance, these are complex contracts and obtaining professional assistance is advised before assuming such a loan.

However, what happens when individuals are unable to make decisions or to communicate their choices? Many nursing home residents suffer from cognitive and physical impairments that affect their ability to reason and to communicate effectively. How does the law protect the rights of individuals who, because of these impairments, cannot protect themselves, and how do they manage their affairs? In such cases the laws provide for surrogates to act. As discussed previously, sometimes older adults have established their own surrogates and granted them the powers required. Sometimes there will be no surrogates appointed, nor family consent laws applicable, and at that time the family or caregivers will have to resort to the laws and courts of the appropriate state and have a surrogate appointed. Such surrogates are called "guardians," or, if the powers are less, "conservators." These surrogates, and how they are appointed, are discussed in the section on guardians and conservators.

Reporting laws

In addition to the statewide registry, all 50 states and the District of Columbia have some form of reporting system for monitoring and responding to abuse, neglect, and exploitation of vulnerable adults. Here again, state approaches vary tremendously. In 42 states the reporting system is mandatory. Of these 42 states, 14 impose a mandatory duty to report on any person with knowledge, or reasonable cause to believe, that a person under the statute has been abused, neglected, or exploited. In other states, only certain designated professionals are under such an imposition of mandatory duty. Generally speaking, in states with mandatory reporting laws, physicians, nurses, and other health care professionals are required to report cases of suspected adult abuse, neglect, and exploitation. There may be criminal penalties ranging from fines to imprisonment for failing to do so. In addition, in 17 states the abuse, neglect, or exploitation of a vulnerable adult is punishable as a criminal offense. These criminal sanctions are in addition to and not in lieu of existing criminal laws dealing with homicide, assault, rape, theft, and fraud. Many state laws protect reporters from liability, provided they have acted in good faith, and most state laws protect the confidentiality of the reporter (American Public Welfare Society and National Association of State Units on Aging, 1986).

In light of the sanctions that may attach, any professional who works with vulnerable adults should become familiar with state law provisions regarding adult protective services. Also, knowledge of how the state's adult protective services program operates may be useful in obtaining needed services for a patient who has been victimized. Many hospitals, nursing homes, and home care agencies provide in-service training to employees regarding these laws. If one of these institutions does not, training should be developed in this area, because ignorance of the law does not excuse a failure to report if indeed a report is required under state law.

Other laws affecting nursing home operation

Two other areas of law that play an important role in defining the rights and obligations of caregivers and residents are the general common law rules of tort law and contract law. They are called "common law" rules because they are court-made rules that have evolved over time through individual case decisions by judges.

Broadly speaking, a "tort" is a civil wrong for which a court will provide a remedy in the form of money damages. A tort may be either intentional or unintentional. An example of an intentional tort is the tort of assault, which occurs when an individual intentionally causes another individual to feel apprehension or fear of bodily injury. Shaking a fist in another person's face would constitute an assault. An unintentional tort occurs when an individual is injured as a result of negligent conduct. Negligence cases constitute the vast majority of lawsuits filed against health care providers.

"Contract law" defines the rights and obligations of institutions and individuals, as established by explicit "bargained-for" agreements between the parties. Generally speaking, a contract is legally enforceable. If one party to a contract fails to perform, the other party can sue to enforce the contract and can obtain money damages to compensate for any loss.

Other laws that relate to the operation of nursing homes, as well as other health care institutions, include certificate-of-need laws and indigent care statutes. These laws are considered tools for health care planning and are considered by some to be necessary to manage scarce resources, to contain costs, and to ensure the availability and accessibility of health care services. Many states have also enacted consumer protection statutes, which can be used to protect consumers from misleading or deceptive advertising. Federal Trade Commission rules concerning misleading trade practices may apply to nursing home chains or other health care providers that operate interstate. In cases where several facilities, a chain, or an association of nursing homes engages in practices that restrict the market in certain ways, such as price fixing, federal antitrust laws may apply. Nursing homes, hospitals, or other health care providers that participate in Medicaid and/or Medicare are also subject to Title VI of the federal Civil Rights Act of 1964, which prohibits discrimination based on race, color, or national origin. Not to be ignored are the numerous state-specific statutes regarding residents' rights, transfer and discharge, and prohibitions barring discrimination against Medicaid recipients.

The long-term care ombudsman program

The long-term care ombudsman plays an important role for residents in long-term care facilities. Under the federal Older Americans Act (1987), every state and the District of Columbia is required to establish and operate a long-term care ombudsman program. The program provides an individual whose full-time job is to investigate and resolve complaints made by or on behalf of residents in long-term care facilities, relating to action or inaction of providers, public agencies, or social service agencies that may adversely affect the health, safety, welfare, or rights of such residents. Many states have enacted or are in the process of enacting authorizing legislation that defines the powers and duties of the ombudsman in greater detail, and that gives the ombudsman access to residents and their records.

The goal of the long-term care ombudsman program is to promote the highest quality of life and care for residents of nursing homes and board and care homes. The primary function of the ombudsman is to act as an advocate for the residents, but in many jurisdictions the office of the long-term care ombudsman also does the following:

- Acts as a clearinghouse for information on long-term care
- Monitors the implementation of legislation and regulations
- Educates providers, residents, and the public on residents' rights
- Trains and supervises volunteers to advocate in nursing homes on behalf of residents

The long-term care ombudsman programs are also authorized under federal law to pursue legal and administrative remedies on behalf of residents. Some operate toll-free telephone numbers that provide access to ombudsmen.

All programs are obligated to protect the anonymity of any person registering a complaint regarding a particular facility.

The preceding discussions reveal the complexity of the various aspects of the demanding task of caring for older adults in the institutional setting. Many laws and regulations must be followed, institutional policies and procedures must be followed and kept up to date, and the practitioner must attempt to learn about significant changes as they occur. This is an area of great flux as the United States attempts to improve its health care delivery system, and the caregiver has a difficult task in staying knowledgeable about these complexities while attempting to give highest-quality patient care.

■ Guardians and Conservators

The previous discussions were addressed to techniques that can be used by older adults fully able to make their own decisions and for whom knowledge of various techniques will be helpful. By encouraging such people to make their desires known through their plans and their surrogates, the caregiver will be providing valuable support and making the older adult's life more comfortable.

However, many individuals who are in nursing homes today already lack the legal capacity to make health care and financial decisions. For these individuals, family members must look to establishing an appropriate and legally authorized person, a surrogate, for giving consent and direction in many matters affecting the older adult, such as obtaining medical care, refusing such care, or managing financial resources. That person is often, but need not be, a family member. It is important to note that "while the intent of guardianship is benevolent, it can result in substantial deprivation of liberty and property" (Thomas, 1994). Keeping this in mind, caregivers can assist older adults and their families by advocating that the decision authority remain with the older adult as long as feasible and that it be given to a surrogate only to the extent necessary.

There are varied legal steps that a family member might take to manage an older adult's affairs and protect that older adult's rights. These steps include discussions of obtaining surrogates for decision making and of legal actions that will empower a surrogate to make various decisions or plans on behalf of the older adult. The emphasis here is on reacting to an incapacity that has not been adequately planned for.

All states and the District of Columbia have a procedure by which courts can appoint a third party to manage the affairs or to make personal decisions for individuals who are unable to care for themselves. The person appointed is usually called a guardian or conservator, although in some states the term *committee* is used. The terms *guardian* and *conservator* are often used interchangeably. However, some courts may distinguish between a person appointed to manage the financial affairs of the incapacitated person (a conservator) and a person appointed to make decisions, as well, about the incapacitated person's personal care, medical treatment, and/or daily activities (a guardian). The incapacitated person is usually referred to as the "ward."

The process for appointment of a guardian or conservator varies greatly from state to state. Generally speaking, a determination of the need for a guardian or conservator requires that the person bringing the action, sometimes referred to as a "petitioner," show first that the proposed ward has a specified mental or physical impairment and, second, that as a result of the impairment, the proposed ward is unable to manage personal and/or financial affairs. The Uniform Probate Code (1983), which is followed by a number of states, defines an incapacitated person as follows:

Any person who is impaired by reason of mental illness, mental deficiency, physical illness or disability, advanced age, chronic age, chronic use of drugs, chronic intoxication, or other cause (except minority) to the extent [that he or she] lacks sufficient understanding or capacity to make or communicate a responsible decision.

If the court finds that the proposed ward is incapacitated, a guardian or conservator will be appointed. Again, who will be appointed depends on the state law. In some states, preference is given to relatives, whereas in others, the court must give priority consideration to the person chosen by the ward, if that information is known. Many states routinely appoint attorneys, banks, social services agencies, or other disinterested persons or entities. Some states have a public guardian. States following the Uniform Probate Code use priorities such as the following for selecting guardians, and a similar list for selecting conservators (Regan, 1996):

1. The incapacitated person's most recent nomination in a durable power of attorney

2. The person's spouse, or a person nominated by will of a deceased spouse or by other writing signed by the spouse and attested to by at least two witnesses
3. The person's adult child
4. The person's parent, or a nominee by will of a deceased parent or by other writing signed by a parent and attested to by at least two witnesses
5. Any relative of the incapacitated person with whom the person has resided for more than 6 months before the filing of the petition
6. A person nominated by the person who is caring for or paying for the care of the incapacitated person

Once guardians and conservators are appointed, their powers vary greatly, also depending on state law. In many states, guardians and conservators exercise "plenary powers," meaning that they have the power to make decisions affecting virtually every aspect of the ward's life. Increasingly, courts and legislatures are recognizing that persons with mental or physical disabilities do not and should not necessarily lose all their rights to exercise personal autonomy. Thus in some states the guardian's powers, as delineated by the court, must be drawn as narrowly as possible, whereas in other states the courts have broad discretion to structure the guardian's or conservator's authority to fit the needs of the individual ward.

A trend, encouraging to those concerned that the older adult's wishes always be followed, is the increasing application of the doctrine of "substituted judgment" in cases where a guardian has been appointed by a court to make a health care decision for an incapacitated person. Under the doctrine of substituted judgment, a surrogate who has been designated to act for an incapacitated person has a duty to determine what choice the incapacitated person would make with respect to medical treatment if the person were competent to make that decision.

Under the doctrine of substituted judgment the surrogate literally stands in the shoes of the incapacitated person and makes decisions based on the incapacitated person's values, motives, and beliefs.

There are numerous problems with the application of guardianship and conservatorship laws for people who are mentally and physically incapacitated. The proceedings may be very costly and time consuming. The person appointed by the court to make and exercise personal choices on behalf of the ward may in fact be a total stranger to the ward. Although many court-appointed guardians and conservators will make an effort to become familiar with the ward and will make conscientious efforts to fulfill their fiduciary obligations, it is not uncommon to hear complaints about guardians and conservators who fail to establish any personal relationship with the ward, who make personal care decisions in a vacuum, and who even fail to ensure that the ward's bills are paid and that basic needs are met. The ability and willingness of courts to monitor guardianships and conservatorships once established also vary greatly from state to state. Although some states monitor guardianships and conservatorships closely, most only require an annual accounting of financial transactions. Few states have the resources necessary to conduct extensive audits of these accounts or to monitor personal care decisions made under a court appointment.

In spite of these concerns, the use of guardianships is widespread to meet the need for effective management of an incompetent older adult's affairs. Caregivers are in a unique position to observe the older adult's capabilities and to help ensure that the most effective, but least intrusive, type of surrogate power is instituted. Often health care professionals, seeing both the need for, and the effects of, guardianships, are spearheading policy changes to have the process better serve older adults (Coker & Johns, 1994).

■ Conclusion

The information presented here is wide ranging and complex. The delivery of health care in today's environment is challenged by constant changes in personnel, resources, and administrative requirements, and by advances in technology. Education is often narrowed to better serve specified audiences at several nursing levels, sometimes failing to provide a broad view of the complexities of assisting the aging person. Federal and state laws and regulations are changing as attempts are being made to improve care delivery while reducing the costs of health care professionals. There is continuity of concern for the older patient and a growing recognition of the patient's need for control and autonomy. The challenge lies in not reducing the quality of care that will be delivered to our nation's older population, but in assisting this population in as many ways as possible. Encouraging such planning techniques as are presented in this chapter is one way of offering such assistance.

REFERENCES

American Public Welfare Society and National Association of State Units on Aging. (1986). *A comprehensive analysis of state policies and practices related to elder abuse* (Vols. 1-4). Washington, DC: Author.

Black's law dictionary (5th ed. abr.), (1983). St. Paul: West Publishing.

Coker, L.H., & Johns, A.F. (1994). Guardianship for elders: Process and issues. *Journal of Gerontological Nursing, 20*(12), 25-32.

Darr, J. (1995). Guardianship and conservatorship. *Journal of Gerontology Nursing, 21,* 10.

Health Care Financing Administration. (1990). *State operations manual.* Washington, DC: U.S. Government Printing Office.

Huntington, S., & Fry-Revere, S. (1991). Provider responsibilities under the patient self-determination act— Living wills, durable powers of attorney and the law. In *Health law trends.* Washington, DC: Arent, Fox, Kintner, Plotkin, and Kahn.

Mewhinney, K. (1994). Legal aspects of geriatric medicine. In W.R. Hazzard, et al. (Eds.), *Principles of geriatric medicine and gerontology.* New York: McGraw-Hill.

Morris, W. (Ed.). (1979). *The American Heritage dictionary, college edition.* Boston: Houghton Miflin.

Older Americans Act Amendments of 1987, Public Law 100-175 (Vol. 101, Stat. 926) (1987, November).

Omnibus Budget Reconciliation Act of 1987, Public Law 100-203 (1987, December).

Regan, J.J. (1996). *Tax, estate and financial planning for the elderly,* rel 20. New York: Matthew Bender.

Sarrassat v. Sullivan, C.A. No. C 88-20161 RPA (D.C. Cal.) (Stipulation of settlement, May 1, 1989).

Stedman's medical dictionary (25th ed.). (1990). Baltimore: Williams and Wilkins.

Thomas, B.L. (1994). Research considerations: Guardianship and the vulnerable elderly. *Journal of Gerontological Nursing, 20*(5), 10-16.

Uniform Probate Code, S5-108, 8 U.L.A. 437 (West 1983).

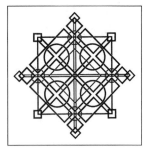

Old age has a great sense of calm and freedom; when the passions have relaxed their hold you have escaped, not from one master but from many.

PLATO, *The Republic*

Ethical Perspectives

■ Learning Objectives

On completion of this chapter, the reader will be able to do the following:

1. Compare and contrast four current approaches to studying and applying bioethics: principle-based ethics, virtue theory, communitarianism, and caring.
2. Critique age-based rationing as a means to achieve intergenerational justice.
3. Counsel older adults who seek assistance in making end-of-life treatment decisions.
4. Describe the advocacy responsibilities and related competencies of gerontologic nurses.
5. Identify strategies to prevent and resolve ethical conflict.
6. Use a process of ethical decision making to resolve moral distress and dilemmas.

■ Moral Competency and Gerontologic Nursing

In a now classic article, physician-ethicist Mark Siegler (1984) describes the three ages of medicine as the age of paternalism, the age of autonomy, and the current age of bureaucratic parsimony. Throughout these ages the principal concern of physicians has changed from the good of individual patients, to the good of the patient's freedom and right of self-determination, to the current balancing of the patient's good against the goods of society, health care institutions, and caregivers. The more the standard decision criteria of medical indications and pa-tient preferences are replaced by quality of life considerations and other external factors, the more vulnerable older adults become. It is no longer unusual to hear intensive care staff (with no knowledge of the patient under consider-ation) question, "What is this old person doing taking up a critical care bed?" Nor is it out of the ordinary to hear youth complain about being taxed to finance Medicare benefits. Those of us who work with older adults know how difficult it is to attract the "best and brightest" in nursing to choose gerontology as a specialty. The knowl-edge and experience of gerontologic nurses po-sition us to advocate effectively for older adults. But to do this well, our moral competence

---

BOX 22-1 THE AMERICAN NURSES' ASSOCIATION CODE OF ETHICS

CODE FOR NURSES

1. The nurse provides services with respect for human dignity and the uniqueness of the client, unrestricted by considerations of social or economic status, personal attributes, or the nature of health problems.
2. The nurse safeguards the client's right to privacy by judiciously protecting information of a confidential nature.
3. The nurse acts to safeguard the client and the public when health care and safety are affected by the incompetent, unethical, or illegal practice of any person.
4. The nurse assumes responsibility and accountability for individual nursing judgments and actions.
5. The nurse maintains competence in nursing.
6. The nurse exercises informed judgment and uses individual competence and qualifications as criteria in seeking consultation, accepting responsibilities, and delegating nursing activities to others.
7. The nurse participates in activities that contribute to the ongoing development of the profession's body of knowledge.
8. The nurse participates in the profession's efforts to implement and improve standards of nursing.
9. The nurse participates in the profession's efforts to establish and maintain conditions of employment conducive to high-quality nursing care.
10. The nurse participates in the profession's effort to protect the public from misinformation and misrepresentation and to maintain the integrity of nursing.
11. The nurse collaborates with members of the health professions and other citizens in promoting community and national efforts to meet the health needs of the public.

From American Nurses' Association. (1985). *Code for nurses with interpretive statements.* Kansas City, MO: Author.

---

must be as fine-tuned as other intellectual, technical, and interpersonal competencies.

Moral competence is not an option for nurses—too much is at stake. How (and whether) we choose to nurse can literally determine the human well-being of those entrusted to our care at vulnerable moments of their living and dying. Recognizing this truth, professional nursing organizations such as the American Nurses' Association (1985) have formulated codes of ethics to regulate practice (Box 22-1). More recently the American Nurses' Association (1991) has published standards of clinical nursing

practice and complemented standards of care with a set of professional performance standards, which includes the injunction that "the nurse's decisions and actions on behalf of clients are determined in an ethical manner" (p. 15). See Box 22-2 for related measurement criteria. This chapter describes elements of moral competency that are essential to excellence in gerontologic nursing. A brief examination of popular approaches to "doing bioethics" will provide a theoretic background for later discussions of broad ethical issues and aging, clinical ethics and nursing, and ethical decision making.

BOX 22-2 THE AMERICAN NURSES'
ASSOCIATION STANDARDS OF
PROFESSIONAL PERFORMANCE

Standard v. ethics: The nurse's decisions and
actions on behalf of clients are determined in
an ethical manner.

MEASUREMENT CRITERIA

1. The nurse's practice is guided by the *Code for Nurses.*
2. The nurse maintains client confidentiality.
3. The nurse acts as a client advocate.
4. The nurse delivers care in a nonjudgmental and nondiscriminatory manner that is sensitive to client diversity.
5. The nurse delivers care in a manner that preserves and protects client autonomy, dignity, and rights.
6. The nurse seeks available resources to help formulate ethical decisions.

From American Nurses' Association Task Force on
Nursing Standards Practice. (1991). *Standards of clinical nursing practice.* Kansas City, MO: Author.

■ Approaches to Ethical Inquiry

PRINCIPLE-BASED APPROACH

Ethical theories are systems of reflection that attempt to explain how we ought to live and why. These theories may be broadly categorized as action-guiding theories that answer the question, What ought I to do? or character-guiding theories that answer the question, What kind of person ought I to be? In the early days of bioethics, attention was focused almost exclusively on action-guiding theory of two types: utilitarian theory, in which the rightness or wrongness of an action depends on the consequences the action produces, and deontologic theory, in which an action is right or wrong independent of the consequences it produces.

From these action-guiding theories, various principles have been derived, such as autonomy (self-determination), beneficence (doing good), nonmaleficence (avoiding harm), justice (treating fairly), veracity (truth telling), confidentiality (respecting privileged information), and fidelity (keeping promises). All of these are held to obligate health care professionals in a prima facie manner (i.e., all things being equal, I am obligated to respect patients, benefit them and cause them no harm, treat all fairly, be truthful, etc.).

Most applications of bioethics involve the resolution of dilemmas involving conflicts between two or more of these principles. Unfortunately, there is no agreed upon hierarchy of principles that specifies which principles may trump others. Moreover, because many of these dilemmas highlight dramatic clinical problems—definitely not of the everyday "to do a terminal wean or not to do a terminal wean" variety—this particular type of principle-based ethics, namely, quandary ethics, has been critiqued as not being sensitive to the everyday ethical concerns of practicing nurses and other health care professionals. Beauchamp and Childress (1994) offer a comprehensive examination of the principle-based approach to bioethics, and Clouser and Gert (1994), a strong critique.

VIRTUE THEORY

Dissatisfaction with action-guiding moral theories that ignore the character of the moral agent has led some ethicists to resurrect virtue theory and attempt new formulations of virtues or human excellences intrinsic to human flourishing. Virtue may be defined as a trait of character that disposes a person habitually to seek excellence with respect to an end, such as human flourishing. Virtue theorists claim that who health care professionals are is as important as what they do. Although many agree with this claim, the harder task is agreeing upon which virtues and excellencies are intrinsic to the practice of good nursing or medicine. In a recent text, Pellegrino and Thomasma (1993) recommend as virtues essential to the practice of medicine the following: fidelity to trust, compassion, phronesis (prudential judgment), justice, fortitude, temperance, integrity, and self-effacement. Nursing has yet to agree upon its core virtues. Even more elusive is determining how (and if) virtue can be taught and whether virtue should be used as a criterion for admission to and advancement in nursing practice. It may be helpful to reflect on and begin to describe the traits of character that enable gerontologic nurses to secure the outcomes they desire for older patients.

COMMUNITARIANISM

Amitai Etzioni (1993), founder of the communitarian movement, sharply portrays the limitations of the rugged individualism for which Americans are famous and proposes a new balance between our rights as individuals and our social responsibilities. Believing that an allegiance to the shared values and institutions that sustain us is possible, in spite of our pluralism, he directs attention to the common good and calls for a revival of the ideal that small sacrifices by individuals can create large benefits for most all of us. As citizens in the United States struggle to reform health care, the communitarian challenge to set aside individual differences and interests to achieve the laudable goals of access for all, high-quality care, and affordable cost assumes a special urgency and one seemingly compatible with nursing's agenda.

Relevant to the preceding comments about virtue theory, communitarians argue that what youngsters require is to develop the basic personality traits that characterize effective individuals and to acquire core values—in a word, character development.

We mean by *character* the psychological muscles that allow a person to control impulses and defer gratification, which is essential for achievement, performance, and moral conduct. The *core values*, which need to be transmitted from generation to generation, contain moral substances that those with the proper basic personality can learn to appreciate, adapt, and integrate into their lives: hard work pays, even in an unfair

world; treat others with the same basic dignity with which you wish to be treated (or face the consequences); you feel better when you do what is right than when you evade your moral precepts (Etzioni, 1994, p. 91).

ETHIC OF CARE

Dissatisfaction with the principle-based approach to nursing ethics, combined with attentiveness to Gilligan's ground-breaking work (1982) in moral development, has led some nurse theorists to begin to articulate an ethic of care (Benner & Wrubel, 1989; Fry, 1989; Watson, 1985). Central to this perspective is the nature of the nurse-patient relationship and attention to the particulars of individual patients viewed within the context of their life's narrative. Rejecting a reductionistic, mechanistic approach to healing, the care perspective calls for a phenomenologic methodology that invites caregivers to empathically enter the patient's world. Characteristics of the care perspective include the following: centrality of the caring relationship, promotion of dignity, respect of patients as people, acceptance of particular patient and health care beliefs, norms of responsiveness and responsibility, and a redefinition of fundamental moral skills (Taylor, 1993). As yet undecided is whether the ethic of care provides sufficient grounding for a distinct theory of nursing ethics.

■ Ethics and Aging

As members of the moral community of health care professionals entrusted with securing the well-being of older adults, gerontologic nurses have a moral obligation to understand and participate in the contemporary moral debate about ethical issues and aging. This chapter highlights four areas of controversy: intergenerational justice, age-based rationing, good dying for older adults, and autonomy and long-term care.

INTERGENERATIONAL JUSTICE

Intergenerational justice is problematic at both the macro and micro levels. When ex–Colorado governor Richard Lamm suggested that older adults have a duty to die to free up resources for younger adults, he sparked a national debate about intergenerational duties. To date there is no consensus about what society as a whole and what individuals owe older adults, nor consensus about what older adults owe society and individuals. For nurses and social workers, the issue often presents itself as a practical question about how much expense and hardship it is reasonable to expect the families of older adults to bear. Can family members refuse to provide care for an older relative who needs assistance with activities of daily living? And conversely, can an older parent refuse to assist an adult child in need of supportive care after discharge? With hospital and long-term care not an option for many older adults because of absent or deficient coverage or finances, home care is becoming a grave problem. Ethicists are beginning to assert the moral relevance of family interests when decisions are being made for individual patients (Blustein, 1993; Hardwig, 1990; Jecker, 1991; Kapp, 1991; Nelson, 1992).

Similar issues present themselves at the policy level as society struggles to distribute the benefits and costs of quality health care. Are older adults entitled to as much health care as they desire, regardless of the costs of this care? To what extent should younger citizens be taxed in order for the government to fund health care for older adults? Are the needs of children being sacrificed to support the entitlements of "greedy geezers"? What degree of sacrifice is reasonable to expect from affluent older adults to provide care for indigent older adults? Philosopher Norman Daniels (1988) offers as one way to avoid intergenerational warfare a "prudential saver" policy of distributive justice. He advocates that we approach the problem of distributing resources between age groups from the perspective of people prudently allocating resources throughout the stages of their own lives, rather than for distinct sets of people. This and other proposals are critiqued by Moody (1992).

Nurses who understand what is at stake for older adults in this dialogue at both the macro and micro levels and who can appreciate the financial and human costs of caregiving have a moral obligation to participate in these debates.

AGE-BASED RATIONING

In a book entitled *Setting Limits,* Dan Callahan (1987), director of the Hastings Center, stimulated public discussion about the future of health care for older adults and shocked many by proposing age as a specific criterion for the allocation and limitation of health care. Urging medicine to give up its relentless drive to extend the lives of older adults and turn its attention instead to the relief of their suffering and an improvement in their physical and mental quality of life, Callahan posits two conditions:

The first condition is that we need, both young and old, to understand that it is possible to live out a meaningful old age that is limited in time, one that does not require a compulsive effort to turn to medicine for more life to make it bearable. The second condition is that as a culture we need a supportive social context for aging and death, one that cherishes and respects the elderly while at the same time recognizing that their primary orientation should be to the young and the generations to come, not to the welfare of their own group (pp. 25-26).

Individuals can agree with Callahan that it is time to rethink the meaning and significance of old age, and yet differ dramatically about what this means for clinical decision making and public policy. Whereas some favor public policy that cites an arbitrary chronologic age as justification for limiting aggressive therapy such as cardiac bypass surgery or dialysis (e.g., no bypass surgery or dialysis for people older than 65 years of age), others prefer to individualize decision making and would only limit treatment for older adults who believe that they have lived their lives and are ready to die. At issue are the questions of who decides when an individual is too old for certain types of care and what criteria are used to make this decision. And whereas attention to the chronic problems of aging is a central theme of Callahan, Battin (1987) has proposed that in an age-based rationing system, direct termination of

Battin, M.P. (1987). Age rationing and the just distribution of health care: Is there a duty to die? *Ethics, 97,* 317-340.

Beauchamp, T.L., & Childress, J.F (1994). *Principles of biomedical ethics* (4th ed.). New York: Oxford University Press.

Benner, P., & Wrubel, J. (1989). *The primacy of caring.* Menlo Park, CA: Addison-Wesley.

Binstock, R.H., & Post, S.G. (Eds.). (1991). *Too old for health care? Controversies in medicine, law, economics, and ethics.* Baltimore: Johns Hopkins University Press.

Blustein, J. (1993). The family in medical decision making. *Hastings Center Report, 23*(3), 6-13.

Callahan, D. (1987). *Setting limits: Medical goals in an aging society.* New York: Simon and Schuster.

Clouser, K.D., & Gert, B. (1994). Morality vs. principlism. In R. Gillon (Ed.), *Principles of health care ethics.* New York: John Wiley and Sons.

Daniels, N. (1988). *Am I my parents' keeper?* New York: Oxford University Press.

Etzioni, A. (1994). *The spirit of community: Rights, responsibilities, and the communitarian agenda.* New York: Crown.

Fry, S. (1989). The role of caring in a theory of nursing ethics. *Hypatia, 4,* 88-103.

Gadow, S. (1980). Existential advocacy: Philosophical foundations of nursing. In S.F. Spicker & S. Gadow (Eds.), *Nursing: Images and ideals—Opening dialogue with the humanities* (pp. 79-101). New York: Springer.

Gilligan, C. (1982). *In a different voice: Psychological theory and women's development.* Cambridge, MA: Harvard University Press.

Hardwig, J. (1990). What about the family? *Hastings Center Report, 20*(2), 5-10.

Jameton, A. (1993). Dilemmas of moral distress: Moral responsibility and nursing practice. *AWHONN's Clinical Issues in Perinatal and Women's Health Nursing, 4,* 542-551.

Jecker, N.S. (1991). *Aging and ethics: Philosophical problems in gerontology.* Clifton, NJ: Human Press.

Kapp, M.B. (1991). Health care decision making by the elderly: I get by with a little help from my family. *Gerontologist, 11,* 619-622.

Moody, H.R. (1992). *Ethics in an aging society.* Baltimore: Johns Hopkins University Press.

Nelson, J.L. (1992). Taking families seriously. *Hastings Center Report, 22*(4), 6-12.

Pellegrino, E.D. (1989). Withholding and withdrawing treatments: Ethics at the bedside. *Clinical Neurosurgery 35,* 164-184.

Pellegrino, E.D. (1991). Ethics [Contempo issue]. *Journal of the American Medical Association, 265*(23), 3118-3119.

Pellegrino, E.D., & Thomasma, D.C. (1993). *The virtues in medical practice.* New York: Oxford University Press.

Siegler, M. (1984). Should age be a criterion in health care? *Hastings Center Report, 14*(5), 24-27.

Smeeding, T.M., Battin, M.P., Francis, L.P., & Landesman, B.M. (Eds.). (1987). *Should medical care be rationed by age?* Totowa, NJ: Rowman and Littlefield.

Taylor, C. (1993). Nursing ethics: The role of caring. *AWHONN's Clinical Issues in Perinatal and Women's Health Nursing, 4*(4), 552-560.

Watson, J. (1985). *Nursing: The philosophy and science of caring.* Boulder: Colorado Associated University Press.

BIBLIOGRAPHY

American Association of Retired Persons. (1989). *A matter of choice: Planning ahead for health care decisions.* Washington, DC: Author.

American Hospital Association. (1991). *Put it in writing: A guide to promoting advance directives.* Chicago: Author.

Berlowitz, D.R., Wilking, S.V.B., & Moskowitz, M.A. (1991). Do-not-resuscitate orders at a chronic care hospital. *Journal of the American Geriatric Society, 8,* 472-476.

Buchanan, A.E., & Brock, D.W. (1989). *Deciding for others: The ethics of surrogate decision making.* New York: Cambridge University Press.

Callahan, D. (1990). *What kind of life: The limits of medical progress.* New York: Simon and Schuster.

Callahan, D. (1993). *The troubled dream of life.* New York: Simon and Schuster.

Collopy, B. (1988). Autonomy and long-term care: Some crucial distinctions. *Gerontologist, 28*(Suppl.), 10-17.

Concern for Dying. (1991). *Advance directive protocols and the Patient Self-Determination Act: A resource manual for the development of institutional protocols.* New York: Author.

Gadow, S. (1984, March 29). Gov. Lamm asserts elderly, if very ill, have "duty to die." *New York Times,* p. A16.

Hastings Center. (1987). *Guidelines on the termination of life-sustaining treatment and the care of the dying.* Bloomington and Indianapolis: Indiana University Press.

President's Commission for the Study of Ethical Problems in Medicine and Biomedical and Behavioral Research. (1982). *Making health care decisions* (Vols. 1-3). Washington, DC: U.S. Government Printing Office.

President's Commission for the Study of Ethical Problems in Medicine and Biomedical and Behavioral Research. (1983). *Deciding to forego life-sustaining treatment: Ethical, medical, and legal issues in treatment decisions.* Washington, DC: U.S. Government Printing Office.

Weir, R.F., & Gostin, L. (1990). Decisions to abate life-sustaining treatment for nonautonomous patients: Ethical standards and legal liability for physicians after Cruzan. *Journal of the American Medical Association, 264,* 1846-1853.

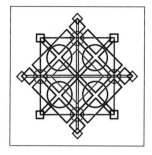

C H A P T E R 23

*The quality of a life's experience cannot
be measured in the same way as its quantity;
numbers of years may have little to do with
satisfactions in living.*

M.B. WEINER, A.J. BROK, AND A.M. SNADOWSKY,
Working with the Aged

The Future

■ Learning Objectives

On completion of this chapter, the reader will be able to do the following:

1. Appreciate the importance of stating ideas and contributing suggestions in public policy discussions to advance professional nursing.
2. Contribute to the refinement of nursing language, including nursing diagnoses, that will improve the understanding of nursing and encourage clear and frequent communication.
3. Emulate models of care that enable improved practice, research, and education to be understood and applied in patient care.
4. Prepare for and be prepared to cope with the adjustments that are anticipated to be imposed in the twenty-first century.

Only if a person were denied access to electronic or print media would that person be unaware of the prevalence of older adults in today's population. No matter the subject for discussion in the current media, it is difficult to ignore the ever-increasing numbers of older adults in social, civic, economic, or other gatherings of people. Awareness of one's surroundings and consciousness of one's associates present a clear message: there are increased numbers of older people in the population today. An examination of the status and the activities of these people—at this, the end of the twentieth century—leads to the question, What will be the status of older adults in the twenty-first century?

There is no magic wand to create situations for the future, nor is there a seer to portray what the future will hold in terms of the numbers of older adults or the status of older adults. The best we can do is to look at some of the events that are occurring today and project *what might be the future* for older adults in the years ahead. This chapter presents some of the ideas that have been suggested by people who have worked with older adults in the recent past and by our discussions and collaborations with others who are equally interested in and concerned about what will happen to older adults in the future. Some of the trends that can now be identified point to the directions that one can expect to be taken in the future.

The availability of educational opportunities and of various and diverse experiences—both personal and professional—and the opening of windows of opportunity around the globe have all contributed to the development of the professional nurse's expertise. As numbers of older people increase in the world, the nurse observes people in various states of health, residing in various settings that are more or less conducive to maintaining health, with full recognition of the responsibility for assisting and/or supporting a few or many of the people who are amenable to the benefits the nurse can offer.

■ Future Roles of Nursing

Few people debate the issues that are ahead in the world of professional nursing. Rather, debate revolves around the "how" of coping with the challenges that will be faced. This chapter considers the debatable issues of coping with the challenges that will occur.

The following statements summarize the present state of affairs and suggest what lies ahead:

Throughout the world, health care is undergoing dramatic transition, perhaps better described as a quiet revolution. And clearly, the health profession most affected by these changes is nursing. The intensely technological components, physician-driven components of health care, will remain in hospitals, while the care, comfort, rehabilitation, education and counseling—the nursing piece—has shifted to community settings along with the nurses who provide it (Dreher, 1995).

The nurses of this latter part of the twentieth century are much more savvy than were the nurses of pre–World War II. They are an articulate group of professionals, and they are knowledgeable about the issues that are critical to their survival and the welfare of the people who will be dependent on their expertise in the twenty-first century. This group of caregivers will be able to use their abilities to speak, analyze situations, and establish priorities that will ultimately benefit the health care givers, as well as the health

care consumers. Recognition of the influence of the political system in the United States will thrust the nurses into that arena to state their cases and to plead for justice in the workplace, as well as justice in the care system for the consumers of health care. A recent report from an attorney and policy analyst suggests five challenges as the new century approaches; it will be important to do the following:

1. Demonstrate that nurses provide cost-effective, high-quality care that can be measured. Good and valid data are needed to illustrate the cost of care, as well as patient outcomes.
2. Adopt uniform licensure and educational requirements for the nursing profession and establish fewer and simpler titles.
3. Overcome the mentality of an oppressed minority. Develop the self-confidence necessary to provide leadership in clinical situations, as well as in positions of administration and government.
4. Accept the reality of job insecurity; other health care givers, besides nurses, will be faced with the same downsizing.
5. Sustain a commitment to lifelong professional learning. This is one of the defining characteristics of professionals (Hadley, 1996).

To emphasize the significance that nursing will achieve in the twenty-first century, Hadley (1996) pays tribute to Florence Nightingale, who used her intellect and her compassion to shape the nursing profession. Nightingale recognized, more than 100 years ago, that nursing outcomes must be measured with good data. The quality of good nursing care must be measured and documented to be valued. The following quotation accompanies a portrait of Florence Nightingale: "To understand God's thoughts we must study statistics, for these are the measure of His purpose." Careful reading of this quote suggests that it expresses the relationship among epidemiology, biostatistics, and the health of populations that is at the heart of public health and managed care. Hadley pleads with nurses to combine this intellectual legacy with the well-known compassion of nursing to master both the political and economic marketplaces (Hadley, 1996).

■ Changes and Transitions in Aging

As one ponders the thought of aging, whether it be the aging of self or of others, it is the optimist's view of aging that is most appealing. A review of all the benefits of aging and careful reflection on the "good life" can produce happy thoughts and good feelings about self and those nearby. Although it is the pessimist's tendency to think negatively, to think of all the wrong things that will occur as "age creeps up," observation of aging people reveals that there are often many more positives than there are negatives about the process of aging.

For example, one of the prevalent fears among older adults is that brain function will be impaired as they age. This fear is especially strong if the aging person has been mentally active and very much involved in multiple cerebral activities. A recent study confirms what some scientists have long believed: brain power decreases very little in healthy people as they age. As a result of a study conducted by Dr. John Morris, it was concluded that impairment of brain function is a result of disease, not age (Crowley, 1996). Reports of studies such as this one are important to share with people who are concerned about what the future might hold.

Literature and conversations about the fears that are faced by older adults often revolve around concern about change; they are fears about the changes that will, or might, occur as people grow older. Some of the concerns are very real—based on factual data that are available now. Some of the concerns are not reality based—they have no basis in fact. One of the approaches to helping the older person cope with these fears is to distinguish between "transition" and "change"; it is helpful in adjusting the perspective of the older person and the caregiver, especially if there is an undue focus on

change. A dictionary definition of *change* suggests that this term means to substitute one thing for another, to adopt one thing in place of another; change tends to be abrupt. The idea of transition, however, suggests a process that occurs over time; there is a sense of flow and movement. For example, a brief, self-limiting illness usually creates some necessary changes. Few people have not experienced an upper respiratory tract infection, and no one looks forward to such an experience. Various changes must be made in work schedules, in activities of daily living, in eating schedules, and in sleeping routines, and these changes usually continue for a number of days. All who experience this type of illness know that an adjustment in living is necessary, but they also know that these changes are not prolonged. Very soon the ill person will be able to return to the usual schedule. At the same time, a chronic illness has been viewed as requiring a process of transition that goes beyond the realm of change. An illness that requires major adjustments in life patterns is viewed as creating a major transition in one's lifestyle. For instance, an occurrence of cancer, bronchiectasis, diabetes, or other major interruption in life pattern will be considered in a different manner than a head cold. A period of change can occur, but most likely, the chronic ailment will require major transitions in living patterns. Internal processes usually make up the process of transition, whereas external processes tend to characterize change (Bridges, 1991; Meleis & Trangenstein, 1994).

■ Changes in Nursing Frameworks

Whether concerned with change or with transition, caregivers need a framework or a structure within which care can be planned and given. To enable universal acceptance of what is the caregiver's responsibility, a clear statement is needed to define the responsibility of the nurse to the patients for whom the nurse cares. Since 1992, the Congress of Nursing Practice has been revising the social policy statement for nursing.

This 3- to 4-year effort on the part of many nurses in the United States has resulted in the acceptance and publication of a social policy statement that represents nursing's commitment to society and to the people who are served by the professionals. It is a document that nurses can use as a framework for understanding "nursing's obligation to those who receive nursing care" (American Nurses' Association [ANA], 1995). With this as a basis for planning the directions for the twenty-first century, nurses can proceed with a sound framework for setting directions for the future.

Significant strides have been made in nursing since midcentury; the twentieth century will be noted for defining the historical development of nursing theory and nursing diagnosis, as well as for providing a clear definition of nursing. In 1980 the ANA defined nursing as "the diagnosis and treatment of human response to actual or potential health problems" (p. 9). At the North American Nursing Diagnosis Association (NANDA) conference inclusive in 1990, a more inclusive definition of nursing was accepted that is more inclusive of the full range of nursing thought and that reflects a wholistic approach to the patient. The following definition was found quite acceptable: Nursing diagnosis is a clinical judgment about an individual, family, or community response to actual or potential health problems or life processes. Nursing diagnosis provides the basis for selection of nursing interventions to achieve outcomes for which the nurse is accountable (NANDA, 1992).

After many years of work and much energy expenditure by many nurses, the NANDA Foundation will be incorporated by the end of 1996. This will enable NANDA to continue the development of a nursing language for the international classification of nursing practice.

Having defined the framework for nursing via *Nursing's Social Policy Statement* (American Nurses Publishing, 1995), the next logical step in defining nursing's responsibility was to accept the *Scope and Standards of Gerontological Clinical Nursing Practice* (ANA, 1995). Once these revised data were discussed and promulgated, they were accepted and the directions were clear for examining and analyzing the essence of nursing in a more profound way than had been done in the past.

It can be predicted that multiple efforts will continue to be pursued to clarify the definition of nursing. One of the more profound discussions that have recently been addressed is that of *data bases*. An appointed group became the ANA steering committee on data bases to support clinical nursing practice. Topics for discussion included the following: electronic information activities; the ways, means, and rationales for linking nursing research language with the clinical language of nursing; and the progress of the International Council of Nurses (ICN) project on an international classification of nursing practice (ICNP). With multiple efforts such as these, coming from multiple sources, the involvement of nurses will be encouraged for many of these data base projects. The National Library of Medicine (NLM) has been examining linkages between the NLM staff nomenclatures and ANA-recognized nursing nomenclatures. One of the major goals is to incorporate the nursing interventions classification (NIC) and the OMAHA system into the metathesaurus. This linkage will assist in the development of a unified nursing language, as well as examining the implications for staff nurses. This is a strategic goal that will bear watching in the immediate future ("Steering Committee," 1995).

Another role for which nurses will be responsible in the not-too-distant future is that of advocacy. Traditionally, nurses have perceived themselves as being the patient's advocate, although this has been more difficult in some places than in others. The ANA position statement on ethics and human rights calls for nurses to value the differences among persons. British epidemiologist Sir Richard Doll considered the

Numeric Identifier_____

MINIMUM DATA SET (MDS) - VERSION 2.0
FOR NURSING HOME RESIDENT ASSESSMENT AND CARE SCREENING

REENTRY TRACKING FORM

SECTION AA. IDENTIFICATION INFORMATION

1.	RESIDENT NAME	
		a.(First) b.(Middle Initial) c.(Last) d.(Jr/Sr)
2.	GENDER	1. Male 2.Female
3.	BIRTHDATE	☐☐ — ☐☐ — ☐☐☐☐ Month Day Year
4.	RACE/ ETHNICITY	1. American Indian/Alaskan Native 4. Hispanic 2. Asian/Pacific Islander 5. White, not of 3. Black, not of Hispanic origin Hispanic origin
5.	SOCIAL SECURITY AND MEDICARE NUMBERS [C in 1st box if non med. no.]	a. Social Security Number ☐☐☐ — ☐☐ — ☐☐☐☐ b. Medicare number (or comparable railroad insurance number)
6.	FACILITY PROVIDER NO.	a. State No. b. Federal No.
7.	MEDICAID NO.[*+* if pending, *N* if not a Medicaid recipient]	
8.	REASONS FOR ASSESS-MENT	[Note-Other codes do not apply to this form] a. Primary reason for assessment 9. Reentry
9.	SIGNATURES OF STAFF COMPLETING FORM:	

a. Signatures		Title	Sections	Date
b.				Date
c.				Date

SECTION A. IDENTIFICATION AND BACKGROUND INFORMATION

4a.	DATE OF REENTRY	Date of reentry ☐☐ — ☐☐ — ☐☐☐☐ Month Day Year
4b.	ADMITTED FROM (AT REENTRY)	1. Private home/apt. with no home health services 2. Private home/apt. with home health services 3. Board and care/assisted living/group home 4. Nursing home 5. Acute care hospital 6. Psychiatric hospital, MR/DD facility 7. Rehabilitation hospital 8. Other
6.	MEDICAL RECORD NO.	

Resident _____   Numeric Identifier _____

MINIMUM DATA SET (MDS) - VERSION 2.0
FOR NURSING HOME RESIDENT ASSESSMENT AND CARE SCREENING
BACKGROUND (FACE SHEET) INFORMATION AT ADMISSION

SECTION AB. DEMOGRAPHIC INFORMATION

1.	DATE OF ENTRY	*Date the stay began. Note - Does not include readmission if record was closed at the time of temporary discharge to hospital, etc. In such cases, use prior admission date*

		Month — Day — Year

2.	ADMITTED FROM (AT ENTRY)	1. Private home/apt. with no home health services 2. Private home/apt. with home health services 3. Board and care/assisted living/group home 4. Nursing home 5. Acute care hospital 6. Psychiatric hospital, MR/DD facility 7. Rehabilitation hospital 8. Other
3.	LIVED ALONE (PRIOR TO ENTRY)	0. No 1. Yes 2. In other facility
4.	ZIP CODE OF PRIOR PRIMARY RESIDENCE	
5.	RESIDEN-TIAL HISTORY 5 YEARS PRIOR TO ENTRY	*(Check all settings resident lived in during 5 years prior to date of entry given in time AB1 above)* Prior stay at this nursing home — a. Stay in other nursing home — b. Other residential facility-board and care home, assisted living, group home — c. MH/psychiatric setting — d. MR/DD setting — e. *NONE OF THE ABOVE* — f.
6.	LIFETIME OCCUPA-TION(S) [Put "/" between two occupations]	
7.	EDUCATION (Highest Level Completed)	1. No schooling 5. Technical or trade school 2. 8th grade/less 6. Some college 3. 9-11 grades 7. Bachelor's degree 4. High School 8. Graduate degree
8.	LANGUAGE	*(Code for correct response)* **a.** Primary Language 0. English 1. Spanish 2. French 3. Other **b. if other, specify**
9.	MENTAL HEALTH HISTORY	Does resident's RECORD indicate any history of mental retardation, mental illness, or developmental disability problem? 0. No 1. Yes
10.	CONDITIONS RELATED TO MR/DD STATUS	*(Check all conditions that are related to MR/DD status that were manifested before age 22, and are likely to continue indefinitely)* Not applicable - no MR/DD (Skip to AB11) — a. MR/DD with organic condition Down's syndrome — b. Autism — c. Epilepsy — d. Other organic condition related to MR/DD — e. MR/DD with no organic condition — f.
11.	DATE BACK-GROUND INFORMA-TION COMPLETED	Month — Day — Year

SECTION AC. CUSTOMARY ROUTINE

1.	CUSTOMARY ROUTINE	*(Check all that apply. If all information UNKNOWN, check last box only.)*
	(In year prior to DATE OF ENTRY to this nursing home, or year last in community if now being admitted from another nursing home)	**CYCLE OF DAILY EVENTS** Stays up late at night (e.g., after 9 pm) — a. Naps regularly during day (at least 1 hour) — b. Goes out 1+ days a week — c. Stays busy with hobbies, reading, or fixed daily routine — d. Spends most of time alone or watching TV — e. Moves independently indoors (with appliances, if used) — f. Use of tobacco products at least daily — g. *NONE OF ABOVE* — h. **EATING PATTERNS** Distinct food preferences — i. Eats between meals all or most days — j. Use of alcoholic beverage(s) at least weekly — k. *NONE OF ABOVE* — l. **ADL PATTERNS** In bedclothes much of day — m. Wakens to toilet all or most nights — n. Has irregular bowel movement pattern — o. Showers for bathing — p. Bathing in PM — q. *NONE OF ABOVE* — r. **INVOLVEMENT PATTERNS** Daily contact with relatives/close friends — s. Usually attends church, temple, synagogue (etc.) — t. Finds strength in faith — u. Daily animal companion/presence — v. Involved in group activities — w. *NONE OF ABOVE* — x. **UNKNOWN** - Resident/family unable to provide information — y.

[END]

SECTION AD. FACE SHEET SIGNATURES

SIGNATURES OF PERSONS COMPLETING FACE SHEET:

a. Signature of RN Assessment Coordinator			Date
b. Signatures	Title	Sections	Date
c.			Date
d.			Date
e.			Date
f.			Date
g.			Date

MDS 2.0 10/18/94N

*American College of Nursing Home
Administrators*
4650 East-West Freeway
Washington, DC 20014

American Council of the Blind
1155 15th Street N.W., Suite 720
Washington, DC 20005
(202) 467-5081

American Diabetes Association
Diabetes Information Service Center
1660 Duke Street
Alexandria, VA 22314
(800) ADA-DISC

*American Federation for Aging Research
(AFAR)*
1414 Avenue of the Americas, 18th Floor
New York, NY 10019
(212) 752-AFAR
(212) 832-2298 (fax)

American Foundation for the Blind, Inc.
National Office
15 W. 16th Street
New York, NY 10011
(212) 620-2000

American Geriatrics Society
770 Lexington Avenue, Suite 300
New York, NY 10021
(212) 308-1414

American Health Care Association
1201 L Street N.W.
Washington, DC 20005-4014
(202) 842-4444

American Heart Association
7320 Greenville Avenue
Dallas, TX 75231
(214) 373-6300

American Lung Association
1740 Broadway
New York, NY 10019-4373
(212) 315-8700

American Medical Association (AMA)
515 N. State Street
Chicago, IL 60610
(312) 464-5000

*American Medical Directors Association
(AMDA)*
10480 Little Patuxeny Parkway, Suite 760
Columbia, MD 21044
(800) 876-2632

American Nurses' Association
600 Maryland Avenue S.W.
Washington, DC 20024-2571
(202) 544-4444

American Parkinson's Disease Association
60 Bay Street, Suite 401
Staten Island, NY 10301
(800) 825-2732

American Public Health Association
1015 15th Street N.W.
Washington, DC 20005
(202) 789-5600

American Red Cross
National Headquarters
430 17th Street N.W.
Washington, DC 20006
(202) 737-8300

American Society for Geriatric Dentistry
211 E. Chicago Avenue, 17th Floor
Chicago, IL 60611
(312) 440-2500. x 2660

*American Society for Parenteral and Enteral
Nutrition*
8630 Fenton Street, Suite 412
Silver Spring, MD 20910-3805
(301) 587-6315

American Society on Aging
833 Market Street, Suite 512
San Francisco, CA 94103-1824
(415) 882-2910

American Speech-Language-Hearing Association
10801 Rockville Pike
Rockville, MD 20852
(301) 897-5700
(800) 638-8255

Arthritis Foundation
1330 West Peachtree Street
Atlanta, GA 30309
(800) 283-7800

Association for Gerontology in Higher Education
1001 Connecticut Avenue N.W., Suite 410
Washington, DC 20036-5504
(202) 429-9277

Catholic Charities U.S.A.
1731 King Street
Alexandria, VA 22314
(703) 549-1390

Catholic Health Association of the U.S.
4455 Woodson
St. Louis, MO 63134-3797
(314) 427-2500

Center for Social Gerontology
2307 Shelby Avenue
Ann Arbor, MI 48103-3895
(313) 665-1126

Children of Aging Parents
1609 Woodbourne Road, Suite 302-A
Levittown, PA 19057
(215) 945-6900

Department of Veteran's Affairs
Veterans Health Administration
Nursing Service Programs (118c)
810 Vermont Avenue N.W.
Washington, DC 20420
(202) 299-4000

Federal Council on Aging
330 Independence Avenue S.W.
Room 4280 HHS-N
Washington, DC 20201

Food and Drug Administration (FDA)
Professional and Consumer Programs
5600 Fishers Lane, Suite 1685
Parklawn Building
Rockville, MD 20857
(301) 443-5006

Foundation for Hospice and Home Care
519 C Street N.E.
Washington, DC 20002
(202) 547-6586

Gerontological Nutritionists
4103 44th Street
Sacramento, CA 95820
(916) 451-7149

Gerontological Society of America
1275 K Street N.W., Suite 350
Washington, DC 20005-4006
(202) 842-1275

Gray Panthers
1424 16th Street N.W., Suite 602
Washington, DC 20036
(202) 387-3111

House Select Committee on Aging
House Office Building
Annex 1, Room 712
Washington, DC 20515

Lighthouse National Center for Vision and Aging
800 Second Avenue
New York, NY 10017
(212) 808-0077

Mountain States (Human Services Organization)
950 N. Cole Road
P.O. Box 6756
Boise, ID 83704
(208) 322-4880

National Association for Hispanic Elderly
3325 Wilshire Boulevard, Suite 800
Los Angeles, CA 90010-1724
(213) 487-1922

National Association for Home Care
519 C Street N.W.
Washington, DC 20002-5809
(202) 547-7424

National Association of Directors of Nursing
Administration in Long-term Care
(NADONA-LTC)
10999 Reed Hartman Highway, Suite 229
Cincinnati, OH 45242
(800) 222-0539

National Association of the Deaf
814 Thayer Avenue
Silver Spring, MD 20910-4500
(301) 587-1788
(301) 587-1789 (TTY)

National Cancer Institute
Office of Communications
Room 10A24
9000 Rockville Pike
Rockville, MD 20892
(800) 4-CANCER

National Caucus and Center on the
Black Aged, Inc.
1424 K Street N.W., Suite 500
Washington, DC 20005
(202) 637-8400

National Citizens Coalition for Nursing Home
Reform
1224 M Street N.W., Suite 301
Washington, DC 20005
(202) 393-2018

National Conference on Geriatric Nurse
Practitioners
P.O. Box 270101
Fort Collins, CO 80527-0101
(303) 493-7793

National Council of Senior Citizens, Inc.
1331 F Street N.W.
Washington, DC 20004-1171
(202) 347-8800
(202) 624-9595 (fax)

National Council on the Aging
(Includes National Institute of Senior Citizens
and National Institute on Adult Day Care)
409 3rd Street S.W., Suite 200
Washington, DC 20024
(202) 479-1200

National Gerontological Nursing Association
c/o Mosby, Inc.
7250 Parkway Drive, Suite 510
Hanover, MD 21076
(800) 723-0560

National Hospice Organization (NHO)
1901 N. Moore Street, Suite 901
Arlington, VA 22202
(703) 243-5900

National Indian Council on Aging
6400 Uptown Boulevard N.E., Suite 510W
Albuquerque, NM 87110
(505) 242-9505

National Institute on Aging
31 Center Drive, MSC 2292
9000 Rockville Pike
Bethesda, MD 20892-2292
(301) 496-1752

National League for Nursing
350 Hudson Street
New York, NY 10014
(212) 989-9393

National Meals on Wheels Foundation
1133 20th Street N.W., Suite 321
Washington, DC 20036
(202) 463-6039

National Osteoporosis Foundation
1150 17th Street N.W., Suite 500
Washington, DC 20036
(202) 223-2226

National Policy Center on Housing and Living
Arrangements for the Older Americans
University of Michigan
2000 Bonisteel Boulevard
Ann Arbor, MI 48109

National Rehabilitation Association
633 S. Washington Street
Alexandria, VA 22314
(703) 836-0850

National Senior Citizens Law Center
1815 H Street N.W., Suite 700
Washington, DC 20006
(202) 887-5280

National Stroke Association
8480 E. Orchard Road, Suite 1000
Englewood, CO 80111-5015
(303) 771-1700

Older Women's League (OWL)
666 11th Street N.W., Suite 700
Washington, DC 20001
(202) 783-6686

Oncology Nursing Society
501 Holiday Drive
Pittsburgh, PA 15220-2749
(412) 921-7373

Senate Special Committee on Aging
Dirksen Senate Office Building
Room 623
Washington, DC 20510
(202) 224-5364

Social Security Administration
6401 Security Boulevard
Baltimore, MD 21235
(800) 772-1213

INDEX